# Migrant architects of the NHS

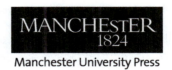

MANCHESTER
1824

Manchester University Press

# SOCIAL HISTORIES OF MEDICINE

Series editors: David Cantor and Keir Waddington

*Social Histories of Medicine* is concerned with all aspects of health, illness and medicine, from prehistory to the present, in every part of the world. The series covers the circumstances that promote health or illness, the ways in which people experience and explain such conditions, and what, practically, they do about them. Practitioners of all approaches to health and healing come within its scope, as do their ideas, beliefs, and practices, and the social, economic and cultural contexts in which they operate. Methodologically, the series welcomes relevant studies in social, economic, cultural, and intellectual history, as well as approaches derived from other disciplines in the arts, sciences, social sciences and humanities. The series is a collaboration between Manchester University Press and the Society for the Social History of Medicine.

*Previously published*

*The metamorphosis of autism: A history of child development in Britain*
Bonnie Evans

*Payment and philanthropy in British healthcare, 1918–48*
George Campbell Gosling

*The politics of vaccination: A global history*
Edited by Christine Holmberg, Stuart Blume and Paul Greenough

*Leprosy and colonialism: Suriname under Dutch rule, 1750–1950*
Stephen Snelders

*Medical misadventure in an age of professionalization, 1780–1890*
Alannah Tomkins

*Conserving health in early modern culture: Bodies and environments in Italy and England*
Edited by Sandra Cavallo and Tessa Storey

*Mediterranean quarantines, 1750–1914: Space, identity and power*
Edited by John Chircop and Francisco Javier Martinez

# Migrant architects of the NHS

## South Asian doctors and the reinvention of British general practice (1940s–1980s)

Julian M. Simpson

Manchester University Press

Published by Manchester University Press
Altrincham Street, Manchester M1 7JA, UK
www.manchesteruniversitypress.co.uk

British Library Cataloguing-in-Publication Data is available

ISBN 978 1 7849 9130 2  hardback

ISBN 978 1 5261 4501 7  paperback

First published by Manchester University Press in hardback 2018

This edition published 2020

The publisher has no responsibility for the persistence or accuracy of URLs for any external or third-party internet websites referred to in this book, and does not guarantee that any content on such websites is, or will remain, accurate or appropriate.

Typeset by Out of House Publishing
Printed in Great Britain
By TJ International Ltd, Padstow, Cornwall

# Contents

# List of tables and figures

## Tables

## Figures

# Preface and acknowledgements

This book is the product of a decade of work inspired by my desire to better understand how Britain's imperial past and the agency of migrants have contributed to shaping modern Britain. My interest in these topics stems from a number of personal experiences and is a reflection of my multiple identities. I spent most of my life up to my mid-twenties crossing cultural boundaries. I was born in the north-east of England, then started school in France before moving to Gabon where I went to high school at the Lycée National Léon Mba. I then returned to France to complete my secondary education and go to university and journalism school, before moving to Romania to do my national service as a French citizen (working for the French Foreign Office). I finally returned to the UK (I am also a British citizen) in my mid-twenties where I went to work on the BBC World Service's broadcasts to French-speaking Africa. I developed through this trajectory an appreciation of the interconnectedness of the world and, through the African teachers at my state school in Libreville, a sense of how the new social realities of independent African countries could nurture a quest for different interpretations of the past, replacing colonial histories with closer engagement with the continent's history. In others words, an understanding that the past is also political.

My family background is also mixed. I have ancestors with roots in Ireland, Germany and the Indian subcontinent. Such trajectories and mixed backgrounds are becoming more common in modern Britain. Yet, histories, including academic histories, continue to remain overly focused on events that occurred within the confines of national borders, rather than exploring the international relationships and movements that have contributed over time to the making of the modern world. This is slowly changing in the world of scholarship but the history of migration remains a marginal pursuit as does writing history that seeks to speak to contemporary debates. This feeling was exacerbated when, having decided to move on from journalism and working as a press officer for the Scottish Refugee Council in the early 2000s, I witnessed the full force of the wave of hostility towards migrants that was then building up and continues to play such an important part in British public life. I was intrigued to find that in a city such as Glasgow, built on imperial trade and the labour of migrants from Ireland and elsewhere, international migration could be perceived by many (not all) as such an alien and unwelcome phenomenon. I felt strongly that a lack of historical awareness was at least partially at the root of such attitudes. I therefore seek to reconnect in these pages with a tradition of writing history that sees it as having as much to tell us about the present as about the past. I was keen though to carry out rigorous research on this topic and not to succumb to the temptation of uncritically celebrating the roles of migrants. I wanted my work to be part of a process of critical engagement with the past that I feel would make a significant contribution to public discourse today.

Having spent a substantial part of my childhood in Howdon, in industrial North Tyneside in the north-east of England (during summer holidays from Africa), I also witnessed at first hand the central part that South Asian doctors played in staffing general practice in working-class areas. To say I was surprised that no historian had sought to tell this story would be an understatement. It offered an ideal opportunity to write a history of migration that was also a history of how Britain came to be what it is today. This was particularly the case in the light of the status of the NHS in the British national psyche—akin to a 'national religion' as the former British Chancellor of the Exchequer Nigel Lawson quipped—and the central position of general practice within the NHS. This is the path that led me to research the movement of these doctors and its impact on the making of modern British healthcare.

Along the way, I have naturally incurred a number of intellectual debts—too many to list. Whilst apologising to those left unnamed, I would like to acknowledge the support and guidance of Aneez Esmail at the University of Manchester without whom this book would not have seen the light of day. His work challenging racism in the British medical profession and his pioneering exploration of the role of migrant

South Asian doctors in the NHS laid a substantial amount of ground-work for the research I present here. He eloquently formulated a number of highly relevant questions about the role of South Asian medical migrants in British medicine that I have here attempted to answer. I was also fortunate to meet Stephanie Snow at an early stage of my time as a researcher at Manchester, which has been my academic base for the last ten years. Her expertise when it comes to the history of the NHS and of British general practice was instrumental in enabling me to produce what is both a discussion of the role of a group of migrants in Britain and a revisiting of the history of British healthcare. Similarly, Virinder Kalra's background in sociology led me to give greater consideration to social theory when seeking to understand the personal and professional trajectories of my research participants and I am grateful to him for encouraging me to go down this road. Thanks are also due to the University of Manchester and the Medical Research Council for providing me with three years of funding to research the history of South Asian GPs in the NHS.

Beyond the confines of the University of Manchester, Joanna Bornat was a constant source of encouragement and constructive criticism and it was always hugely enjoyable to discuss my research with her and her colleagues on the Open University's South Asian Geriatricians project, Parvati Raghuram and Leroi Henry. I am also grateful to the anonymous reviewers of the manuscript and the editor of the social histories of medicine series, Keir Waddington, for his meticulous engagement with my work. I would like to thank all at Manchester University Press for their initial interest in my research and their efforts in bringing this project to its conclusion. I am indebted too to the late Alex Cowan who offered me a place on the Northumbria University History MA programme and to Howard Wickes who supervised my dissertation at Northumbria and helped me set out on the path of historical research.

This book would not have been written without the cooperation and goodwill of those who gave up their time and often invited me into their homes to talk about their lives and their work in the NHS. In many cases research participants provided me with documents and photographs which cast further light on their experiences; some of them are reproduced on these pages with their permission. A number of participants also went out of their way to put me in touch with potential interviewees. I am deeply grateful to Dr Dipak Ray, Dr Rooin Boomla, Dr Darius

Preface and acknowledgements

Boomla, Dr Krishna Korlipara, Dr Sri Venugopal, Dr Shiv Pande, Dr Muhammad Noorul Islam Talukdar, Dr S. K. Ahuja, Dr L. R. M. Kamal, Dr M. A. Salam, Dr Rupendra Kumar Majumdar, Dr Arup Chaudhuri, Dr Mohammed Abu Khaled, Dr Ruban Prasad, Dr Hasmukh Joshi, Dr P. L. Pathak, Dr Urmila Rao, Dr Raman N. Rao, Dr N. R. Shah, Dr Anup Kumar Sen, Dr M. F. Haque, Sir Netar Mallick, Dr S. A. A. Gilani, Dr F. B. Kotwall, Dr M. S. Kausar, Dr Hira Lal Kapur, Dr Raj Chandran, Sir Donald Irvine, Dr K. S. Bhanumathi, Sir Liam Donaldson, Dr S. M. Qureshi, Mr Ajeet Gulati, Mr Jangu Banatvala and the twelve participants who chose to remain anonymous. I sincerely hope that my work does justice to the wealth of information that they entrusted me with. Dr Steve Watkins, Dr Michael Taylor, Professor Julian Tudor Hart, Dr Alan Rowe, Dr Irvine Loudon and Dr Satya Chatterjee and Mrs Chatterjee spoke to me informally about my research and I am equally grateful to them for their time. I would also like to thank the following people who assisted in the recruitment of participants: Dr Judith Ramsay, Dr Roseanna Mohammed, Naheed Asghar, Dr Umesh Chauhan, Dr Satya Chatterjee and Mrs Chatterjee, Professor Aneez Esmail, Professor Julian Tudor Hart, Liz Watson of the 'More than a curry' project, Claire Jackson of the Royal College of General Practitioners and Moira Auchterlonie of The Small Practices Association.

The interactions with participants were complemented by archival research. I benefited from the assistance of expert staff who often went beyond the call of duty in locating relevant documents. My numerous visits to the archives of the British Medical Association would have yielded little without the patient guidance of the BMA archivist Lee Sands. Claire Jackson and Sharon Messenger provided similarly precious advice at the Royal College of General Practitioners as did Judy Vaknin at the Runnymede Collection of the University of Middlesex. I am also very appreciative of the efforts of staff at the National Archives, the British Library Sound Archive and Newspaper Archive, the General Medical Council, Manchester Central Library and the Churchill Archive in Cambridge who facilitated my access to relevant documents.

Some of the arguments I develop here were presented in earlier forms in journal articles and in a chapter included in an edited volume on the migration of physicians. I would like to thank the University of Toronto Press and the publishers of *Oral History, Diversity and Equality in Health and Care*, the *British Journal of General Practice* and the *Journal of the Royal Society of Medicine* for allowing me to revisit those articles here. The British Medical Association kindly granted me permission to reproduce the image of Ralph Lawrence.

I would also like to express my gratitude to those friends and family who offered support and advice during a period when I have spent many hours researching and writing this book. Judith Ramsay in particular gave me the encouragement I needed to pursue my research interests at the outset and helped me through the times when the enormity of the task I had undertaken felt overwhelming.

Finally, a note on the style of this book, which in accordance with the task I set myself, seeks to build bridges between academic research and the concerns of a broader readership. My aim was to produce a text that would be both a scholarly work of serious research that contributes to future thinking about the history of the NHS and one that remains accessible to a wider readership interested in exploring a different understanding of the role of migration in the making of Britain. In presenting my conclusions, I have tried to achieve a balance between writing in a scholarly fashion, referencing claims and engaging with existing literature and debates whilst at the same time producing an account of this history that might speak to a broader audience not just of non-historians but of readers interested in engaging with the significance of this history. It is in this spirit that I have also allowed space for the voices of the participants in this project to be heard, both to provide evidence of the claims I am advancing and to enable readers to immerse themselves in these accounts.

I believe this to be a logical approach consistent with my aim to write history that is of relevance in the public domain and that it is possible, indeed necessary, to seek out new ways of connecting academic research to a broader readership.[1] A particular source of inspiration in this respect was the anthropologist Paul Stoller's account of his dialogue with one of his principal informants when he was writing his classic study of traditional beliefs in West Africa, *In Sorcery's Shadow*. Adamu Jenitongo enjoined him to 'Produce something that will be remembered, something that describes me and you, something that my grandchildren and your grandchildren will use to remember the past, something they will use to learn about the world'.[2] Scholarly work can surely only be improved by following this advice.

## Notes

1 For a detailed discussion of these issues see A. Bammer & R.-E. Boetcher Joeres, (eds), *The Future of Scholarly Writing: Critical Interventions* (Basingstoke: Palgrave, 2015).

2 P. Stoller, 'Looking for the right path', in Bammer & Boetcher Joeres (eds) *The Future of Scholarly Writing*, p. 104.

# Abbreviations

| | |
|---|---|
| BMA | British Medical Association |
| *BMJ* | *British Medical Journal* |
| DHSS | Department of Health and Social Security |
| FPC | Family Practitioner Committee |
| FRCP | Fellowship of the Royal College of Physicians |
| FRCS | Fellowship of the Royal College of Surgeons |
| GMC | General Medical Council |
| GMSC | General Medical Services Committee |
| GP | General Practitioner |
| LMC | Local Medical Committee |
| MRCGP | Membership of the Royal College of General Practitioners |
| MRCP | Membership of the Royal College of Physicians |
| MRCS | Membership of the Royal College of Surgeons |
| NAEMD | National Association of Ethnic Minority Doctors |
| ODA | Overseas Doctors' Association |
| PLAB | Professional and Linguistic Assessment Board |
| RCGP | Royal College of General Practitioners |
| SRN | State Registered Nurse |
| TRAB | Temporary Registration Assessment Board |
| TUC | Trades Union Congress |
| WHO | World Health Organization |

# Introduction: writing the history of the 'International' Health Service

The histories of the National Health Service (NHS) and of British general practice are profoundly intertwined with the history of the imperial legacy and of medical migration. This book shows that the NHS, which was established in 1948, would not have been what it had become by the 1980s without being able to draw on the labour of migrant South Asian[1] doctors. When it comes to the history of the NHS, the migration of South Asian doctors cannot be treated as a side issue. An appreciation of its importance is essential to our understanding of the history of British healthcare. These doctors made it possible for British general practice to take on a role as the so-called 'cornerstone' of the NHS, the function of which was to control access to other (more expensive) treatments and provide care in community settings.

By the 1980s, over 4,000 general practitioners (GPs) working in the NHS had been born in India, Pakistan, Bangladesh or Sri Lanka.[2] They accounted for around 16 per cent of the GP workforce[3] and were the first point of contact in the UK's healthcare system for one-sixth of the population—some nine million people.[4] These GPs were overwhelmingly concentrated in parts of Britain that the majority of locally trained doctors deemed less attractive. In the early 1990s, over half of the GPs working in Walsall, an industrial town in the English Midlands, had qualified in South Asia. In predominantly rural Somerset in the South of England, the equivalent figure was of less than 1 per cent.[5]

South Asian GPs were instrumental to the delivery of care in industrial and inner-city areas. Their presence was a central dimension of the working class experience of healthcare. M. A. Salam, a GP who worked in a mining community in South Wales, thus told me of the surprise of one of his young patients at encountering a white doctor for the first time: 'One little boy was born in my practice. He saw me all the time and at the age of ten he had to go to hospital for tonsillectomy … When British doctors came to see him he was astonished: he thought all the doctors look like Dr Salam!'[6]

This account of a patient seeing a Bangladeshi doctor as being a member of something akin to a caste of practitioners at the service of the NHS is illustrative of the extent to which South Asian medical graduates were key to the functioning of the British healthcare system. Practitioners such as Dr Salam were working with populations that had historically found access to medicine difficult and that the NHS had been set up to serve, in a field that brought them in contact with a broad cross-section of the population. Aneurin Bevan, the radical Welsh politician who, as Minister of Health, presided over the introduction of the NHS, talked about the need to root out the 'evil' that was the link between the provision of medical care and the ability of the patient to afford it.[7] The establishment of the NHS sought to remove this barrier by making access to care free. Recourse to migrant labour enabled the British government to achieve this aim.

In the chapters that follow I explore the impact that South Asian migrant doctors had on British medicine and more generally British society. In so doing, I seek to draw on history's ability to inform our understanding of the present and to contribute to a reflection around the role of immigration in modern Britain. The marginalisation of migrants in historical accounts of Britain's past is not just an unfortunate oversight that deprives us of a better understanding of a particular dimension of history. It supports contemporary political narratives that construct migrants as outsiders and obscures the fact that migrants have been essential to the functioning of the societies in which they live.[8]

This is not to say that this is a celebratory history: it engages critically with archival evidence and oral history interviews in order to offer a new perspective on the history of the National Health Service. Whether the NHS's reliance on migrants is a cause for celebration or not is debatable. For instance, I highlight the fact that many British-trained doctors shunned general practice in areas where demand for healthcare was greatest and show that local populations were served by marginalised doctors who moved into these roles because of a lack of alternatives. This does not offer an ideal model of how to run a health service. Moreover, although South Asian GPs worked in areas of great need, it could be argued that there was an even greater need for their medical expertise in their countries of origin. The point is that we should recognise that the transnational movement of doctors fundamentally shaped an important dimension of life and death in post-war Britain.

In the following sections of this Introduction, I begin with an outline of how this study builds on current understandings of the histories of the NHS, empire, migration and more specifically medical migration. I then explain the rationale behind my focus on South Asian GPs during this period and go on to discuss how the study was conducted, as well as the conception of history which underpins it. I conclude by outlining the structure of the book.

## Putting imperial legacies and medical migration centre stage

Around a third of doctors in the UK today are overseas-born.[9] Migrant nurses and other healthcare workers have also been instrumental to the development of the NHS since its establishment.[10] The role of medical migration has however remained marginal both to accounts of the organisation's development and to work on the history of general practice.[11] Historians of South Asian immigration and of the impact of the imperial legacy on life in Britain have for their part devoted little attention to the post-war migration of doctors.[12]

Approaches to the history of the NHS are not untypical in marginalising the impact of migration. Over the last thirty years, historians working within academia and beyond its confines have simultaneously highlighted the importance of empire and international population movement to the history of the UK and other European nations and critiqued the lack of attention that has been devoted to it.[13] Alexandre Afonso has thus drawn attention to the relative lack of scholarly research into the history of Portuguese migrants in Switzerland and has noted their over-representation in areas such as hospitality and construction.[14] Leo Lucassen has written of the absence of 'Ellis Islands' (i.e. spaces that explicitly recognise the historical importance of immigration in European countries) and attributes this state of affairs to European preoccupations with notions of stable and homogenous nation states that have influenced the work of historians.[15] Tony Kushner offers a not dissimilar argument regarding forced migration in his book *Remembering refugees: Then and now* where he notes the lack of historical attention paid to the movement of some 250,000 Belgian refugees to Britain during World War I and contrasts it with what he calls the 'near obsession' with racist and fascist groups in British history.[16] Gérard Noiriel has shown how discussing migration as an internal dimension of the development of European nations rather than an external part of contemporary societies can serve to fundamentally reframe historical understandings by pointing out that between World War II and the late 1980s, immigrants to France built half of all new housing and 90 per cent of the motorways.[17] The silences of NHS history are symptomatic of what Noiriel has described as a 'collective amnesia' with respect to the role of immigration.[18] Of course, histories of migrants are being written, but as Panikos Panayi has pointed out, the need to ground wider histories in an understanding of population movement is still not widely appreciated by the mainstream of British academic history.[19]

Recent work pertaining to Britain has shown the utility of adopting the type of perspective that Panayi has argued for. Anandi Ramamurthy's work on British Asian youth movements and Linda McDowell's research into female migrants in the British workplace show that there is much to be gained by looking at the interaction between migrants and their social environments, rather than focusing exclusively on culture, experiences of exile and generally what makes migrants different.[20] Jamil Sherif, Anas Altikriti and Ismail Patel have further contributed to our understanding of these questions by exploring the impact of Muslim voters and organisations on electoral participation in British general elections.[21]

Naturally, if migration has tended to remain marginal to the preoccupations of historians in British and European contexts, other historical traditions have taken different approaches, which can support a shift in perspective when it comes to British history. Whilst the American paradigm of the 'nation of immigrants' is not unproblematic and can serve as a basis for the exclusion of certain groups (not least those who were forced to migrate as slaves) it has nevertheless compelled historians to engage with migration as a key dimension of US national histories.[22] In Argentina, international population movement is portrayed as a central dimension of the country's economic development.[23] Similarly, in Australia and New Zealand, migration appears more naturally as part of national stories.[24]

The growing body of transnational history has also contributed to further enhancing our appreciation of the need to pay greater attention to population movement, its effects and its regulation. Of particular relevance to the specific context discussed in this book, Anna Greenwood and Harshad Topiwala have shown how taking a transnational approach to the history of medicine and empire can bring to light the neglected roles of particular groups of physicians such as Indian doctors in Kenya under British rule.[25]

This study also builds on historical work which has underscored the importance of what Andrew Thompson refers to as the 'after-effects' of empire in contemporary Britain—in other words the ways in which the history of empire and colonialism has left its mark on present day society.[26] Georgina Sinclair and Chris A. Williams have demonstrated how the development of policing in Britain was influenced by colonial law enforcement, and argued that more attention should be paid to such concrete effects of the link between Britain and its empire.[27] Richard Whiting has made the case for the need to consider British politics and in particular the role of Britain in the world in the light of attitudes and perspectives connected to imperial dynamics.[28] Roberta Bivins has linked new approaches to imperial history to the history of the NHS by examining the ways in which responses to different patient groups influenced the development of healthcare in post-war Britain.[29]

This book adds to our understanding of the after-effects of empire by documenting their impact on the development of the British medical profession and therefore the structure of the NHS. Understanding modern Britain involves exploring the extent to which it has been and continues to be shaped by its imperial past. As Antoinette Burton has noted, this requires engaging with Franz Fanon's contention that Europe is literally the product of the Third World.[30] Drawing on the insights offered by these different strands of research enables a revisiting of the history of South Asians in Britain as a central part of the national story and can support the emergence of an alternative narrative of the making of modern Britain.[31]

### The significance of the international movement of doctors

Although overarching histories of the NHS tell us little about the role of migrant doctors, since the beginning of the twenty-first century, researchers have started to recover the history of migrant doctors in the NHS and have provided indications of how this task might serve to shape our understanding of the history of British healthcare. An essay published in 2007 by Aneez Esmail[32] set out a clear research agenda along these lines. He pointed out that although approximately a third of doctors practising in the NHS are from overseas, very little is known about their contribution to British medicine and to specific fields such as geriatrics, psychiatry and general practice where many of them found work. Esmail also outlined the importance of understanding the impact of discrimination against migrant doctors and of the legacies of empire on the development of healthcare provision in the UK.

Some answers to these questions have since been provided by oral history research on migrant South Asian geriatricians. Geriatrics formed a professional niche for South Asian doctors who exploited the unpopularity of the field of geriatrics to build careers in an organisation where they faced discrimination.[33] The specialty thus developed in a social context where both migrant practitioners and ageing patients were marginalised.[34] As one South Asian doctor put it: 'without racism there would be no discipline of geriatrics'.[35] Research on black and minority ethnic healthcare workers employed in the Manchester area between 1948 and 2009 provided additional evidence that migrants were essential to the staffing of the NHS in (post-) industrial northern cities: in 1972, over 80 per cent of doctors occupying the junior medical position of senior house officer in the Manchester Regional Hospital Board's area were from overseas.[36] Their testimony bore witness to their ability to engage with and shape the environments that they found, by setting up specialised clinics or simply through choosing to build careers in the NHS rather than leaving the UK.[37] The memoirs of a small number of doctors and of at least one doctor's wife contain additional evidence of the individual and collective roles of South Asian medical migrants.[38] Film makers,[39] community groups[40] and the race equality think tank the Runnymede Trust[41] have also explored this topic in ways which underscore the importance of this history and its relevance to ways in which we think of migrants in the present day.

Work on other groups of medical migrants in the UK and elsewhere also hints at the relevance of their professional trajectories to the development of global healthcare. Medical migrants are numerous; there is also evidence that in different locations and at different points in time, they have tended to cluster in particular roles and specific geographical areas. Several thousand medical refugees from Nazism settled in the UK and were an important part of the NHS workforce when it was launched in 1948.[42] They faced obstacles, including xenophobia and anti-Semitism, but also played a structural role in providing care to other Central European migrants and in some cases made significant contributions to medicine: Max Glatt, for example, was a pioneer of the rehabilitation of people with alcohol dependency.[43] According to Paul Weindling, specialisms such as psychiatry and pharmacology were particularly 'accommodating' to refugees.[44] Refugee doctors were in some cases directed towards locations in British colonies and dominions such as Newfoundland, Hong Kong or Burma that were seen as remote and where there was an undersupply of doctors.[45] Just over two thousand Irish general practitioners were working in Britain in 1965.[46] Alongside Scottish-trained doctors, they were often to be found working in general practice in industrial English cities.[47]

The United Kingdom is far from unique in being dependent on migrant medical labour. In 1972, 140,000 of the world's doctors were not living in the country they had been born in, with three quarters of these medical professionals working in the United States, the United Kingdom, Canada, the Federal Republic of Germany and Australia.[48] In 1997, 81 per cent of doctors in Saudi Arabia were migrants.[49] There is also evidence that the tendency for medical graduates who have moved from their country of origin to be disproportionately represented in the parts of the service that local graduates deem less desirable is not confined to the NHS. Indian doctors working in Riyadh reported being discriminated against when applying for managerial positions and being underpaid; the majority of them attributed this state of affairs to their geographical origins.[50] In Australia, services for the Aboriginal population and in areas far from major centres of population have historically relied on overseas graduates.[51] A study of medical migration to Canada between 1954 and 1976 found that less affluent provinces such as Newfoundland and Saskatchewan were the earliest and most active recruiters of migrant doctors.[52] Abraham Verghese's account of his work as a migrant doctor in deprived areas and 'under siege'[53] city hospitals in the USA paints a similar picture of dependency on international medical graduates to provide services to the local population:

> The effect of having so many foreign doctors in one area was at times comical. I had once tried to reach Dr Patel, a cardiologist, to see a tough old lady in the ER whose heart failure was not yielding to my diuretics and cardiotonics. I called his house and his wife told me he was at 'Urology Patel's' house, and when I called there I learned that he and 'Pulmonary Patel' had gone to 'Gastroenterology Patel's' house. Gastroenterology Patel's teenage daughter, a first-generation Indian-American, told me in a perfect Appalachian accent that she 'reckoned they're over at the Mehta's playing rummy', which they were.[54]

This vignette provides us with an intriguing insight into the realities of medical provision in the Appalachian Mountain range on the east coast of the USA, which is, of course, the scene of some of the most entrenched poverty in the country.

It is to be expected, though, that as we learn more about different groups of medical migrants, we will also learn more about how their experiences varied across time and space and according to their nationality, gender, ethnic origin and other factors. John Armstrong's research into the migration of doctors from New Zealand to the UK and the advantages that they derived from this movement on their return in the form of involvement in medical networks provides an insight into the experiences of white doctors in the NHS and an indication that this history is not necessarily one of marginalisation and disadvantage.[55] Although doctors who migrated to Canada were initially over-represented in particular geographical areas, there is also evidence that they were able to forge careers in the more prestigious fields.[56]

As well as adding to the history of the NHS, this book is therefore a contribution to the development of a contemporary history of the international movement of doctors and to the understanding of the role of migrants in healthcare systems in the Global North.[57]

## The making of the NHS: 1940s–1980s

General practice in the first 40 years of the NHS offers a particularly fertile ground where these questions of the impact of migration on the mainstream of society, the legacies of empire and the influence of medical migrants on the development of healthcare can be explored. Up to the late 1940s, the NHS was but a political idea. By the 1980s, it had established itself as a pillar of British society. As I will show in Chapter 1, at the beginning of this period, general practice was seen as in crisis and marginal. By the end of it, it was an indispensable part of the NHS and key to its workings. The process of dismantling the formal British Empire began in earnest with the independence of India in 1947, and by the 1980s Zimbabwean independence had marked its virtual end. As the formal Empire was dismantled, shifts in immigration policy and the regulation of the medical profession made it harder for former British subjects to move to the metropole.

The movement of South Asian doctors to Britain cannot be properly understood without reflecting on the legacy of empire. During the decade that followed independence and the partition of India in 1947, South Asian doctors who had been trained in English in schools shaped by the British model of medicine were able to move relatively freely within the former British Empire. This freedom was gradually eroded by new immigration laws from the 1960s onwards; by the withdrawal of recognition of medical degrees awarded on the Indian subcontinent as well as the introduction of professional and linguistic tests in the 1970s and finally by the establishment of compulsory specialised professional training for general practitioners in 1980 (until then any holder of a medical degree recognised by the General Medical Council (GMC) could become a GP).[58] By the 1980s, the relationship between British general practice and migration from the Indian subcontinent had been radically altered. Doctors who had qualified when subcontinental degrees were still recognised or who had passed the required tests and successfully undertook training could still enter general practice. The impact of South Asian medical migration on the NHS and general practice was however no longer on the same scale. The number of South Asian doctors working in the UK grew dramatically during the first four decades of the NHS—from up to 1,000[59] immediately after its inception to 10,000[60] by the end of the 1970s, making them the main group of international medical graduates working in the NHS. The percentage of South Asian-born doctors in the GP workforce peaked in the 1980s before beginning to decline in the 1990s.[61] Between the 1940s and the 1980s, the NHS was taking shape and establishing itself as a viable healthcare system as opposed to a political vision. The fact that it remains in existence today should not be retrospectively taken for granted: there was a strong current of opposition to it, which persisted throughout much of this period.[62] By the 1980s, the need to preserve the NHS had however become part of the political consensus.[63] Margaret Thatcher, whose governments were uncompromising about the virtues of wholesale privatisation in other domains, felt compelled to reassure voters that 'The National Health Service is safe with us'.[64]

I will show in this book that the NHS's ability to provide access to general practice services in all parts of Britain[65] was fundamentally dependent on the work of the South Asian doctors who contributed to its development as a field of medicine which was itself at the heart of the evolving structure of the NHS between the 1940s and the 1980s. As I will discuss in Chapter 1, general practice went through a period of fundamental change at this time, from being perceived as marginal to becoming central to the NHS and benefiting from an enhanced professional status. The College of General Practitioners was formed in 1952 and became a Royal College in 1972. Having been traditionally looked down upon by hospital specialists as the application of medical knowledge at a less in-depth level, general practice was by the 1980s formally recognised as a form of medical expertise in itself. It was also more than a newly defined specialty. Practitioners were at the heart of the British medical system. They managed care in community settings (thus containing the cost of specialised treatment) and controlled access to specialists in their role of 'gatekeepers'. GPs' direct contact with the population at large sets them apart from the majority of hospital specialists.[66] If a third of practitioners in a major urban conurbation were South Asian-born, this signifies that around a third of the people living in that area were dependent on these doctors as a first point of contact with the NHS. If it might be possible to argue that the NHS would have continued to exist in a recognisable form with, say, 30 per cent fewer geriatricians in a particular area, the absence of 30 per cent of GPs would have posed a problem of a different magnitude.

## Writing an oral history of a 'marginalised elite'

The argument that I develop in the following pages is based on an analysis of the forty-five oral history interviews that I conducted in the course of my research and a diverse array of archival material. It is also founded on a conception of history which views it as having the potential to enhance our understanding of society, rather than solely being concerned with interpreting the past.[67] In adopting this approach, I build on a tradition of historical scholarship that uses history to engage with contemporary questions.[68] As Eric Hobsbawm has noted, the flight of numerous historians from 'big questions' of social transformation towards culture, ideas and individual historical experiences is one of recent decades rather than a fundamental characteristic of social history.[69] He points out that historians can be stimulated not just by the methods used by social scientists but also by the questions they pose.[70] He attributes for instance the multiplication of historical studies of the British industrial revolution to the concerns of economists regarding the processes that shape industrial revolutions.[71] It should not be forgotten that E. P. Thompson's *The Making of the English Working Class*, one of the pioneering texts of British social history, was written, according to the author's preface, with a view to making a contribution to the understanding of class structures (through the examination of the history of ordinary people towards whom posterity had in his view shown 'enormous condescension').[72] In her preface to *Hidden from History*, her pioneering text of women's history, Sheila Rowbotham explicitly states that the inspiration for the book came from a desire to inform ongoing discussions about women's liberation.[73] It is worth restating that history provides useful tools for understanding the world that we live in and that using contemporary questions to formulate research questions has the potential to open up rich new seams of historical enquiry.

My work is also influenced by the arguments that a number of scholars have made in favour of the integration of historical perspectives into policy-making processes.[74] Virginia Berridge and John Stewart have argued that history is not necessarily solely concerned with the past and that it should also be seen as a social science that supports us in reflecting on social processes more generally.[75] As John Tosh has argued, history's emphasis on a holistic approach to evidence that unlike, say, economic or sociological research, is not informed by a problem-solving agenda driven by theory can serve to generate 'unexpected and illuminating' insights.[76] Historical reflection naturally offers a different perspective rather than clear instructions on how to proceed.[77] Its strength lies in its ability to generate different ways of thinking about current concerns.[78] Attempts to discuss history's policy relevance are of course subject to contestation and debate as is all historical knowledge. There are moreover limitations to such an approach: in addition to questions around the nature of historical knowledge, the extent to which understanding can be transferred across space and time is subject to debate and decontextualised historical knowledge has the potential to be misused.[79] It remains that reference to the past is in any case made in the context of policy debates and that historians can contribute to these ongoing discussions by using their training to provide a counterpoint to more simplistic recourses to history.[80] What I offer here is therefore a critical history of a group of migrants that I believe speaks to contemporary immigration debates.

This agenda naturally shaped my approach to the research I conducted for this book. Oral history, which involves drawing historical understanding from an engagement with people who lived through a particular period, can play a crucial role in helping to understand the interactions between migrants and the social mainstream. This approach builds on Rob Perks's critique of what he describes as British oral historians' central preoccupation with histories of ordinary people to the detriment of 'elite oral history', which he describes as being viewed with 'deep suspicion'.[81] According to Perks, the political origins of British oral history as a radical alternative to histories of male elites make historians ideologically averse to engaging with those who cannot be described as 'voiceless'.[82] He argues that this helps to explain the lack of attention that British oral historians devote to business and corporate culture.[83] Sjoerd Keulen and Ronald Kroeze have built on Perks's argument to make the case for the relevance of oral history to leadership and organisational research.[84] As they put it, oral historians tend to pay insufficient attention to important historical actors who are viewed as 'elites' because there is a presumption that they have already had ample opportunities to make their voices heard.[85] Perks retains a dichotomy between elite and marginalised histories which can at times be problematic: South Asian GPs were at times professional leaders and socially influential but they were also marginalised and have tended to remain hidden from history. Alongside Keulen and Kroeze, he does however point the way to a different approach to oral history by encouraging oral historians to strive to develop what he describes as a 'better understanding of our wider society'.[86]

As is the case with oral history generally, the focus of much of the history of immigration to the UK on experience and identity can be attributed at least in part to the intellectual roots of studies of migrant and black experiences conducted from the 1970s which were influenced by the emergence of a 'history from below' approach.[87] Cynthia Brown's analysis of recordings from the East Midlands Oral History Archives led her to conclude that it was time to 'move on from questions about settling in Britain or food and festivals to others that are more directly relevant to an understanding of experiences and relationships in the twenty-first century'.[88] She notes in particular that the influence of ethnic minority city councillors in Leicester is a subject that would merit detailed investigation.[89] It is in the fulfilling of this type of role that migrants might be described as marginalised elites. Medical migrants in some respects found themselves in subaltern positions but they also formed part of a group of professionals that was in a position to shape the NHS. Historians have much to gain from questioning the notion that there are rigid boundaries between the margins and the centre. Adopting this position supports the production of a more rounded account of the history of general practice and of the NHS, which incorporates the influence of marginalised practitioners on the development of the discipline and of British healthcare.

When assessing the ability of a group of migrants to exert influence on the system in which they were working, it is perhaps particularly important to be aware of the potential synergies between interviews and archival evidence. South Asian doctors have left traces in traditional archives as members of medical organisations, through the dealings that groups that they established had with government and as a result of their position in communities. They also preserved documents themselves in their personal or organisational archives and wrote to (and for) medical journals and the national media. Evaluating the impact of South Asian general practitioners on their field has therefore involved consulting a number of relevant sources such as newspapers, UK government records and the archives of professional medical bodies. The documents located in the process complement the interviews, providing details that many interviewees could not recall decades later and additional evidence of the agency revealed by participants' accounts of their lives. Interviews also served to help locate material in the archives, for instance when doctors discussed efforts to lobby government.

It is through a holistic engagement with this broad range of sources that a sense of how South Asian doctors contributed to shaping British general practice was developed. Finding relevant archival documents that provided information about the specific nature of the roles played by South Asian migrant doctors involved consulting a wide range of material and gradually building up a picture of their influence by drawing on a range of qualitative material and relevant statistics compiled at different times. I came to the conclusion quite early on in my research that this was the only logical way to proceed. As will be apparent, this is not the story of an official programme to import GPs that was centrally monitored. Nor does monitoring the degree to which migrants were able to exert agency necessarily figure high on the list of government priorities. Doctors did leave traces in government records, studies were at times carried out to determine their numbers and migrant doctors were discussed in the medical and mainstream media but I am unaware of the existence of any official files pertaining to a systematic monitoring of their deployment and their roles. In this book, I am often interpreting a range of materials and seeking to make a case beyond reasonable doubt rather than attempting to offer some form of immediate 'proof' of my claims. I believe in fact that this rounded approach has ultimately served to provide a more accurate picture than simply relying on government records and other official documents. For instance, as I will detail in this book, the Home Office during this period was publishing statistics on the migration of doctors that at least one of its officials believed were deliberately misleading.

It should of course be recognised that by proposing an interpretation of the past based on a human interaction located in the present, oral history is undoubtedly engaged in a task which differs from the endeavours of historians who remain solely focused on documents. This should naturally lead to a reflection around how best to conduct interviews and engage with their content. Kirby provides a useful summary of some of the main issues involved in collecting and analysing these data:

> How can the interviewer ask relevant, informed questions yet still provide an atmosphere that will not improperly influence the informant's responses? How can the historian evaluate the responses of the informant, which can be tainted in a variety of ways? And related to both of these is the larger issue of the objectivity or subjectivity of all historical data, indeed of all historical knowledge.[90]

Kirby's point about the relative nature of all historical knowledge is key to the oral history approach used in this study. Dealing with such concerns in respect of oral history is a not dissimilar process to the one advocated to make the broader case for the value of a historical approach in the context of this study. The historical methodology which has been adopted here involves essentially treating other sources such as printed materials with just as much caution. If the relationship between interviewer and interviewee can shape the content of an interview, then decisions made by historians when using archival material, the availability of material and the choices made by those who produced the documents equally shape the context and therefore the content of their work. Interviews contain statements which can be evaluated and provide information in the way that other sources do. If historians are able to critically engage with written sources as subjective as the records of the Inquisition or police reports on youth movements and produce historical accounts that are deemed credible, the same principle can be applied to oral sources.

The attachment of some historians to documentary sources over oral sources can in fact, as Pat Thane has pointed out, be seen as paradoxical, particularly given that many written documents are themselves reliant on oral sources or memory.[91] Paul Thompson, whilst recognising that all recollections are subjective, emphasises the relative nature of such concerns, mentioning that much of the process of memory shaping takes place in the immediate aftermath of an experience, thus influencing contemporaneous documentation such as newspapers, correspondence and official reports.[92] He also notes that oral history has the advantage of being able to engage with protagonists who may well express themselves more frankly as a result of the passage of time.[93] In addition, one of the neglected contributions that oral history makes to history is that it often enables researchers to gain access to printed material that has been preserved by individuals and would otherwise not have been available.[94] Oral sources can be used along with other sources, with the interaction between the two leading to the gathering of additional information and the development of new lines of enquiry.[95] The approach to oral history adopted here therefore involves seeing it as a natural component of a contemporary social history aimed at enhancing our understanding of the past and of the present through what Thompson describes as 'reconstructive cross-analysis'.[96]

It is also open to the insights that the subjective engagement of participants with the research project might produce and to drawing on the subjective nature of memory as a resource.[97] As Alessandro Portelli has argued, even factually inaccurate statements can contain a psychological truth that can be just as important as any narrative based on established facts.[98] Kirby's advocacy of the recourse to phenomenological principles (which focus on perceptions of the world) in oral history provides a useful reminder that:

> When the informant's memory seems vague or unreliable, the interviewer keeps in mind that all the 'real facts' cannot be known under even the best circumstances and looks rather for truths of understanding, of spirit, of cultural values, that tell the story of the historical event or era … often the goal should be to suggest possibilities rather than draw conclusions.[99]

This is not to say, as Portelli himself has pointed out, that oral history should be solely defined as an exercise in analysing subjectivity.[100] It also reveals 'unknown events or unknown aspects of known events'[101] and casts 'new light on unexplored areas of the daily life of the non-hegemonic classes'.[102] Both of these dimensions of oral history are relevant in the context of gaining a greater understanding of the role of South Asian doctors in the development of general practice and the NHS. They have enabled me to explore the interface between medical migration and the development of the British healthcare system.

At times, engagement with subjectivity predominated and I have drawn historical understanding from themes that emerged from the interviews. This was the case for instance when it came to reflecting on the ways that doctors described their relationship to the UK or with their patients (see Chapters 3 and 6). In other cases, I have heavily relied on contemporary media coverage or archival research, such as when trying to understand the evolution of British general practice and of migration policy (see Chapters 1 and 2). Elsewhere, oral history is interpreted alongside archival evidence. Although there was at times a greater reliance on one or the other, I viewed interviews and archival research as forming part of the same process that served to cast light on a past I was seeking to better understand. The conclusions of this research are therefore founded on an exploration of a range of evidence examined critically in different ways with the aim to gradually develop an understanding of the question being explored. Theory in this context was used when appropriate to provide an explanatory framework, for instance when using the concept of 'dirty work' (i.e. work that is perceived as lacking in dignity and prestige) in the context of medicine to understand how migrants came to be over-represented in particular roles or referring to 'heterophobia' (i.e. hostility towards difference) to seek to understand the discriminatory environment provided by the NHS.[103]

The findings presented here are based on forty-five oral history interviews (forty with South Asian GPs and five with other witnesses to this period, i.e. two medical politicians and three children of South Asian GPs) and extensive archival research (a list of sources is included in the bibliography). I sought to avoid being over-reliant on particular personal and professional networks and aimed to speak to male and female doctors from different parts of the subcontinent, who had worked in different parts of Britain. I recruited participants through various means, from attending gatherings of South Asian doctors to using the internet to locate doctors whose names appeared in the course of archival research, recourse to medical directories and reliance on personal contacts of people who agreed to participate. Obtaining consent to participate involved a negotiation process and in order to encourage participation I frequently promised to limit interviews to around ninety minutes—sometimes one hour in the case of doctors who continued to work long hours. This inevitably shaped the interviews as with limited time I tended to devote most of my questioning to doctors' lives and careers in medicine, which was the central focus of my research. At the end of the interviews participants were given the opportunity to frame a photographic portrait of themselves in a way that they felt represented them appropriately, choosing the setting and background. I believed that this would be a useful exercise in that it would produce a photographic record of the first generation of South Asian GPs to work in the NHS but also that doctors' engagement with this exercise might help cast light on the history I was researching.[104] All but three of the doctors interviewed received their initial medical training in the Indian subcontinent. I chose to not exclude South Asian-born and British-trained doctors from the study as I felt it would be useful to record their experiences and reflect on the extent to which they differed from those of their South Asian-trained counterparts. I also wanted to explore connections with pre-NHS medicine: the British-trained doctors I interviewed were all children of South Asian GPs. My aim in interviewing South Asian doctors was in any case not to claim that they formed a homogenous group; they clearly differ in many ways. It was rather to explore how the fact that the mainstream constructed them as different contributed to the development of medicine in the UK. When participants asked to remain anonymous, I refer to their quotations as being from an anonymous participant. I have refrained from the temptation to use different names or assign participants a number in an effort to ensure they cannot be recognised in a study that draws on biographical information. Some readers might for instance have been able to make an accurate educated guess concerning the identity of 'participant number 20' based on the content of several interview extracts that are attributed to the same person (i.e. one that identified them as having been active in local politics, another saying they trained in Calcutta and yet another detailing their passion for sport). A note finally on the transcripts of the interviews which accurately reflect the words and expressions used by participants. I have used ellipses ( ... ) to shorten passages and when people hesitated or stumbled on words. I have however refrained from anglicising extracts of interviews, preferring to remain faithful to the South Asian English used by many of the people I spoke to.

## The chapters

The book is divided into three parts.

The first two chapters place the history of migrant South Asian doctors in its wider context. Chapter 1 deals with the relationship between the migration of South Asian doctors, the development of general practice and the establishment of the NHS. It outlines my argument concerning their role in underpinning what came to be seen as a 'cornerstone' of the British healthcare system. Chapter 2 relates this history to the history of the British presence in the Indian subcontinent and situates it in relation to post-war immigration to the UK.

The second part of the book shows how imperial legacies and professional discrimination were central dimensions of the development of general practice. Chapter 3 draws on the narratives of South Asian doctors to bring to the fore the persistence of a deep-seated connection with the former metropole which is relevant to our understanding of the movement of doctors to Britain. Chapter 4 looks at the role of professional discrimination in shaping doctors' professional trajectories. Chapter 5 outlines how the limited choices available to doctors in a discriminatory environment led to them having a significant structural effect on the staffing and development of British general practice.

The third part of this book (Chapters 6–8) examines the impact that this group of migrants had on British society and medicine once they had taken up posts as GPs. Chapter 6 reflects on the nature of the relationships that doctors developed with their patients, be they white working class, South Asian or members of other ethnic minority groups. Chapter 7 charts the influence that South Asian doctors had on British medicine as a whole through individual and collective initiatives—such as for instance the establishment of the Overseas Doctors' Association. Chapter 8 focuses more specifically on their impact on the nascent specialty of general practice. In my conclusion, I explore how this history might inform contemporary thinking about the role of migrants in medicine and in wider British society.

## Notes

1  It is recognised that the term 'South Asian' does not do justice to the diversity of the group of people it encompasses. It is also the product of a contemporary framework of analysis rather than a reflection of the language used at the time. It is used here in the interests of clarity and simplicity to designate people born in present-day India, Pakistan, Bangladesh and Sri Lanka. It should hopefully be apparent by the end of this book that the shared professional experiences and comparable roles that medical migrants from the Indian subcontinent had in the NHS justify the collective approach adopted in this study. The term 'Asian', which appears at times in interviews with participants and references to other sources, is synonymous in the UK.

2  P. S. Gill, 'General practitioners, ethnic diversity and racism', in N. Coker (ed.), *Racism in Medicine: An Agenda for Change* (London: King's Fund Publishing, 2001), pp. 107, 111. The figure given by Gill is of 4,366

unrestricted GP principals. The expression refers to doctors who provide a full range of general medical services and whose list is not limited to a particular type of person. It excludes some GPs, for instance GP assistants, and salaried GPs. It is indicative of the prominent role that South Asian doctors took on in the GP workforce but does not tell us exactly how many of them worked in general practice at the time.

3  Gill, 'General practitioners'.

4  This estimate is calculated on the basis that the average GP patient list at the time was approximately 2,200 (British Medical Association Archives, London (henceforth, BMA), Executive Committee of Council, 1978–1979, Report of a working party on medical manpower, staffing and training requirements, 9 May 1979). Again, this figure is indicative. It is possible that South Asian doctors had smaller patient lists although given that they were generally to be found working in areas of high demand with an under-supply of doctors the reverse is more likely.

5  D. H. Taylor & A. Esmail, 'Retrospective analysis of census data on general practitioners who qualified in South Asia: Who will replace them when they retire?', BMJ, 318 (1999), pp. 307–8.

6  M. A. Salam interview with author, 18 March 2010.

7  Hansard, vol. 422 cc. 43–142, HC Deb, 30 April 1946 [online]. Available at: http://hansard.millbanksystems.com/commons/1946/apr/30/national-health-service-bill#S5cv0422PO-19460430-hoc-7 (accessed 24 May 2013).

8  J. M. Simpson, A. Esmail, V. S. Kalra, S. J. Snow, 'Writing migrants back into NHS history: Addressing a "collective amnesia" and its policy implications', Journal of the Royal Society of Medicine, 103:10 (2010); J. M. Simpson, 'Reframing NHS history: Visual sources in a study of UK-based migrant doctors', Oral History, 42:2 (2014).

9  OECD, International Migration Outlook 2015 (Paris: OECD Publishing, 2015), p. 111.

10 L. Doyal, G. Hunt, J. Mellor, 'Your life in their hands: Migrant workers in the National Health Service', Critical Social Policy, 1 (1981); L. Ryan, 'Who do you think you are? Irish nurses encountering ethnicity and constructing identity in Britain', Ethnic and Racial Studies, 30 (2007); E. L. Jones & S. J. Snow, Against the Odds: Black and Minority Ethnic Clinicians and Manchester, 1948 to 2009 (Lancaster: Carnegie, 2010).

11 See for instance C. Webster, The Health Services Since the War, Vols I & II (London: HMSO, 1988, 1996); G. Rivett, National Health Service History

[online]. Accessed 30 April 2012 at: www.nhshistory.net/; M. Gorsky 'The British National Health Service 1948–2008: A review of the historiography', *Social History of Medicine*, 21:3 (2008); I. Loudon, J. Horder, C. Webster (eds), *General Practice under the National Health Service 1948–1997* (London: Clarendon Press, 1998); G. Smith, F. Ferguson, E. Mitchell, M. Nicolson, G. C. M. Watt, *Speaking for a Change: An Oral History of General Practice*. School of Health and Related Research (ScHARR), University of Sheffield. ScHARR Report Series No.17, 2007 [online]. Available at: http://personal.rhul.ac.uk/usjd/135/indexgp.htm (accessed 1 May 2012).

12  See M. H. Fisher, S. Lahiri, S. Thandi (eds), *A South Asian History of Britain: Four Centuries of Peoples from the Indian Sub-Continent* (Oxford and Westport, Connecticut: Greenwood World Publishing, 2007); A. Thompson, *The Empire Strikes Back? The Impact of Imperialism on Britain from the Mid-Nineteenth Century* (Harlow: Pearson Education Limited, 2005).

13  See for example C. Holmes, *John Bull's Island: Immigration and British Society 1871–1971* (Basingstoke, London: Macmillan Education, 1988); G. Noiriel, *Le Creuset Français* (Paris: Editions du Seuil, 1988) (French); R. Visram, *Asians in Britain: 400 Years of History* (London: Pluto Press, 2002); L. Lucassen, *The Immigrant Threat: The Integration of Old and New Migrants in Western Europe since 1850* (Urbana and Chicago: University of Illinois Press, 2005); T. Kushner, *Remembering Refugees: Then and Now* (Manchester, New York: Manchester University Press, 2006); A. Burton, *After the Imperial Turn: Thinking with and Through the Nation* (Durham, North Carolina and London: Duke University Press, 2003); P. Panayi, *An Immigration History of Britain: Multicultural Racism since 1800* (Harlow: Pearson, 2000); D. Olusoga, *Black and British: A Forgotten History* (London: Macmillan, 2016).

14  A. Afonso, 'Permanently provisional: History, facts and figures of Portuguese immigration in Switzerland', *International Migration*, 53:4 (2015).

15  Lucassen, *The Immigrant Threat*, pp. 13 & 19.

16  Kushner, *Remembering Refugees*, pp. 6–7. Kushner noted that only one major study of the Belgian refugee movement had been conducted whereas nearly one hundred studies of the British Union of Fascists and of its leader Oswald Mosley had been published.

17  Noiriel, *Le Creuset Français*, p. 312.

18  Noiriel, *Le Creuset Français*, p. 19; Simpson et al., 'Writing migrants'.

19  Panayi, *Immigration History*, p. 6.

20  A. Ramamurthy, *Black Star: Britain's Asian Youth Movements* (London: Pluto Press, 2013); L. McDowell, *Working Lives: Gender, Migration and Employment in Britain, 1945–2007* (Chichester: Wiley-Blackwell, 2013).

21  J. Sherif, A. Altikriti, I. Patel, 'Muslim electoral participation in British general elections: An historical perspective and case study', in T. Peace (ed.), *Muslims and Political Participation in Britain* (Abingdon: Routledge, 2015).

22  P. Spickard, 'Introduction: Immigration and race in United States history', in P. Spickard (ed.), *Race and immigration in the United States* (New York: Routledge, 2012), pp. 1–12; B. O. Hing, *Defining America Through Immigration Policy* (Philadelphia: Temple University Press, 2004).

23  R. Benencia, 'Apéndice: La inmigración limítrofe', in F. Devoto *Historia de la inmigración en la Argentina* (Buenos Aires: Sudamericana, 2009) (Spanish), p. 433.

24  See for instance C. Coleborne, *Insanity, Identity and Empire: Immigrant and Institutional Confinement in Australia and New Zealand, 1873–1910* (Manchester: Manchester University Press, 2015); A. McCarthy, 'Migration and madness at sea: The nineteenth- and early twentieth-century voyage to New Zealand', *Social History of Medicine*, 28:4 (2015).

25  A. Greenwood & H. Topiwala, *Indian Doctors in Kenya, 1895–1940: The Forgotten History* (Basingstoke: Palgrave, 2015).

26  Thompson, *The Empire Strikes Back?*, p. 203.

27  G. Sinclair & C. A. Williams, '"Home and away": The cross-fertilisation between "colonial" and "British" policing, 1921–85', *The Journal of Imperial and Commonwealth History*, 35:2 (2007), pp. 221–2.

28  R. Whiting, 'The Empire and British politics', in A. Thompson (ed.), *Britain's Experience of Empire in the Twentieth Century* (Oxford: Oxford University Press, 2016).

29  R. Bivins, *Contagious Communities: Medicine, Migration and the NHS in Post-War Britain* (Oxford: Oxford University Press, 2015).

30  Burton, *Imperial Turn*, p. 1.

31  R. Ranasinha, 'Introduction', in R. Ranasinha (ed.), *South Asians and the Shaping of Britain 1870–1950* (Manchester and New York: Manchester University Press, 2012), p. 1.

32  A. Esmail, 'Asian doctors in the NHS: Service and betrayal', *British Journal of General Practice*, 57 (2007).

33  P. Raghuram, J. Bornat, L. Henry, 'Ethnic clustering among South Asian geriatricians in the UK: An oral history study', *Diversity in Health and Care*, 6 (2009).

34  P. Raghuram, J. Bornat, L. Henry, 'The co-marking of aged bodies and migrant bodies: Migrant workers' contribution to geriatric medicine in the UK', *Sociology of Health and Illness*, 33: 2 (2011).

35  Raghuram et al., 'Ethnic clustering', p. 295.

36  Jones & Snow, *Against the Odds*, p. 36.

37  Jones & Snow, *Against the Odds*, pp. 87 & 94.

38  A. Sayeed, *In the Shadow of my Taqdir* (Stanhope: The Memoir Club, 2006); S. Chatterjee, *All my Yesterdays* (Stanhope: The Memoir Club, 2006); R. A. A. R. Lawrence, *A Fire in his Hand* (London: Athena Press, 2006); B. Bhowmick, *You Can't Climb a Ladder with your Hands in Your Pockets* (Warboys, Cambridgeshire: Biograph, 2006); S. Chowdhary, *I Made my Home in England* (Basildon: published by Savritri Chowdhary and printed by Grant-Best Ltd, 1962?).

39  J. Foot, *Time Shift: From the Raj to the Rhondda*, BBC, 2003; S. Suri, *'I for India'*, Fandango and Zero West, 2005.

40  Eastside Community Heritage, *Living in Barking: Hidden from History*, 2010 (?).

41  D. Weekes-Bernard (with interviews by Klara Schmitz, Saher Ali, Valentina Migliarini), *Nurturing the Nation: The Asian Contribution to the NHS since 1948* (London: The Runnymede Trust, 2013).

42  P. Weindling, 'Medical refugees in Britain and the wider world, 1930–1960: Introduction', *Social History of Medicine*, 22:3(2009), p. 454.

43  P. Weindling, 'The contribution of Central European Jews to medical science and practice in Britain, the 1930s–1950s', in W. E. Mosse, J. Carlebach, G. Hirschfeld, A. Newman, A. Paucker, P. Pulzer (eds), *Second chance: Two Centuries of German-Speaking Jews in the United Kingdom* (Tübingen: J. C. B. Mohr (Paul Siebeck), 1991), pp. 247 & 253; P. Weindling, 'Medical refugees and the modernisation of British medicine, 1930–1960', *Social History of Medicine*, 22:3 (2009), pp. 504–6; A. Winklemann-Gleed & J. Eversley, 'Salt and Stairs: A history of refugee doctors in the UK', in N. Jackson & Y. Carter (eds), *Refugee Doctors: Support, Development and Integration in the NHS* (Oxford and San Francisco: Radcliffe Publishing, 2004), pp. 15–17.

44  Weindling, 'Modernisation', p. 505.

45  Weindling, 'Introduction', pp. 455–6.

46  O. Gish, 'Emigration and the supply and demand for medical man-power: The Irish case', *Minerva*, 7:4 (1969), p. 669.

47  Esmail, 'Asian doctors', p. 834; A. Digby, 'The British National Health Insurance Act, 1911', in M. Gorsky and S. Sheard (eds), *Financing Medicine: The British Experience since 1750* (Abingdon, New York: Routledge, 2000), p. 186; J. S. Collings, 'General practice in England today: A reconnaissance', *The Lancet*, 255: 6604 (1950), p. 580.

48  D. Wright, N. Flis, M. Gupta, 'The "brain drain" of physicians: Historical antecedents to an ethical debate', *Philosophy, Ethics and Humanities in Medicine*, 3:24 (2008).

49  S. I. Alkhudairy, 'International labour migration to Saudi Arabia: A case study of the experiences of medical doctors in Riyadh' (PhD dissertation, University of Essex, 2001), p. 8.

50  Alkhudairy, 'International labour migration to Saudi Arabia', pp. 141–2 & 152.

51  M. T. Gilles, J. Wakerman, A. Durey, '"If it wasn't for OTDs, there would be no AMS": Overseas-trained doctors working in rural and remote Aboriginal health settings', *Australian Health Review*, 32:4 (2008); R. Iredale, 'Luring overseas trained doctors to Australia: Issues of training, regulating and trading', *International Migration*, 47:4 (2009).

52  S. Mullally & D. Wright, 'La grande séduction? The immigration of foreign-trained physicians to Canada c. 1954–76', *Journal of Canadian Studies*, 41:3 (2007).

53  A. Verghese, *My Own Country: A Doctor's Story of a Town and its People in the age of AIDS* (London: Phoenix, 1995), p. 12.

54  Verghese, *My Own Country*, p. 17.

55  J. Armstrong, 'A system of exclusion: New Zealand women medical specialists in international medical networks, 1945–1975', in L. Monnais and D. Wright (eds), *Doctors Beyond Borders: The Transnational Migration of Physicians in the Twentieth Century* (Toronto: University of Toronto Press, 2016).

56  D. Wright & S. Mullally, '"Not everyone can be a Gandhi": South Asian-trained doctors immigrating to Canada, c. 1961–1971', *Ethnicity and Health*, 21:4 (2016), p. 346.

57  See L. Monnais & D. Wright (eds), *Doctors Beyond Borders: The Transnational Migration of Physicians in the Twentieth Century* (Toronto: University of Toronto Press, 2016).

58  Changes to medical regulations will be discussed in detail in Chapter 2.

59  C. Kondapi, *Indians Overseas 1838–1949* (New Delhi, Bombay, Calcutta, Madras, London: Indian Council of World Affairs, Oxford University Press, 1951), p. 360. The figure of 1,000 Indian doctors in the UK that Kondapi provides should be treated with caution as the author does not state how this figure was calculated. It is however clear that the presence in Britain of a substantial community of South Asian doctors predates the establishment of the NHS (see in particular Lahiri, *Indians in Britain: Anglo-Indian Encounters, Race and Identity, 1880–1930* (London: Frank Cass, 2000) and Visram, *Asians in Britain*).

60  Simpson et al., 'Writing migrants', p. 392.

61  R. Jones & S. Menzies, *General Practice Essential Facts* (Abingdon: Radcliffe Medical Press, 1999), p. 43; Taylor & Esmail 'Retrospective analysis of census data', pp. 307–8.

62  See for instance, C. Webster, *The National Health Service: A Political History* (Oxford, New York: Oxford University Press, 1998), pp. 140–55; D. Seaton, 'Against the "Sacred cow": NHS opposition and the Fellowship for Freedom in Medicine, 1948–72', *Twentieth Century British History*, 26:3 (2015).

63  Webster, *Political History*, pp. 140–55.

64  Margaret Thatcher, Speech to Conservative Party Conference, 14 October 1983 [online]. Accessed 17 April 2017 at: www.margaretthatcher.org/document/105454. Her statement is often misquoted as 'The NHS is safe in our hands'.

65  The focus of this research has been on Great Britain rather than on the whole of the UK, to the exclusion of Northern Ireland. This is for two reasons—no evidence regarding South Asian GPs in Northern Ireland was located in the course of this study and the specific dynamics of the relationship between medicine in Northern Ireland and the Republic of Ireland has served to guard against any temptation to simply extrapolate the conclusions of this study to the whole of the UK. According to one estimate, between 10 and 15 per cent of GPs working in Northern Ireland in May 1968 were from the Republic of Ireland (Gish, 'The Irish case', p. 670). I have used the term Britain to refer to Great Britain. I refer to the UK when I am quoting from studies that focused on the UK or when discussing the actions of the UK government.

66  Accident and emergency constitutes a partial exception in this respect.

67  V. Berridge & J. Stewart, 'History: A social science neglected by the other social sciences (and why it should not be)', *Contemporary Social Science: Journal of the Academy of Social Sciences*, 7:1 (2012).

68  See for instance S. Lynd, 'Historical past and existential present', in T. Roszak (ed.), *The Dissenting Academy: Essays Criticising the Teaching of the Humanities in American Universities* (London: Pelican, 1969), p. 91.
69  E. Hobsbawm, *How to Change the World: Tales of Marx and Marxism* (London: Little, Brown, 2011), p. 392.
70  E. Hobsbawm, 'From social history to the history of society', *Daedalus*, 100:1, p. 25.
71  Ibid.
72  E. P. Thompson, *The Making of the English Working Class* (London: Penguin Books, 1991), pp. 10 & 12.
73  S. Rowbotham, *Hidden from History: 300 Years of Women's Oppression and the Fight Against It* (London: Pluto Press, 1977).
74  See for instance R. A. Stevens, C. E. Rosenberg, L. R. Burns (eds), *History and Health Policy in the United States: Putting the Past Back In* (New Brunswick, New Jersey and London: Rutgers University Press, 2006); S. Szreter, *Health and Wealth: Studies in History and Policy* (Rochester: University of Rochester Press, 2007); J. Tosh, *Why History Matters* (Basingstoke: Palgrave Macmillan, 2008); D. Drakeman, *Why we Need the Humanities: Life Science, Law and the Common Good* (Basingstoke, New York: Palgrave Macmillan, 2016); M. Woolcock, S. Szreter, V. Rao, et al., 'How and why does history matter for development policy', *Journal of Development Studies*, 47:1 (2011); P. Cox, 'The future use of history', *History Workshop Journal*, 75:1 (2013); A. Green, 'History as expertise and the influence of political culture on advice for policy since Fulton', *Contemporary British History*, 29:1 (2015); A. Green, *History, Policy and Public Purpose: Historians and Historical Thinking in Government* (London: Palgrave, 2016); G. Noiriel, *Introduction a la socio-histoire* (Paris: Editions La Découverte, 2006) (French).
75  Berridge & Stewart, 'History: a social science'.
76  Tosh, *Why History Matters*, pp. 22, 38 & 41.
77  L. Jordanova, *History in Practice* (London: Hodder Arnold, 2006), p. 3.
78  Tosh, *Why History Matters*, pp. 22 & 41; L. Delap, S. Szreter, P. Warde, 'History and policy: A decade of bridge-building in the United Kingdom', *Scandia*, 80:1 (2014), pp. 100–1.
79  Woolcock et al., 'How and why does history matter', p. 73.
80  V. Berridge, 'Public or policy understanding of history?', *Social History of Medicine*, 16:3 (2003), p. 75.

81  R. Perks, 'The roots of oral history: Exploring contrasting attitudes to elite, corporate, and business oral history in Britain and the US', *The Oral History Review*, 37:2 (2010), p. 215.

82  Perks, 'The roots of oral history', pp. 215 & 220.

83  Perks, 'The roots of oral history', p. 215.

84  S. Keulen & R. Kroeze, 'Back to business: A next step in the field of oral history – The usefulness of oral history for leadership and organisational research', *The Oral History Review*, 39:1 (2012).

85  Keulen & Kroeze, 'Back to business', p. 16.

86  Perks, 'Roots of oral history', p. 220.

87  T. Kushner, 'Great Britons: Immigration, history and memory', in K. Burrell & P. Panayi (eds), *Histories and Memories: Migrants and Their History in Britain* (London, New York: Tauris Academic Studies, 2006), p. 22.

88  C. Brown, 'Reflections on oral history and migrant communities in Britain', *Oral History*, 34:1 (2006), p. 69.

89  Brown, 'Reflections on oral history', p. 72.

90  R. K. Kirby, 'Phenomenology and the problems of oral history', *The Oral History Review*, 35:1 (2008), p. 24.

91  P. Thane, 'Oral history, memory and written tradition: An introduction', *Transactions of the Royal Historical Society*, 6:9 (1999), p. 161.

92  P. Thompson, 'Oral history and the history of medicine: A review', *Social History of Medicine*, 4:2 (1991), p. 374.

93  Ibid.

94  V. E. Harrington, 'Voices beyond the asylum: A post-war history of mental health services in Manchester and Salford' (PhD dissertation, The University of Manchester, 2008), p. 15.

95  Thompson, 'Oral history and the history of medicine', p. 377.

96  P. Thompson, *The Voice of the Past: Oral History*, third edition (Oxford: Oxford University Press, 2000), pp. 270–1.

97  A. Thomson 'Making the most of memories: The empirical and subjective value of oral history', *Transactions of the Royal Historical Society*, 6: 9 (1999), p. 54.

98  A. Portelli, 'What makes oral history different?', in R. Perks & P. Thomson, *The Oral History Reader*, second edition (London and New York: Routledge, 2008), p. 37.

99  Kirby, 'Phenemonelogy', pp. 33–5.

100  Portelli, 'Oral history', p. 36.

101  Ibid.
102  Ibid.
103  Simpson et al., 'Providing "special" types of labour'; J. M. Simpson &
     J. Ramsay, 'Manifestations and negotiations of racism and "heteropho-
     bia" in overseas-born South Asian GPs accounts of careers in the UK',
     *Diversity and Equality in Health and Care*, 3–4 (2014).
104  I discuss these portraits and their significance in more detail in Simpson,
     'Reframing NHS history'.

Part I

# Healthcare and migration in Britain during the post-war period

# 1

# The making of a cornerstone

Before exploring in detail the way in which migrant South Asian doctors shaped general practice and the NHS, I first want to situate their story within the broader context of the history of British healthcare, empire and of post-war migration to the UK. The role of migrant doctors in the NHS is not confined to general practice. They were disproportionately represented in junior positions, less prestigious types of medicine and in geographical areas that were unpopular with local medical graduates. I will say more about the legacies of empire in the context of labour shortages in the NHS and post-war medical migration in Chapter 2. However, the presence of South Asian GPs in the NHS was about much more than the simple provision of additional labour. Additional labour can be seen as a convenient benefit that an organisation could do without if necessary. But if the South Asian GPs who accounted for 16 per cent of practitioners working in the NHS by the 1980s had been taken out of the system, it would not simply have continued to function at a slightly reduced capacity. In their absence, recruitment problems in the NHS would have had a debilitating effect on its ability to provide general practice services in areas of high need. General practice might have been able to function with 16 per cent fewer GPs across Britain but imagining the service continuing without between a third and half of its practitioners in unpopular industrial locations is another matter. Migrant doctors were providing 'special labour', as migrants frequently do in other parts of the economy—doing jobs that are unpopular with the indigenous population.[1]

Understanding the importance of the presence of South Asian GPs in the NHS involves engaging with the fact that they were enabling the continued existence of a service that by the 1980s was widely acknowledged by politicians and practitioners to be a cornerstone of the NHS and to some was even the 'jewel' in its crown.[2] It involves reflecting on the significance of something that did not happen: an acute crisis in British general practice caused by the lack of graduates from British medical schools willing to become GPs in particular areas given the pay and conditions on offer in the NHS and the decisions of these graduates to migrate. Thousands of British doctors left the country during this period rather than take up the jobs that their over-seas-trained counterparts ended up doing. In order to appreciate the impact of South Asian GPs on their field of medicine and on the NHS it is important to have a sense of how precarious the future of general practice was during this period, how it was reinvented and established itself as a core part of the NHS and to acknowledge the degree to which it remained an unpopular and fragmented field. It retained credibility as a means of delivering care because the scale of medical migration disguised the gap between the aspirations of British doctors and the needs of the NHS. When the NHS was launched in 1948, its long-term viability was far from guaranteed and the future and relevance of gen-eral practice was in question. The thousands of South Asian doctors who became general practitioners were also, because of the nature of the field, placed in a position where they often had a great deal of pro-fessional autonomy and therefore had a significant impact on the provi-sion of care on a day-to-day basis.[3]

I will seek here to give a sense of the radical changes that took place in British general practice during the first forty years of the NHS; I will emphasise the challenges that general practice faced in terms of its status and the profession's ability to recruit British doctors; and will make the case for the need to write histories of the profession that reflect its fragmented nature and reintegrate the role played by migrants. I start by situating the history of general practice within the wider context of the history of the NHS. I then describe the problems that general practice faced following the establishment of the NHS, the scepticism that many British doctors expressed towards the new healthcare system and the scale of the exodus of British-trained doc-tors from the UK. I will then outline how the parallel processes of the professionalisation of general practice following the establishment of the College of General Practitioners in 1952 and government moves to rely on GPs to deliver more care in community settings combined to consolidate general practice's status at the heart of British health-care provision. Finally I will discuss the fragmented nature of British general practice during these years, the variations between geograph-ical areas, the lack of a precise sense of what being a GP involved and the loose relationship between the state and GPs. I will argue that this meant that migrant doctors working in the system were not only underpinning provision but also by definition contributing to defin-ing the nature of general practice as the field was at the time made up of the sum of the individual understandings of those working in it, rather than being a set of practices and procedures followed by all doctors.

## The NHS, 'special' labour and westernised medical systems

Aneurin Bevan and the post-war Labour government, which came to power after its victory in the 1945 general election, abolished the exist-ing system of health insurance, which provided cover for just over 40 per cent of the pre-war population, replacing it with a centrally funded body.[4] Although other western governments also became more directly involved in healthcare between the 1940s and the 1960s, the British state was atypical in placing itself at the centre of the funding and deliv-ery of provision.[5] This commitment inevitably brought with it financial pressures. As Charles Webster puts it: 'The National Health Service had barely begun before it was overtaken by the crisis over expenditure.'[6] Access to the service was free at the outset but in the face of mounting costs, discussions around the introduction of charges took place as early as the late 1940s.[7] Charges for prescriptions, dental and ophthalmic services were introduced in 1951.[8] The establishment of the Guillebaud Committee, which reported on the financing of the NHS in 1956, has been described by John Stewart as 'indicative of a deep-rooted politi-cal and Treasury scepticism about social welfare expenditure'.[9] In fact the Committee did not serve the agenda of the Conservative govern-ment of the time as it concluded that the NHS was providing value for money and indeed required a higher level of expenditure.[10] It remains that keeping the NHS going while containing costs is a key preoccupa-tion of governments.

Although there were divergences between England, Wales and Scotland when it came to the organisation of the delivery of care between the 1940s and the 1980s, the NHS was characterised by its so-called 'tripartite' structure. Separate administrative structures governed family practitioner services (including general practice but also dentists, pharmacists and opticians), personal social services and public health, and the hospital service.[11] This set-up was criticised within medical policy circles for being inefficient and uncoordinated: general practitioners were providers of services to the NHS and retained their independence, public health was the responsibility of local authorities and hospitals were under the control of central government.[12] Critics also pointed out that although health ministers were nominally in full control of health policy, in fact, much power resided with local bodies.[13] This allowed the medical profession scope to pursue its own agendas.[14] A major structural reform aimed at improving the functioning of the NHS was introduced in 1974, but without fundamentally altering these dynamics nor the tripartite structure.[15]

The fact that the NHS is regarded as a distinctively British organisation and that it has survived until the present day should not lead us to believe from the vantage point of the present that its continued existence into the 1980s was inevitable. Scepticism towards it persisted within the medical profession during the first four decades of its existence.[16] Questions about how it should be funded continued to be asked. The introduction of an alternative funding system reliant on insurance was seen as a potential policy option following the Conservative victory in the 1979 election.[17] It was as late as 1989 that Margaret Thatcher made a firm commitment to preserving existing arrangements, her foreword to the White Paper *Working for Patients* making it clear that the 'National Health Service will continue to be available to all, regardless of income, and to be financed mainly out of general taxation.'[18] Rethinking the history of the NHS should therefore involve acknowledging the challenges it has faced and documenting the ways in which they have been met. It also necessitates engaging with the diverse range of social forces that shaped the organisation rather than solely focusing on top-down political initiatives, as indeed historians have begun to do by examining for instance the roles of patient organisations.[19] The NHS's reliance on medical migrants and the growth in prestige of general practice can both be connected to successive governments' cost-containment agendas and are interconnected.

### The ongoing crisis of general practice and the exodus of British doctors

Six months before the NHS was established in July 1948, the British Medical Association held a vote to gauge the views of general practitioners concerning the new system. It revealed that 84 per cent of them were opposed to its introduction.[20] This scepticism did not simply fade away in the years that followed. Many GPs continued to be unhappy with their lot and thousands of newly qualified British doctors left the country. The gradual change in the status of general practice did make a difference in this respect but discontent persisted. Conditions within the NHS, particularly in industrial areas, contributed to this. General practice as a whole was also perceived within the medical profession, particularly at the beginning of this period, as a subordinated form of medicine and one practised by those who had failed to build successful careers in hospital medicine. The former president of the Royal College of Physicians and personal physician to Winston Churchill, Lord Moran, notoriously ridiculed the notion that general practitioners could be compared to hospital consultants, saying that GPs were those who had 'fallen off the ladder' that the more talented hospital specialists had succeeded in climbing.[21] The importance of the role of South Asian GPs in respect of general practice in the NHS can only be properly understood with reference to this context. British general practice was simply not self-sustaining during this period: it could not rely on British-born and trained doctors to support the new system and do the work that was required.

*The state of general practice in 1950: 'bad and still deteriorating'*
The future of general practice following the establishment of the NHS was deemed at best uncertain. According to the historian of the NHS Charles Webster, 'There was a real danger that general practice might retreat into its ghetto, deteriorate, and ultimately face extinction'.[22] The notion that general practice might have ceased to exist as a distinct area of medicine is debatable. There continues to be a demand around the world for doctors who are the first port of call in community settings and it is hard to imagine the UK representing an exception in this respect.

Nevertheless, Webster is undoubtedly correct to draw attention to the extent of the challenges facing the field at the time. In 1950, the medical journal *The Lancet* published a report entitled 'General Practice in England Today' which suggested that it was an ill-defined field, under pressure because of the extension of access to care under the NHS, that too little was done to establish and maintain standards and that practitioners were becoming demoralised.[23] Its author, Joseph Collings, an Australian-trained doctor who had been granted a Harvard Fellowship to study general practice in the UK, visited fifty-five practices in England (and a number in Scotland for the purpose of comparison). His report came at a time when doubts were emerging about the NHS's ability to address long-standing issues in British general practice, particularly given the decline in its prestige at a time when GPs' roles in the hospital system were perceived as becoming increasingly marginal.[24] The document's conclusions were scathing:

> The working conditions (surgeries and equipment, organisation and staffing) of many general practices are unsatisfactory. Some are bad enough to require condemnation in the public interest. In some cases— particularly in industrial areas—the working conditions are so bad as to override the abilities and skills of the individual doctor … The over-all state of general practice is bad and still deteriorating.[25]

What Collings saw led him to conclude that the present and future of general practice looked 'grim' and that the field was 'becoming an unattractive proposition' for young doctors.[26] His report was greeted with anger at the time but came to be accepted as an accurate description of the state of the field in the aftermath of the inception of the NHS.[27] The editorial that accompanied the report in *The Lancet* is also indicative of the uncertainty surrounding the future of general practice at the time:

> Within the profession there is indeed a very real, if unavowed, difference of opinion: on the one hand are those who see no future for the general practitioner except as an appendage to the hospital service, while on the other are those who believe he must be brought back to his former position as a highly responsible doctor. Somewhere between these opposites are those who hold, by no means unreasonably, that ideally the practitioner should concern himself less with organic disease and more with elementary psychotherapy and preventive medicine.[28]

In 1950, it appeared far from inevitable that general practice would become a central part of the NHS system. There were tensions connected to the gap between the professional and personal aspirations of medical professionals and the characteristics of the new healthcare system. In the late 1950s, the possibility that doctors might withdraw from the NHS was still being given serious consideration by the General Medical Services Committee (GMSC)—the national body closely associated with the British Medical Association (BMA) responsible for matters pertaining to general practice.[29] In 1965, this ambivalence towards the NHS and the work that it offered GPs took the form of a threat of mass resignation by GPs demanding new terms and conditions.[30]

### Disillusionment persists

Even though a new contract was eventually agreed, discontent about pay and conditions persisted. In 1974, a letter sent to the BMA by the wife of a single-handed GP who had a patient list of nearly 3,000 stated that her husband:

> has none of the 'perks' of General Practice viz: Clinics, Factories, Insurance companies etc so in order to make a living he cannot afford to cut down his list and has to slog away at the ever-increasing burden of providing a good, conscientious service ... So here is your single-handed G.P. sweating his guts out with a list well above the recommended average, with the prospect of only 3 weeks holiday a year, and never more than 2 weeks at a stretch. He is a hard-working, conscientious chap much loved by his patients ... but because of the pressures of work, and the mounting FINANCIAL [sic] pressures ... he is looking into the possibility of taking up superannuation and doing locums ... I have been my husband's Nurse-receptionist, after seeing general practice from the house and telephone for the last 27 years ... frankly I wonder why all G.P.s are not locked up in lunatic asylums.[31]

The fact that this bleak assessment of the realities of a particular GP's day-to-day existence has survived as an appendix to the minutes of the rural practices subcommittee of the GMSC suggests that this account resonated with other doctors. Writing in the medical magazine *Pulse* in 1977, a GP in Essex, in south-east England, lamented the decline in

social status and purchasing power that he believed general practitioners had suffered in the course of his lifetime:

> When I first came into practice, my teachers at university had Daimlers,
> Bentleys and the occasional Rolls. My established colleagues in general
> practice had Rovers and Jaguars. Recently I looked around as I was get-
> ting into my car after a meeting at the local postgraduate centre. The cars
> that filled the car park were not only far less illustrious names ... but
> even more disappointing, they were usually several years old, and one
> or two were in obvious states of disrepair.[32]

Whilst the plight of British doctors reduced to relying on humdrum
modes of transportation might not elicit a great deal of sympathy, this
comment—and the fact that the writer and the magazine presumably
thought that doctors would identify with the sentiments expressed—
helps to explain why so many doctors left the UK at the time. If the
NHS was seen as offering an environment where the status of doctors
was diminished, working in other parts of the world could naturally be
perceived as a tempting alternative.

The testimony of doctors did not contradict this picture. It might be
expected that oral history interviews would to a degree reflect dominant
professional narratives of general practice as being in crisis in the early
years of the NHS before gaining in prestige and becoming recognised
as a specialty.[33] Such narratives are attractive as they make it possible for
doctors to present themselves as succeeding professionally in spite of
overwhelming challenges and successfully contributing to the survival
and development of general practice. Nevertheless, a clear sense of the
marginal and undesirable nature of work as a general practitioner in the
NHS emerges from the two following accounts. There is little sense of
any excitement at being part of the newly formed NHS, nor of general
practitioners being at the heart of developments from the outset. Anup
Kumar Sen, a South Asian doctor who moved to Britain in the early
1950s and became a GP in a Yorkshire mining village in the north of
England, remembers a widespread sentiment of apathy towards working in the NHS amongst British-trained colleagues:

> When I came there was a lot of talk about how doctors were poorly paid
> and many were giving up here and going to America, Canada, Australia.
> It soon stopped. Government increased the pay and the doctors settled
> down here. At one time, a lot of people were leaving because they were

dissatisfied with the pay they were receiving. *In what year would this have been?* I can't be certain, about mid-sixties. *These were British trained doctors, GPs?* Yes, leaving England or Britain and going. Mainly Australia, Canada, USA.[34]

Sir Donald Irvine trained as a doctor in the 1950s and worked as a GP in the Northumberland mining village of Ashington in the north-east of England from 1960. He was a prominent medical politician, who chaired the Council of the Royal College of General Practitioners in the 1980s and subsequently became President of the GMC. Whilst someone closely involved in professional changes might be expected to describe severe problems that were successfully addressed through appropriate interventions, his account does not diverge significantly from evidence gathered in the archives. It is also noteworthy that he does not simply describe general practice as a field encountering difficulties but recalls that emigration seemed a logical option for many of his colleagues in the years before the Family Doctors' Charter of the 1960s:

> The ... government of the day embarked on a massive expansion of specialist medicine, a wholly appropriate thing to do ... Specialist medicine was on the ascendancy, it could conquer everything. Remember the new medicine, the new science, the glamour, it was all new—penicillin was only ten years old at that time. An unstoppable surge put ... final paid to general practice as it had been pre-war and through the war ... The clamour was to get into specialist medicine ... added to this was the huge expansion in the numbers of specialists and recruitment to general practice automatically fell. Then, on top of all that, a lot of very good GPs said (sighs) 'There's no future here for me, we'll never get on top of the awful reputation we've got as a ... branch of medicine which nobody respects any more. General practice and life overseas ... Australia, New Zealand, Canada, America, it all looks much more rosy—I'm going there'. The overall result ... a catastrophic collapse in manpower recruitment.[35]

Interestingly, both A. K. Sen and Sir Donald Irvine suggested that the situation improved from the 1960s, a perspective consistent with the narrative of 'renaissance' of general practice that I will come to in the next section. The evidence for this is more nuanced. The field was gaining in prestige and government investment was forthcoming but a number of problems remained deeply entrenched.

Archival evidence suggests that scepticism and dissatisfaction persisted well beyond the 1960s. A document prepared for a meeting on general practice at the BMA in 1975 argued that British GPs were paid around a third of what their counterparts in the Netherlands and West Germany earned and that given that they would soon benefit from freedom to practice within the European Economic Community:

> The relevant question is not whether UK doctors are in some sense paid 'too much' at present but how much more they will have to be paid to retain even the barest of medical services in this country.[36]

As late as the mid-1970s, the sustainability of British general practice and therefore of the NHS was a subject for debate rather than something to be taken for granted from the perspective of members of the main representative body of British doctors. This was also the view of the government's Chief Medical Officer Henry Yellowlees, as expressed in a letter sent in 1977 to the President of the Royal College of General Practitioners, Ekkehard von Kuenssberg:

> During recent years disquiet has been expressed in several quarters about the future of primary health care in the central parts of our large conurbations. The negotiators of the General Medical Services Committee told us some months ago that they feared a complete breakdown of primary care in Central London in the near future if action is not taken to improve the situation.[37]

### The uneven distribution of doctors

The general sense of dissatisfaction connected to remuneration, working conditions and the status of general practice, which persisted throughout this period, was particularly acute in industrial and inner-city areas. The problem of the hugely uneven distribution of doctors in England and Wales predated the NHS. In the 1930s, the Yorkshire spa town of Harrogate had 2.66 doctors per 1,000 people as compared to 0.08 doctors per 1,000 people in the industrial setting of Abersychan in South Wales.[38] Similar patterns persisted after the establishment of the NHS.[39] Medical Practices Committees (one for England and Wales, one for Scotland) were given responsibility for attempting to address these imbalances by restricting doctors' right to practice in areas deemed 'over-doctored' and encouraging them to go to work in areas of high need (at times through the provision of financial incentives).[40] By the late 1970s, they had not succeeded in bringing about significant change.[41] A study published in 1975 found that when considering future career moves, general practitioners 'would pay closest attention to the educational facilities of an area, its rural or coastal location, its social and cultural amenities, and the practice conditions.'[42] Industrial areas were obviously less likely to provide GPs with the type of middle-class lifestyle that they aspired to. General practice in areas such as these with high proportions of less affluent working-class patients also generated a greater workload.[43]

It could also be difficult for GPs who at the time had to take responsibility for the out-of-hours provision of care to meet this requirement in working-class areas without ending up being permanently on-call and having to regularly see patients in the evenings, during the night, and at weekends. Rupendra Kumar Majumdar who worked as a GP in the working-class Welsh Valleys pithily summarised the factors that according to him kept many UK-trained doctors away from the area: 'No out-of-hours, no good school, no college, no tennis ground, no bowling centre, no wives' big [hairdressing] salon.'[44] Areas such as South Wales in the decades following the establishment of the NHS offered general practitioners a professionally demanding environment and one that was socially and culturally alien.

The work pressures and class values that came into play in the staffing of general practice are outlined quite explicitly in the Chief Medical Officers' report for 1976. The fact that doctors found work in inner-city areas unattractive was simply noted as a reality that required to be accommodated:

> The profession's representatives urged that few young doctors and their families would live in inner city areas; while not advocating that GP principals should provide a solely office hours service they insisted that an efficient deputising service is a necessity in inner city areas.[45]

Nearly thirty years after the establishment of the NHS, there was still a significant gap between the aspirations of the new system to make healthcare accessible to all and the reality of how British doctors wanted to earn a living.

*The post-war exodus of British doctors*
Disillusionment with the new NHS and the opportunities that it offered in general practice was undoubtedly a factor in the large-scale emigration of British doctors in the post-war period. If specific areas were under-doctored, it was not just that insufficient numbers of physicians had been trained in British medical schools, it was also because significant numbers of British doctors chose to work overseas rather than within the British healthcare system. There was a shortage of graduates being trained in British medical schools in the immediate postwar period. This is partly because some policy-makers and medical politicians underestimated the needs of the NHS in the 1950s and as a result did not make plans to train more doctors.[46] However, on its own, this factor does not explain the availability of the posts that migrant doctors took up. It is perfectly possible that in the absence of changes to career structures and conditions in the NHS and in general practice, an increase in the numbers of British-trained doctors would simply have resulted in a significant proportion of additional new graduates leaving the UK.[47]

The emigration of general practitioners trained in Britain was already a concern in the late 1950s when a memorandum produced by the Medical Practices Committee noted that seventy-six (i.e. just over five per thousand doctors) established GP principals in England and Wales had left the country in 1957.[48] The number of general practitioners born in Great Britain or Ireland leaving Great Britain was 170 in the year from September 1964 to September 1965, 120 in 1967/68 and 60 in 1970/71.[49] [50] Between 1960 and 1968 there was a drop of over 1,000 in the total number of active GPs.[51]

The numbers of GPs leaving Britain do not of course reflect the whole extent of the impact of the emigration of medical graduates on the field. The exodus of British doctors became a politically contentious issue in the 1960s as it was connected to debates around the long-term sustainability of the NHS and the way medical staff were trained and deployed.[52] There were tensions between the structure of medical training, which conceived of hospital jobs as staging posts on the way to a consultant's job, and the needs of the system for doctors to fill junior roles and work in general practice.[53] It was in this context that the social administration expert Brian Abel-Smith based at the London School of Economics, was given funding to conduct a study aimed at providing greater insights into the dynamics of this movement and attempting to measure its scale in a more precise way. The study he published in 1964 with Kathleen Gales looked at a 5 per cent sample of doctors born and trained in Great Britain and registered with the General Medical Council between 1925 and 1959. They found that around 12 per cent of them were living abroad.[54] A fifth of British-born and -trained doctors in their sample who registered in the 1950s were living overseas in 1962.[55] Doctors most frequently made the decision to migrate three to six years after registering.[56] They were often leaving junior positions in hospitals and going overseas rather than entering general practice which was perceived as low status.[57] Britain was therefore not just losing general practitioners, it was also being deprived of the junior doctors who were not making the progress they would have wished to make in hospital careers and might have been expected to move into general practice.

In addition to being debated by researchers and politicians concerned about the sustainability of the NHS, the emigration of British-trained doctors and immigration of doctors to Britain also attracted the attention of scholars concerned with mapping the so-called 'brain drain' from the Global South to the Global North.[58] The healthcare policy expert Oscar Gish published a large amount of work on the international movement of doctors at the time. Of the emigration of British-based doctors he noted that:

> The greatest part of all the emigrants had not yet established themselves in permanent medical posts in Britain; this is not because the possibility to do so did not exist—at least in general practice. Evidently, many hospital doctors between the ages of 30 and 40 preferred emigration to going into general practice as it is now constituted in this country.[59]

Between 1962 and 1967 the number of UK- or Irish-born doctors leaving Britain exceeded the number of those returning by an average of just under 400 a year.[60] Of these emigrants, 92 per cent were born in the UK; 19 per cent went to Canada, 13 per cent to the USA, 13 per cent to Australia and 4 per cent to New Zealand.[61] Within the same timeframe, the UK gained an average of 500 overseas-born doctors; the outflow of UK-based doctors was thus on a similar scale to the influx of overseas doctors.[62] Significant numbers of doctors continued to leave Britain in the 1970s and 1980s. A study published in 2001 looked at the professional trajectories of different cohorts of doctors trained in British medical schools. It estimated that of those who qualified in 1974 and had their family homes in Great Britain before entering medical school, just under 10 per cent were practising abroad a decade later.[63]

A letter to the British Medical Journal (BMJ) from one doctor who had left to work in general practice in Singapore gives an additional insight into what was behind the movement of at least some of these doctors:

> We have a group practice of eight doctors, each with his particular interest. We have x-rays, a laboratory, etc., and three private hospitals in which to admit and look after our patients. The beds range from free ones to luxury single private rooms. We can run our practice just as we like and there is no interference from outside. There are plenty of good consultants to call on when required. We find the practice of medicine a joy and infinitely more rewarding (in both senses) than in this abominable N.H.S. in Britain. What beats me is not why 400 doctors a year leave Britain but why any stay behind.[64]

Naturally, doctors who had made the decision to leave had every reason to describe their new way of life as idyllic. Doctors have also always formed part of an international profession and have always migrated. The possession of a UK medical degree in effect places its bearer on an international jobs market. We should not assume that decisions to migrate were always motivated by scepticism towards the NHS and its aims, but there can be little doubt that such attitudes played a part. By the 1970s, the UK was both a major exporter and importer of medical labour, being among the top ten countries in the world on both counts.[65] This is in contrast to countries such as the USA, which mainly imported international medical graduates.[66] A study of migrant British doctors who went to work in Canada between the 1950s and the 1970s found that 'among the host of issues that motivated a physician to leave the NHS, the inflexibility and hierarchy of the structure of British medicine loomed very large as a factor behind emigration'.[67] Medical migration served as a way of addressing shortages in the NHS but there was not necessarily a shortage of doctors in absolute terms, rather a shortage of doctors willing to remain within the NHS and do certain types of work.

## The emergence of the 'jewel in the crown of the NHS'

It is important to recognise that not all British-trained doctors were of the view that the NHS was 'abominable' and some of those who had their reservations thought that it was nevertheless reformable and that general practice could be improved. Governments throughout this period were also keen to contain the growing cost of providing free healthcare and, particularly from the 1960s onwards, sought to ensure that more care was provided in community settings as opposed to the more cost-intensive environment offered by hospitals. Professional and political agendas thus dovetailed and contributed to enhancing the status of general practice and radically reshaping the field. By the 1980s, general practice had gained recognition as a medical specialty and was accepted as a key part of the NHS.

Although general practice undoubtedly changed and established itself as central to the NHS during this period, it remained a varied and ill-defined field of practice, affected by structural problems and within which GPs enjoyed a great deal of professional freedom. There are in fact multiple histories of general practice, shaped as it was by the different geographical and social contexts in which medicine was practised and by the approaches of practitioners. As I will show in Chapters 6–8 the role of South Asian GPs in this context is not solely one of providing labour. They also participated in what has been termed a 'renaissance' of general practice and defined the forms that it took.

In the next section, I describe the evolving position of general practice within the British healthcare system and relate it to the budgetary constraints that the NHS has faced throughout its history. This is key to understanding the position migrant South Asian GPs occupied in the NHS. I will also argue that doing justice to the history of general practice involves paying heed to the different forms that it took, and in this context to the ability of migrant doctors to shape their working environment.

### General practice and the NHS's 'crisis of expenditure'

In spite of the difficulties I have described, it is during this period that general practice established itself as the so-called 'cornerstone' of provision in the NHS, where the majority of interactions with patients take place and where GPs act as gatekeepers who refer patients for specialist treatments. As Brian Abel-Smith noted in 1979, the UK was one of a minority of industrial countries where general practice represented the 'normal' point of entry into the system.[68] He went on to point out that:

> One fact about the British system of organizing and financing health care is beyond dispute. It is cheap. The proportion of gross national product spent on health service [sic] is one of the lowest among highly industrialised countries. And the strong role of general practice undoubtedly contributes to this low cost.[69]

It is widely accepted by policy-makers and historians that general practice has played a central and distinctive role in Britain and that what Graham Smith and Malcolm Nicolson term a 'structural emphasis upon primary care' helps to explain the relative cost efficiency of the NHS.[70]

That general practice by the late 1970s was performing a cost-containing role and central to the British model of care was no coincidence. By the 1950s, governments were already convinced of the importance of managing expenditure by limiting recourse to hospital treatments through the provision of care in community settings and investment in prevention.[71] The subsequent history of the NHS has been shaped by financial constraints as growing public demand and the rising costs of delivering healthcare put pressure on a service that received relatively little investment from central government.[72] The NHS employed 500,000 staff in 1948 and public expenditure on the new system accounted for 4 per cent of national resources.[73] By 1979, the workforce numbered one million with the health service budget accounting for 5.5 per cent of national resources.[74] It is hard to disagree with Webster's conclusion that:

> The British National Health Service demonstrated more successfully than most of its Western counterparts that the most pressing obligations of health care could be met within a system admitting only limited increases in resources.[75]

The NHS's ongoing 'crisis of expenditure' provides the backdrop for the increasingly central role that general practice took on in the UK health system between the end of the 1940s and the beginning of the 1980s. Governments concerned to contain rising costs in the NHS believed that an increased reliance on primary care could help to achieve this aim.[76]

The enhanced status of British general practice was symptomatic of a worldwide movement towards greater emphasis on primary health-care, which involved adopting a community-based approach to medicine emphasising prevention and cost-effective interventions outside of hospitals. At the World Health Organization (WHO) Conference held in Alma Ata in the USSR in 1978, this approach was presented as a means of enabling the provision of healthcare for all whilst avoiding an exponential rise in expenditure.[77] Initially developed in the context of less affluent countries where high-technology medicine was misaligned with the needs and finances of local populations and governments, it came to be seen to have merits in the industrialised world as well as being a means of containing the rising costs of healthcare.[78]

In the UK, general practice was central to successive governments' moves to place a renewed emphasis on the delivery of treatment in community settings.[79] The 1966 GP charter was an important step towards increased government investment in general practice.[80] Between the end of the 1940s and the end of the 1970s as the number of general practitioners increased, list sizes reduced and health centres multiplied.[81] It is during this period that general practice consolidated its position as the cornerstone of the NHS, taking on not just a role of controlling access to secondary care but also forming part of a wider programme of increased emphasis on primary care. The history of general practice and the history of the NHS during this period are therefore indissociable. They are also indissociable from the history of medical migration. The London GP John Horder, a prominent medical politician and President of the Royal College of General Practitioners from 1979 to 1982, noted that by the late 1980s, general practice was seen as the 'jewel in the crown of the National Health Service'.[82] The imperial connotations of the phrase are almost certainly unintentional but they point to a central aspect of this history. If India was the Jewel in the Crown of the British Empire, the Jewel in the Crown of the NHS was dependent on medical labour from the former Raj. Medical migration enabled governments to develop a strategy of cost containment based around primary care in which general practice, underpinned by the labour of medical migrants, played a key part.

Recourse to migrant doctors and the strengthening of primary care thus enabled governments to offer at least a partial response to Rosemary Stevens' pertinent question when she highlighted the impact that economic reality has had on the development of the NHS: 'Is it possible to provide a world-class service, on an equitable basis, to all members of the population in a capitalist democracy, for 6 percent of the GDP [gross domestic product]?'[83] These official strategies, influenced by budgetary concerns, coincided with the professional agendas of a number of doctors and led to what has been termed a 'renaissance' of general practice.

### 'Renaissance' doctors

It would be inaccurate to suggest that the changes that occurred in general practice between the publication of the Collings report in 1950 and the 1980s were solely the result of a top-down political process. Although it suited governments to strengthen the role of general practice, GPs themselves formulated new conceptions of their work. Not only was the way in which care was provided changing but efforts were being made to give general practice a higher status amongst the medical profession. British general practice was reinvented as a result of a process of professionalisation. As well as establishing itself as central to the NHS, it developed a new identity.

The discipline became recognised as a medical specialty in its own right as opposed to representing the application of knowledge from other fields at a more superficial level.[84] The College of General Practitioners was established in 1952, became a Royal College in 1972 and took on an important role in British medical politics.[85] Greater emphasis was placed on the importance of research in primary care.[86] From 1965, membership of the College of GPs was obtained through examination.[87] Professional vocational training for GPs was introduced and became compulsory for doctors wanting to become GP principals from 1980.[88] Departments of general practice were established in universities.[89] The influential 'biopsychosocial' approach to general practice drew on the work of the Hungarian psychoanalyst Michael Balint, a refugee from Nazi-dominated Europe. It refuted the mind/body dichotomy characteristic of many medical belief systems and formed an important part of the argument in favour of the distinctive nature of general practice that was developed by the College of GPs following its establishment.[90] As Charles Webster put it, 'a new and self-confident ideology of general practice developed distinct from the hospital model of medical care'.[91]

The shift in notions of what general practice should be was in evidence in surgeries and in the structure of delivery of general practice as well. The Family Doctors' Charter of 1966 encouraged GPs to work together in larger practices by providing incentives for the recruitment of other members of staff and making it less attractive to build up large lists of patients.[92] There was, as a result, a trend away from single-handed or small practices,[93] towards larger practices, often based in health centres.[94] Wages for staff such as administrators and nurses were subsidised by government, rent for suitable practice buildings was reimbursed and doctors were given incentives to work together.[95] The Marxist GP and medical politician Julian Tudor Hart, an influential advocate of preventive medicine and critic of the uneven distribution of healthcare resources,[96] went to work in the South Wales mining village of Glyncorrwg in 1961. He described these initiatives as having had a significant impact when it came to changing the context in which GPs practised:

> Eventually, this almost wiped out two common features of industrial general practice; the seedy front-parlour surgery in the GP's own home, and the squalid shop on the high street with a half-painted glass front, staffed only by a harassed GP's wife.[97]

The notion of a healthcare team in primary care came to the fore and general practice became part of a multi-disciplinary setting: doctors worked more closely in their surgeries with other professionals such as nurses and health visitors.[98] This arguably involved recreating a (cheaper to run) hospital system in a community environment: GPs tended to take on a leading role, not dissimilar to that of consultants in hospitals.[99] The boundaries of primary and secondary care were redefined, with GPs taking on responsibilities that had previously been the preserve of hospitals.[100] They for instance devoted less time to home deliveries and increasingly developed areas of specialisation such as hypertension or diabetes.[101] General practitioners also became more likely to take on appointments in specialist units in NHS hospitals.[102]

These changes in professional status and practice organisation have been described as characteristic of a golden age of British general practice. Writing in 1998, in the conclusion to a history of general practice in the NHS, John Horder noted that:

> In all the chapters of this volume, in which different writers have discussed different aspects of general practice and primary care under the NHS, a single underlying theme can be found, expressed sometimes overtly, sometimes by implication. This is that there has been, since the end of the Second World War, a revival—a renaissance—in this part of the service, after a period of stagnation.[103]

It is important however to broaden our frame of reference and seek to understand not just how politicians, civil servants and those involved in medical politics at a national level conceived of professional and political change but also how it was implemented and experienced at a local level, in surgeries. This is particularly important in the case of general practice, as between the 1940s and the 1980s, doctors retained a great deal of freedom to practice in the way that they saw fit: the majority of GPs were independent contractors rather than employees.[104] In the 1960s, their contract stipulated that they were to provide 'all necessary personal medical services of the type usually provided by general practitioners'—a remarkably fluid definition of their function in the British healthcare system.[105] General practice was not a unified and homogenous service, rather it was the sum of the work and conceptions of individual practitioners. It is worth remembering that by 1986 the Royal College of General Practitioners (RCGP) had only 13,000 members; one GP in three had chosen to join the new body.[106] If general practice changed a great deal in this period, according to Julian Tudor Hart, many doctors at the time simply wanted 'to be left alone'.[107] John Horder himself expressed a degree of scepticism towards the narrative of renaissance when he noted that two national studies of doctors and their patients carried out by Ann Cartwright in 1964 and 1977 (the second with Robert Anderson) did not provide any evidence of a radical improvement in patient satisfaction.[108] Attempting to understand how British general practice was reinvented during this period, what made change possible and the extent of its impact involves recognising the multifaceted nature of the field.

### The complex nature of British general practice

General practice was not at the time a unified field. To understand how it was shaped by South Asian doctors, we need to pay attention to how they underpinned the existence of the discipline by helping to avoid a staffing crisis and creating a context within which a new general practice could emerge. It is also important to acknowledge that during this period a range of methods and approaches to medicine were employed in general practice, and the speciality often took on different forms from one location to the next.

Joseph Collings, in his 1950 report which was highly critical of the state of English general practice, noted that 'General practice ... is accepted as being something specific, without anyone knowing what it really is.'[109] Although the reinvention of general practice that I have described attempted to address this issue, the fundamental question of how to define general practice remained relevant up to the 1980s and beyond. At least five models of general practice have been inventoried: the biomedical model which privileges the application of empirical biological understandings of the human body, a humanist model more concerned with the doctor/patient relationship, a public health approach emphasising prevention, general practice as a business with patients seen as customers, and the GP as family doctor.[110] To these might be added the GP as activist and advocate, involved in politics and social action.[111] Yet another strand is provided by GPs who work as single-handed doctors or as a member of a small practice—a model which overlaps with the concept of a family doctor caring for patients rather than dealing with diseases and offering continuity of care.[112] The latter approach to general practice can be linked to alternative conceptions of the role of the general practitioner which were still relevant during this period, with the family doctor being seen as someone who had acquired scientific training but who would need to spend most of their time in an 'unscientific manner ... looking after his flock, like a parson in his parish'.[113]

The pressures of industrial general practice were also different to those of other areas and led to variations in patterns of work. Contrasting the nature of general practice provision he witnessed in the East Midlands in the early 1950s in the market town of Kettering with the steel-manufacturing town of Corby, Julian Tudor Hart argued that there was a fundamental division in medicine which he saw as corresponding to the two nations of British society.[114] He also described his own experience of working in the coalfield communities of South Wales:

> Acting as a locum in Ferndale, Rhondda, in 1960, I saw about 60 patients in the morning session, another 60 in the evening, and visited 25 patients at home. Most doctors qualifying before 1960 who have worked in industrial areas have had similar experiences.[115]

Having a professional interaction with nearly 150 patients in one day at a range of locations would naturally contribute to defining the nature of doctors' work. In a collection of interviews with doctors, one inner-city GP stated that 'I would suspect that a GP from a prosperous area who came and worked here for a week would seriously question whether I was doing my job properly, because it wouldn't be recognizable.'[116] Up to the 1980s, concerns continued to be raised about inner-city practice where doctors were more likely to find themselves working alone from poor-quality premises and dealing with high workloads.[117]

To complete this picture of general practice as mosaic rather than monolith, it is essential to recognise that migrant doctors, even when trained according to western methods, brought with them a cultural and social background that had the potential to inform their approach to medicine. Claire L. Wendland's ethnographic study of a medical school in Malawi provides compelling evidence that local medical cultures can have a profound effect on the practice of medicine, even in a profession where knowledge is deemed to be international.[118] She shows how local cultural contexts shape the nature of biomedical practices and that medicine can take specific forms in the Global South.[119] Given its exposure to overseas practitioners, general practice in Great Britain has to be seen, to a greater or lesser extent, as the product of the cultural influence that they brought to bear on the system they found. In the light of this, it is important to approach the history of general practice with a sense of the multidirectional and contested nature of change and of the impact that individual doctors could have at the level of their surgeries. The fruitfulness of such an approach is hinted at by research focused on general practice in the town of Paisley, near Glasgow, which emphasises the importance of understanding local cultures of care and touches upon the importance of the hidden local histories of medical politics and the activities that doctors undertake on a voluntary basis.[120]

Writing the history of general practice in fact involves attempting to provide an account of the evolution of what has been described as a 'post-modern' specialty defined by uncertainty, the existence of different voices and experiences of reality and multifaceted understandings of what constitutes 'truth'.[121] The reinvention of British general practice as a medical specialty and a cornerstone of the NHS was a reality of post-war Britain. It is, however, a complex and multi-layered reality that migrant practitioners played a key part in shaping. Migrant doctors contributed to creating the conditions in which this 'renaissance' could take place by playing a significant part in the staffing of general practice. Moreover, as I will show, some of them were closely involved in driving forward these changes, others facilitated their implementation, whilst another set of doctors limited the impact of these developments by resisting them and remaining on the margins. Understanding and recognising such dynamics is key to the reintegration of the role of medical migrants into the history of general practice.

## Notes

1  S. Castles & M. J. Miller, *The Age of Migration: International Population Movements in the Modern World*, fourth edition (Basingstoke: Palgrave Macmillan, 2009), p. 242.

2  J. Horder, 'Conclusion', in I. Loudon, J. Horder, C. Webster (eds), *General Practice under the National Health Service 1948–1997* (London: Clarendon Press, 1998), p. 283.

3  J. Lewis, 'The medical profession and the state: GPs and the GP contract in the 1960s and the 1990s', *Social Policy and Administration*, 32:2 (1998).

4  Webster, *Health Services*, Vol. I, p. 11; V. Berridge, *Health and Society in Britain since 1938* (Cambridge: Cambridge University Press, 1999), pp. 17 & 23.

5  Berridge, *Health and Society*, p. 23.

6  Webster, *Health Services*, Vol. I, p. 133.

7  Webster, *Health Services*, Vol. I, p. 143.

8  Webster, *Health Services*, Vol. I, pp. 178–83.

9  J. Stewart, 'The political economy of the British National Health Service, 1945–75: Opportunities and constraints?', *Medical History*, 52:4 (2008), p. 461.

10 Ibid.

11  R. Baggott, *Health and Healthcare in Britain*, third edition (Basingstoke & New York: Palgrave Macmillan, 2004), pp. 89–90.

12  Baggott, *Health and Healthcare in Britain*, p. 89; Jones & Snow, *Against the Odds*, p. 6.

13  Baggott, *Health and Healthcare in Britain*, p. 91.

14  Ibid.

15  Baggott, *Health and Healthcare in Britain*, pp. 89–90.

16  See for instance Seaton, 'Against the "sacred cow"'.

17  Webster, *A Political History*, p. 155.

18  Ibid.

19  Seaton, 'Against the "sacred cow"', p. 427; A. Mold, *Making the Patient-Consumer: Patient Organisations and Health Consumerism in Britain* (Manchester: Manchester University Press, 2015).

20  D. Morrell, 'Introduction and overview', in Loudon et al. (eds), *General Practice under the National Health Service*, p. 1.

21  N. Bosanquet & C. Salisbury, 'The practice', in Loudon et al. (eds), *General Practice under the National Health Service*, p. 45.

22  Webster, *A Political History*, p. 51.

23  Collings, 'General Practice in England', pp. 578–9.

24  Webster, *Health Services*, Vol. I, pp. 356–7.

25  Collings, 'General practice in England', p. 568.

26  Collings, 'General practice in England', p. 579.

27  Webster, *A Political History*, p. 51.

28  'The Collings Report', *The Lancet* 255: 6604 (25 March 1950), p. 548.

29  BMA, General Medical Services Committee, minutes of General Medical Services Committee 1958–1959, Alternative Service Subcommittee, meeting of 26 November 1958; Webster, *Health Services*, Vol. 1, p. 252.

30  Lewis, 'The medical profession and the state', p. 132; Webster, *Health Services*, Vol. II, p. 265.

31  BMA, General Medical Services Committee 1974–75, General Medical Services Committee Rural Practices Subcommittee, meeting at BMA House, 16 October 1974, Appendix VIII.

32  T. C. Mayer, 'Tomorrow's doctors: The educated poor', *Pulse* (12 March 1977), p. 5.

33  Loudon et al. (eds), *General Practice under the National Health Service*.

34  A. K. Sen interview with author, 10 June 2010.

35  Sir D. Irvine interview with author, 7 April 2011.

36 BMA, Minutes of The General Medical Services Committee 1974–75, General Purposes Subcommittee of the General Medical Services Committee, meeting at B.M.A House, 3 April 1975, Appendix III Draft: Medical Remuneration.

37 Archives of the Royal College of General Practitioners, London (Henceforth, RCGP), ACE J 32-2 Primary Care in Inner Cities 1977–1981/ACE J 32-3 Symposium on Problems of Care in Inner Cities 1980, File 20/2, H. Yellowlees to E. von Kuenssberg, 28 January 1977.

38 M. Powell, 'Coasts and coalfields: The geographical distribution of doctors in England and Wales in the 1930s', *Social History of Medicine*, 18:2 (2005), p. 258.

39 M. Hann & H. Gravelle, 'The maldistribution of general practitioners in England and Wales: 1974–2003', *British Journal of General Practice*, 54 (2004); M. J. Buxton & R. E. Klein, 'Population characteristics and the distribution of general medical practitioners', *BMJ*, 1 (1979); M. Goddard, H. Gravelle, A. Hole, G. Marini, 'Where did all the GPs go? Increasing supply and geographical equity in England and Scotland', *Journal of Health Services Research Policy*, 15:1 (2010); P. L. Knox, 'The intraurban ecology of primary medical care: Patterns of accessibility and their policy implications', *Environment and Planning A* (1978). Much of the available evidence pertaining to this subject relates to England and Wales. The latter article suggests that the pattern of distribution of doctors may have been slightly different in Scotland with some deprived inner-city areas being described as well provided whilst new and severely deprived council estates in peripheral areas of urban centres were extremely under-doctored.

40 Knox, 'Intraurban ecology', p. 417.

41 Knox, 'Intraurban ecology', p. 418.

42 J. R. Butler & R. Knight, 'The choice of practice location', *Journal of the Royal College of General Practitioners*, 25 (1975), p. 496.

43 Y. Ben-Shlomo, I. White, P. M. McKeigue, 'Prediction of general practice workload from census based deprivation scores', *Journal of Epidemiology and Community Health*, 46 (1992).

44 R. K. Majumdar interview with author, 18 March 2010.

45 Great Britain. Department of Health and Social Security, *On the state of public health: the annual report of the Chief Medical Officer of the Department of Health and Social Security for the year 1976*. London: HMSO, 1977, p. 68.

46  Webster, *Health Services*, Vol. II, p. 283; D. Wright, S. Mullally, M. C. Cordukes, '"Worse than being married": The exodus of British doctors from the National Health Service to Canada, c. 1955–75', *Journal of the History of Medicine and Allied Sciences*, 65:2 (2010); Jones & Snow, *Against the Odds*, pp. 11–12; B. Abel-Smith & K. Gales, *British Doctors at Home and Abroad* (Welwyn, England: Published for the Social Administration Research Trust by the Codicote Press, 1964) p. 7.

47  O. Gish, 'British doctor migration 1962–67', *British Journal of Medical Education*, 4 (1970), p. 288.

48  BMA, General Medical Services Committee 1958–59, Memorandum by the Medical Practices Committee on emigration of established general practitioners.

49  BMA, Department of Health and Social Security, Joint medical manpower fact finding group, Basic statistical information, medical manpower fact-finding group.

50  Gish, 'British doctor migration', p. 288.

51  O. Gish, *Britain and the Immigrant Doctor* (Institute of Race Relations, 1969), p. 8.

52  Wright et al., '"Worse than being married"', pp. 547 & 556–8.

53  Wright et al., '"Worse than being married"', pp. 553–5.

54  Abel-Smith & Gales, *British Doctors*, pp. 19 & 28–30.

55  Abel-Smith & Gales, *British Doctors*, p. 59.

56  Abel-Smith & Gales, *British Doctors*, p. 57.

57  Abel-Smith & Gales, *British Doctors*, pp. 43, 51 & 57; Gish, 'British doctor migration', p. 288.

58  Wright. et al., 'The "brain drain" of physicians'.

59  Gish, 'British doctor migration', p. 288.

60  Gish, 'British doctor migration'.

61  Gish, 'British doctor migration', pp. 280–3.

62  O. Gish, 'Overseas-born doctor migration 1962–66', *British Journal of Medical Education*, 5 (1971), p. 108.

63  M. J. Goldacre, T. W. Lambert, J. M. Davidson, 'Loss of British-trained doctors from the medical workforce in Great Britain', *Medical Education*, 35 (2001), p. 341.

64  C. H. A. Hoy, 'Emigration of doctors', *BMJ*, 1: 5436 (1965), p. 721.

65  Wright & Mullally, ' "Not everyone can be a Gandhi"'.

66  A. Mejia, 'Migration of physicians and nurses: A world wide picture', *International Journal of Epidemiology*, 7: 3 (1978), p. 209.

67  Wright et al., "'Worse than being married'", p. 553.
68  B. Abel-Smith, 'Foreword', in F. Honigsbaum, *The Division in British Medicine: A History of the Separation of General Practice from Primary Care 1911–1968* (London: Konan Page, 1979), p. xiii.
69  Abel-Smith, 'Foreword', p. xv.
70  G. Smith & M. Nicolson, 'Re-expressing the division of British medicine under the NHS: The importance of locality in general practitioners' oral histories', *Social Science and Medicine*, 64 (2007), p. 939.
71  Webster, *Health Services*, Vol. II, pp. 109–11. Primary care refers to care provided in community settings (as opposed to secondary care, in hospitals) by a range of healthcare professionals.
72  Webster, *Health Services*, Vol. II, pp. 2 & 6.
73  Webster, *Health Services*, Vol. II, p. 2.
74  Ibid.
75  Webster, *Health Services*, Vol. II, p. 758.
76  Berridge, *Health and Society*, p. 42.
77  Rivett, *National Health Service History*.
78  Berridge, *Health and Society*, p. 42.
79  Berridge, *Health and Society*, pp. 42 & 77.
80  J. T. Hart, *A New Kind of Doctor: The General Practitioner's Part in the Health of the Community* (London: Merlin Press, 1988), pp. 10–11.
81  Webster, *Political History*, p. 131.
82  Horder, 'Conclusion', p. 283.
83  R. A. Stevens, 'Fifty years of the British National Health Service: Mixed messages, diverse interepretations', *Bulletin of the History of Medicine*, 74:4 (2000), p. 809.
84  D. Pereira Gray, 'Postgraduate training and continuing education', in Loudon et al. (eds), *General Practice under the National Health Service*, pp. 182–93.
85  Berridge, *Health and Society*, p. 43.
86  J. Howie, 'Research in general practice: Perspectives and themes', in Loudon et al. (eds), *General Practice under the National Health Service*, pp. 147 & 164.
87  Pereira Gray, 'Postgraduate training', p. 189.
88  Horder, 'Conclusion', p. 283.
89  J. Fry & G. McLachlan, 'The future', in J. Fry, Lord Hunt of Fawley, R. J. F. H. Pinsent (eds), *A History of the Royal College of General Practitioners – The First 25 Years* (Lancaster, Boston, The Hague: MTP Press Limited, 1983), p. 246.

90   Berridge, *Health and Society*, p. 43.
91   Bosanquet & Salisbury, 'The practice', p. 61.
92   Bosanquet & Salisbury, 'The practice', p. 46.
93   I have used David Smith's (*Overseas Doctors in the National Health Service* (London and Thetford: Policy Studies Institute, 1980), p. 109) definition of a small practice as being one staffed by no more than one or two doctors.
94   Fry & McLachlan, 'The future', p. 246.
95   Hart, *New Kind of Doctor*, pp. 10–11.
96   R. Moorhead, 'Hart of Glyncorrwg', *Journal of the Royal Society of Medicine*, 97 (2004).
97   Hart, *New Kind of Doctor*, p. 11.
98   Berridge, *Health and Society*, p. 43; Fry & McLachlan, 'The future', p. 246.
99   M. Jefferys & H. Sachs, *Rethinking General Practice: Dilemmas in Primary Medical Care* (London & New York: Tavistock Publications, 1983).
100  Berridge, *Health and Society*, p. 43.
101  I. Loudon & M. Drury, 'Some aspects of clinical care', in Loudon et al. (eds), *General Practice in the National Health Service*, pp. 112 & 123.
102  Fry & McLachlan, 'The future', p. 246.
103  Horder, 'Conclusion', p. 278.
104  Lewis, 'The medical profession and the state', p. 133.
105  Lewis, 'The medical profession and the state', p. 137.
106  Hart, *New Kind of Doctor*, p. 89.
107  Ibid.
108  Horder, 'Conclusion', p. 282.
109  Collings, 'General practice in England', p. 555.
110  D. Hannay, 'Undergraduate medical education and general practice', in Loudon et al. (eds), *General Practice under the National Health Service*, pp. 180–1.
111  P. Hutt, I. Heath, R. Neighbour, *Confronting an Ill Society: David Widgery, General Practice, Idealism and the Chase for Change* (Oxford and San Francisco: Radcliffe Publishing, 2005), pp. 75–81.
112  M. Taylor, *Statement to the Shipman Enquiry*, 2003. Accessed 1 May 2012 at: www.the-shipman-inquiry.org/getdocument.asp?docid=wt1600004.
113  P. Ferris, *The Doctors* (London: Victor Gollancz, 1965), p. 101.
114  Hart, *New Kind of Doctor*, pp. 3–4.
115  Hart, *New Kind of Doctor*, p. 59.

116 H. Matthews & J. Bain, *Doctors Talking* (Edinburgh: Scottish Cultural Press, 1998), p. 95.

117 Baggott, *Health and Healthcare in Britain*, p. 246.

118 C. Wendland, *A Heart for the Work: Journeys through an African Medical School* (Chicago and London: The University of Chicago Press, 2010).

119 Wendland, *A Heart for the Work*, pp. 21–4.

120 Smith et al., *Speaking for a Change*, pp. 28–31; Smith & Nicolson 'Division of British medicine', p. 939.

121 N. Mathers & S. Rowland, 'General practice – a post-modern specialty?', *British Journal of General Practice*, 47 (1997), p. 178.

# 2

# Empire, migration and the NHS

The establishment and development of the NHS in the post-war period coincided with the dismantling of the British Empire. Colonial-era language or parallels have been used at times to describe the relationship between the NHS and the migrant labour it has relied on.[1] However, the development of the British healthcare system and the impact and legacy of the Empire are two closely linked phenomena that historians have rarely considered together.[2] The same can be said of the history of post-war migration to the UK and the movement of doctors.[3]

In this chapter, I argue that seeing the development of the NHS through the prism of empire and its legacies is key to understanding how it came to be so reliant on migrant South Asian doctors. This reflection draws on the work of historians who have argued that closer attention should be paid to the ways in which Britain's imperial past have shaped its present. It also builds on the insights of post-colonial theorists who argue that the impact of imperialism is an essential dimension of the modern world that cannot be ignored.[4] Adopting such an approach involves, in particular, placing the role of imperial power and the persistence of attitudes and relationships shaped by empire at the heart of historical understanding.[5]

The migration of doctors and the making of British general practice also form part of a broader framework of post-war British social and political history marked by the end of empire and the movement to the former colonial power of hundreds of thousands of people from the Indian subcontinent. The dynamics set in motion by the British Empire outlasted its political structures. While the Empire slowly ebbed away, migrants settled in the UK in significant numbers. By the 1980s, changes in immigration law and in medical regulations had made it much harder for migrant South Asian doctors to become GPs. A shift from a relatively open post-imperial space to a more clearly defined national UK space that denied access to non-white former British subjects had taken place.[6] By then, however, the movement of doctors, first to the UK, and subsequently into general practice had had a major impact on the development of the NHS. It is also important to note that this shift to a post-imperial space was gradual and slow to have a significant effect on doctors.

In this chapter, I will first outline the imperial backdrop to the relationship between migration from the Indian subcontinent and the NHS. The post-war migration of doctors to Britain is not a spontaneous phenomenon—it is connected to the long history of British medicine in South Asia. It also represents a continuation (albeit on a different scale) of the pre-NHS movement of doctors from the Indian subcontinent to the then colonial metropole. I will then give an indication of the scale of the dependency of the NHS on migrant doctors and other healthcare workers, exploring how existing colonial networks were drawn upon to meet the staffing needs of a new and expanding organisation. Finally, I will discuss the evolving nature of the social and political space in which doctors migrated and how it was shaped by post-war debates around 'race'[7] and migration. There was a time lag between the formal end of the British Empire and the (partial) dismantling of its legacies such as the freedom of doctors to move to the UK and their ability to gain recognition for their qualifications (and therefore be in a position to establish themselves as GPs). The arrival in Britain of South Asian doctors who subsequently became GPs was the product of a very specific post-imperial context which existed in the forty years following the establishment of the NHS.

## 'Medical dependency' in colonial India

At the time of the founding of the NHS in 1948, medicine in the Indian subcontinent had been shaped by an imperial history that stretched back over a period in excess of one hundred years. Medical colleges were founded in Calcutta and Madras in 1835, Bombay's Grant Medical College was established ten years later and the Lahore Medical College followed in 1860.[8] The next addition was King George's College Lucknow in 1906 and another five colleges were set up in the following twenty years in Delhi, Belgachia (Calcutta), Vizagapatam, Patna and Bombay.[9] In addition to these medical colleges, by 1938, there were twenty-seven medical schools established to train subordinate medical staff.[10] In present-day Sri Lanka, the Ceylon Medical College came into existence in 1870.[11] The subcontinent constituted an exception to most colonial contexts in that a substantial section of the local population was able to access medical education.[12] It is of course important to acknowledge that western ideas were shaped by local contexts and practices and that empire did not simply represent the wholesale transposition of fully formed ideas to colonies.[13] It remains that the history of medicine in the Indian subcontinent is indissociable from the history of the British Empire. It was shaped by imperial priorities and by British approaches to medicine.[14]

Roger Jeffery has argued that by the late 1930s, the dominance of western conceptions of how medicine should be practised and the desire to gain international recognition for Indian training had resulted in the 'institutionalisation of medical dependency': medical education in the Indian subcontinent mirrored British norms rather than being aligned to local needs and embracing indigenous traditions.[15] Senior posts in Medical Colleges were frequently held by Europeans.[16] In 1892, the GMC first recognised an Indian medical degree as entitling the holder to have their name on the British register.[17] A Bengal branch of the BMA was established in 1863.[18] Although it was disbanded in 1867, other Indian branches were set up in the late nineteenth and early twentieth centuries.[19] From the mid-nineteenth century onwards, Indian medical students were travelling to Britain to gain qualifications and returning to build successful careers.[20] The notion that degrees obtained in the metropole would offer better prospects encouraged this movement.[21] In 1900, thirty Indians were studying medicine in Britain and in 1927 the total number of Indian students in Britain (including other fields such as law) reached 1,800.[22] Experiencing life in Britain had come to be seen as an essential element of a 'gentleman's education.'[23] As Mel Gorman puts it:

> The educational sojourn in England is important for its three-fold effect. First, it showed in a dramatic and conclusive manner that Indians could master science and medicine on a level with Europeans. Second, after these students received their degrees from the University of London

and their diplomas from the Royal College of Surgeons and returned to India, they served as disseminators of modern science and became role models for future Indian scientists. Lastly, their example set the stage for a veritable flood of Indian students to England for study in all fields, a movement which continues to this day. The British had invaded and conquered India politically and geographically, but now the Indians had done so in England academically.[24]

The actual numbers of doctors who travelled to Britain before the partition of India and Ceylon's independence were relatively small but the significance of this flow should not be underestimated. Not only did they provide an example for subsequent generations of doctors to follow, but those who had been to Britain were more likely to become influential members of their profession on their return.[25] In the words of Roger Jeffery, 'The Indian doctors who collaborated with colonial rule were the ones who stepped into positions of power after 1947: by then their socialization into the model of western medicine was already complete'.[26] Independence did not mark an abrupt rupture with these imperial dynamics. As will be shown in the next chapter, the post-independence movement of South Asian doctors to Britain for further studies is linked to this long history.

## Medical migrants at the time of the Raj

In the absence of detailed statistics, the precise number of doctors and medical students from the Indian subcontinent who worked in Britain before the NHS was established is hard to gauge. A survey of 'Indians overseas' published in 1951 put their number at 'no less than 1,000' practising across Britain but the lack of an explanation regarding the provenance of this figure means that it can only be treated as a rough guide.[27] If it is difficult to say precisely how many doctors formed part of the South Asian medical diaspora in Britain in the 1940s,[28] it is possible to develop a sense of the significance of this community. Some information pertaining to the presence of doctors working in the British healthcare system up to the 1940s and 1950s was obtained through interviews conducted for this project and recordings from previous oral history projects. One participant in this study, Rooin Boomla, was himself working as a GP by 1948, having migrated as a child and taken over the practice run by his father, Faridoon Boomla (see Figure 1) who was a GP in South

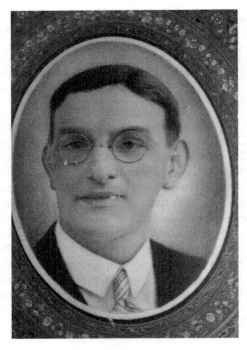

**Figure 1** Faridoon Boomla, a GP in Plumstead, South East London from the 1920s to the early 1940s.

East London from the late 1920s to the early 1940s.[29] Rooin Boomla recalled the existence of a Parsee medical network, which facilitated his father's move into practice in Britain.[30] He believes that his father would have relied on the Indian Medical Association, which he describes as 'quite extensive at the time' and Parsee community networks to recruit assistants.[31] His recollections chime with those of Shirin Kutar, another Parsee doctor who worked as a GP in South East London from the 1940s (as did her husband, also a South Asian doctor).[32] She described how her husband arrived during the war after having been contacted by the Boomla family.[33] She also recalled that there were a number of Parsee doctors based in working-class districts of London. Four participants in this study remembered their fathers' careers in general practice in working-class communities of East London and the north of England, which started before the NHS was set up.[34] A number of the GPs interviewed also recalled entering general practice alongside doctors who had come to Britain before the NHS was created or talked about other doctors who were already in practice nearby when they started working as general practitioners. Savitri Chowdhary's memoirs mention a number of South Asian doctors who helped her husband Dharm Sheel Chowdhary (1902–1959) in his practice in Essex including a Dr Banarji who left for Calcutta, a Dr Naqvi, who had come to England to obtain a Diploma in Public Health and was supporting himself by working as an assistant, and a Dr Madan.[35] Dr Bala Prasad set up a surgery in Barking, in Greater London, in the 1930s.[36]

Evidence that South Asian medical graduates made up a small community of doctors rather than simply finding themselves working in Britain as isolated individuals is also provided by Savitri Chowdhary's reference to receiving a phone call from London with news of Baldev Kaushal, Dharm Sheel Chowdhary's cousin, whose house in Bethnal Green, in industrial East London, had been badly damaged by a bomb.[37] A number of practitioners were prominent figures. Kaushal was awarded an MBE for 'gallant conduct' during the Blitz.[38] Chuni Lal Katial was a GP and councillor in Finsbury in North London where he worked to help establish its pioneering Health Centre in the 1930s.[39] Jainti Saggar came to Britain from the Punjab in 1919 to study medicine at St Andrews University, before setting up as a doctor in Dundee where he also became a local councillor[40] as did Harbans Lall Gulati, a GP in Battersea for forty years until his death in 1967.[41] Another Battersea doctor, Abdul Majid Shah committed suicide by gassing himself in 1935.[42] The actor Sir Ben Kingsley is the son of Rahimtulla Bhanji, a South Asian doctor from East Africa who became a GP in Northern England before World War II.[43] Dhani Prem, who became a councillor in Birmingham and was a prominent advocate of migrant and minority rights migrated to the UK in the 1930s.[44] In 1925, Sureswar Sarkar, an Indian doctor living in Sheffield, was sentenced to five years of penal servitude for 'serious offences against servant girls at his house'.[45] Another doctor traceable because of his encounter with the judicial system is Buck Ruxton (1899–1936). Ruxton, a Lancaster GP from India who had changed his name from Buckhtyar Rustomji Rantanji Hakim, was executed in 1936 for the murder of his wife and his maid.[46]

The obituaries pages of the *BMJ* provide further ample evidence of the movement of South Asian doctors to Great Britain, some staying permanently and building careers, others returning after training, and others living their working lives across two continents. Lieutenant-Colonel Sohrab Shapoorji Vazifdar (1883–1971) thus received his initial medical education in Bombay before going to St Bartholomew's Hospital in London and obtaining the English Conjoint Diploma (which entitled Indian doctors to practise in Britain) in 1907. He served in World War I in East Africa, Mesopotamia and Persia after which he worked in hospitals in Bombay, becoming professor of medicine at Grant Medical College. He returned to England after retiring in 1938 and subsequently worked until 1965 as an assistant to his son who was a GP.[47] Ahmed Ismail Toorawa (1912–1989) was born in India, educated at Royal College, Mauritius, came to the UK in 1933 to train at University College, London and qualified from the Welsh National School of Medicine in 1940 before becoming a GP in the Greater Manchester area during World War II.[48] Dorothy M. Satur (1902–1981) graduated from Madras Medical College in 1928, then trained in Britain before entering the All India Women's Medical Service and becoming professor of obstetrics and gynaecology at Lady Hardinge Medical College in Delhi, then head of the department of obstetrics and gynaecology in Lucknow.[49] Although our understanding of the South Asian medical community in Britain in imperial times remains fragmented, the movement of doctors to Britain was an established and significant phenomenon before the NHS was created.

## Entry into general practice

As already hinted at by the examples just given, the members of this medical community who settled permanently in Britain were frequently to be found working in industrial areas where demand for services was high. The obituaries column of the *BMJ* is again a useful guide to where South Asian GPs were based. A. I. Toorawa (1912–1989) worked in Bolton and Manchester,[50] S. K. Sen (1905–1974) in Birmingham, Walsall and West Bromwich,[51] K. C. Sarkar (1902–1982) in West London and Lewisham,[52] H. V. Sankarayya entered general practice in Birmingham at the end of the second world war,[53] D. Saklatvala went to work in West Bromwich after qualifying in London in 1933,[54] Yadu Nandan Lal (1897–1975) was a general practitioner in the Old Kent Road, London[55] and Krishnan Kumar was an assistant in general practice in County Durham before entering general practice in Newcastle-upon-Tyne.[56] Abdul Wasi Khan (1909–1977) was active in the Solihull and Birmingham area,[57] Home Khurshed Fozdar went into practice in 1925 in the Bilston and Coseley areas of Wolverhampton,[58] Kiran Chandra Bhattacharyya was a GP in the King's Cross area of London for half a century until he retired in 1979.[59] Jadoonanun Bhageerutty, born in Mauritius in 1913, qualified from Edinburgh in 1941 and settled in general practice in the Staffordshire mining village of Norton Canes[60] and Kaiku Ardeshir Anklesaria (1887–1969) became a GP in Walthamstow in London in 1937.[61]

Not all South Asian doctors had practices serving working-class communities and industrial areas. Buck Ruxton in Lancaster and Alfred Barnes Gunasekara, a GP in Hampstead in London from 1918 to 1971,[62] would most likely have been serving a mixed population with a number of middle-class patients. Nevertheless, the overwhelming majority of them do seem to have found work providing primary care to the least affluent sections of the population. After World War I, the dean of the London School of Tropical Medicine tellingly noted that Indian doctors were 'very popular with miners and other classes of workmen'.[63]

General practice was one of the few avenues open to South Asian doctors who wanted to work in Britain before the NHS started. The cost of acquiring a practice could be a factor (at the time doctors could buy and sell them). According to Rooin Boomla this explains why his father went to work in a surgery in South East London: he could not afford to buy into a more desirable area.[64] British hospitals traditionally offered scant opportunities for promotion for doctors perceived as outsiders.[65] Sir Netar Mallick and Ajeet Gulati, both sons of South Asian GPs and NHS consultants, described how entry into general practice was the only option open to their fathers if they wanted a career in medicine in Britain. They felt it would have been quasi impossible for Indian doctors to build careers in the pre-NHS hospital system.[66] Whilst to a degree this might be explained by local cultures in hospitals, which could also be hostile to incomers trained in other British medical schools and hospitals, there can be no doubt that discrimination played a part in shaping the distribution of doctors. Upendra Krishna Dutt, who qualified in 1884 after coming to the UK in the 1870s, for instance described being turned down for various posts and for jobs as a doctor's assistant in spite of a strong academic record.[67] A letter sent to *The Lancet* in 1915 by Dr Chowry Muthu, an Indian doctor who was an authority on tuberculosis and ran a sanatorium in Somerset, provides an insight into the functioning of recruitment processes in British hospitals in the early twentieth century.[68] Muthu argued that in the light of the Indian contribution to the war effort, discrimination against Indian doctors should cease but only in the event that there was no viable English candidate:

> Seeing that the Indians are just now proving their mettle in the battlefield and fighting side by side with the British, it is time the old prejudice against them, like many other fallacies which the war has exposed, should be adjusted and modified according to present conditions and needs. Only two or three weeks ago the appointment of an Indian to the post of house surgeon somewhere in Cornwall was cancelled at the very last moment, after it had been duly made, because of his nationality … One can quite understand, and even justify, the preferment of an Englishman when he is competing for a post with an equally able and efficient Indian candidate but one feels prejudice has triumphed over justice when an Indian is rejected even though he is proved superior in talents and ability to his English rival. Especially now, when all the world is praising the bravery of the Indian troops, their wonderful patriotism in rallying round the British flag, their devotion in giving freely their lives and treasure, the least the hospital authorities and governors can do is to give the Indian an opportunity to compete on equal terms with others (he asks for no favour), without prejudicing his candidature because of his colour or nationality.

Muthu's letter is of interest as a South Asian view of discrimination at the time but its publication in a prestigious medical journal is also an indication of at least a degree of recognition that such practices existed and were deemed acceptable. This is also reflected in the fact that the author stops short of arguing against all discrimination—accepting that it might be understandable to favour white candidates if their non-white counterparts are not more skilled. There was therefore already, prior to the NHS, a well-established pattern of movement to Britain of South Asian doctors who faced professional discrimination and frequently ended up working as GPs in unpopular areas, as happened on a much more significant scale later.

## Dependency and discrimination: the NHS and migrant labour

*NHS staff shortages and the intensification of (post-) imperial flows*
The movement of significant numbers of South Asian doctors to Britain in the four decades following the establishment of the NHS should be understood as the amplification of an existing phenomenon rather than the beginning of a new one. The NHS in its first forty years can be seen as a typically post-colonial institution: run by white people and dependent on labour from parts of the world that Britain had colonised. This parallel is even more striking when one considers that managers and consultants were generally white, a large proportion of doctors working in unpopular medical specialties and geographical areas were South Asian and that significant numbers of nurses came from the Caribbean. That there were fewer African doctors and nurses and that little is known about other Africans working in the NHS and the positions that they occupied completes this picture of an organisation neatly replicating imperial hierarchies.

From the moment it was set up, as well as facing a crisis of expenditure as discussed in the previous chapter, the NHS faced a crisis of recruitment. The NHS has never been self-sufficient when it comes to its medical workforce and has over the years been reliant on the labour of doctors from the Republic of Ireland, Central Europe, South Asia and elsewhere.[69] If there were variations when it came to the main sources of medical graduates, the British healthcare system has always been and remains structurally reliant on the labour of migrant doctors.

In fact, the need for additional medical personnel was apparent before the NHS was established. In 1946, a letter from the Home Office to the BMA referred to the 'undoubted scope for [the employment of 'alien' doctors] in an expanded medical service' and made the case for these doctors being able to continue practising without British qualifications as they had been allowed to under wartime regulations.[70] Whilst wartime conditions clearly created an exceptional environment, these discussions are indicative of a gap between the output of British medical schools and the staffing needs of the NHS, which remained in existence throughout the twentieth century. The following year, parliament passed the Medical Practitioners and Pharmacists Act, which allowed migrant doctors resident in the UK to apply for registration.[71] The Minister of Health, Aneurin Bevan, estimated that around 3,500 doctors would be in a position to apply but that between 1,500 and 2,000 might be expected to do so.[72] Many of these practitioners were refugees who had fled Nazi-dominated Central Europe.[73] In 1957, the Willink Committee on medical manpower found that 12 per cent of doctors in a random sample taken from the medical directories of 1953 and 1955 had done most of their training abroad.[74] The new service also relied on a significant workforce of Irish doctors who at the time were not necessarily viewed as overseas graduates.

South Asian doctors formed a small but not negligible proportion of the British medical workforce during the first decade of the NHS and rapidly took on an increasingly important role. As early as 1946, the *Guardian* newspaper reported that hundreds of Indian doctors were coming to London with a view to pursuing specialist training.[75] That post-imperial links could be put to use to help staff the British healthcare system was already apparent to medical politicians in the immediate aftermath of the inception of the NHS. In September 1948, the Empire Medical Advisory Bureau and the International Medical Visitors Bureau of the BMA noted that a number of overseas doctors required employment in order to gain practical experience and that they could be used to fill vacancies in regional hospitals.[76] The final stages of medical training overlap with the early stages of medical careers so doctors travelling to pursue training were also helping to staff hospitals. In 1949, the BMA received 101 enquiries from Indian doctors and 12 from Pakistan, figures which had risen to 125 and 33 respectively by 1951. In response, the Empire Medical Advisory Bureau observed that if Indian doctors encountered more success in obtaining hospital appointments, 'there would undoubtedly be many more enquiries and visitors from that country where the need for large numbers of very well trained practitioners is very great indeed'.[77]

As staff shortages persisted, those additional visitors did indeed materialise. In 1953, vacancies in junior hospital posts for instance were running at 20 per cent in Sheffield with some areas reaching 50 per cent.[78] The figures for Newcastle-upon-Tyne and Leeds were of 32 per cent and 30 per cent respectively.[79] Industrial parts of the country became dependent on migrant doctors who mostly came from India and Pakistan.[80] By 1960, 40 per cent of junior hospital posts were filled by doctors from overseas.[81] According to the Ministry of Health's figures for 1965, there were 2,799 doctors from India and 438 doctors from Pakistan working in hospitals or as GPs in England and Wales (out of a total NHS medical workforce of 43,825).[82] By the end of the 1970s, the numbers of South Asian-born doctors working in the UK was approximately 10,000 and they formed the principal group of migrant doctors in the NHS, accounting for around half of the overseas doctors it employed.[83] In the early 1980s, one-third of hospital doctors and one-fifth of general practitioners were overseas-born.[84] Although I have not located any figures that provide a breakdown of this number by gender, a significant proportion of doctors (16 per cent of GPs and 18 per cent of hospital doctors) in a survey of migrant doctors published in 1980 were women.[85] Nor should it be assumed that the majority of these female overseas doctors were white: in 1971 in India the ratio of female physicians and surgeons in the medical workforce was of 6.1 per 100 men.[86]

This influx of medical graduates was central to the development of the NHS, which was expanding while large numbers of British-trained doctors were emigrating. The government's evidence to the Committee of Enquiry into the Regulation of the Medical Profession in the 1970s outlined the dynamics at play:

> The staffing of the National Health Service requires annual increases in the numbers of doctors. The Todd Royal Commission, in estimating the required rate of increase, used a formula (related partly to population growth) which worked out at about 2% a year, or about 1,400 extra doctors a year in Great Britain. This has been reached or exceeded in recent years. Only a proportion—up to the present, less than half— of this increase comes from the output of British medical schools (the actual number varies considerably from year to year, because it depends not only on the numbers of new graduates which are fairly predictable, but also on the less predictable number of British doctors leaving the country and returning to it year by year, and on numbers moving into and out of NHS employment within the country). Up to the present, maintenance and development of the Service has taken up an annual net addition to the numbers of overseas doctors here of 700 a year or more. Allowing for the fact that many overseas doctors leave every year—in

the region of 2,000—maintenance of the development of the National
Health Service at present involves the admission of a total of between
2,500 and 3,000 overseas born doctors a year.[87]

It was in this context that a Ministry of Health official expressed concern in the 1960s that NHS hospitals could face 'paralysis within
weeks' in the event of an armed conflict between India and Pakistan
that would result in those countries asking their British-based doctors to return.[88] Doctors were initially migrating to take on junior
posts and subsequently either leaving Britain, building hospital
careers, often in unpopular specialties, or moving into general practice. They worked alongside substantial numbers of migrant nurses.
31,000 Irish-born nurses were employed in Britain in 1971, accounting for 12 per cent of the nursing personnel at the time.[89] There were
also substantial numbers of nurses from the Caribbean: by the mid-
1960s between 3,000 and 5,000 Jamaican nurses were employed in
British hospitals.[90] Just under a thousand work permits and permis-
sions were issued to nurses from Malaysia in 1975 alone.[91] Although
little is known about migrant caterers, cleaners and other NHS staff,
they also played a major part in staffing the NHS. A study for the
South West Thames Regional Health Authority in 1974 estimated
that one-third of domestic and catering staff in the area were from
overseas.[92]

*Professional and geographical hierarchies*
The NHS's substantial migrant workforce was not evenly distributed
within the organisation. Migrant doctors were disproportionately
concentrated in junior roles, unpopular medical specialties and, as has
already been stated, geographical locations viewed as less desirable.[93]
They were not just providing additional labour, they were, as migrants
frequently do, taking on roles that were deemed less prestigious. They
were doing what can be termed medical 'dirty work', i.e. forms of
labour that were undervalued within the British medical profession.[94]
Although medicine as a whole is a high-status profession, there are significant variations when it comes to the status of particular roles within
medicine. This is partly to do with the location of the work and the aspirations of doctors as middle-class professionals. A study of British GPs
published in 1973 noted that there appeared to be a widespread belief

amongst the medical profession that areas with shortages of family doctors were 'a kind of third world—worthy to receive general medical services, but scarcely fit places in which sensible people would voluntarily
choose to live'.[95] In 1966, *The Times* reported that migrant doctors:

> are not distributed evenly and in Northern hospitals they make up
> between 50 and 90 percent of the lower grade staff. It is said that in
> some places English doctors have not been seen in these posts for many
> years.[96]

It is in these junior posts that South Asian doctors frequently found
their first jobs in the NHS. In his memoirs, the Leicester GP Akram
Sayeed, one of the leading members of the Overseas Doctors'
Association (ODA), which was established in the 1970s to work on
behalf of migrant doctors, summarised the post-imperial trajectory of
thousands of medical migrants:

> Most of them ended up in the peripheral and district hospitals, where
> the service demand was enormous. There was hardly any provision
> made for education and training. They were simply used as a 'pair of
> hands'—A phrase … which was repeated time and time again by profes-
> sional colleagues and the media.[97]

Taken in isolation, it would be possible to see this account as politically motivated and it is indeed aligned with the ODA position of the
1970s and 1980s. This perception was, however, shared by Sir Donald
Irvine. Irvine, one of the leading British medical politicians of the late
twentieth century, believed there was little doubt that the early NHS
gave scant consideration to the training needs and career progression
of junior doctors:

> The steeply pyramidal career structure of NHS medicine needed
> an ample supply of newly qualified people—technically in training
> posts—actually to be 'pairs of hands'. It didn't desperately matter what
> their quality was like, or whether they were taught well or not, because
> they were always going to be in supervised practice whilst in hospital
> and at the end of the day they could be extruded from the system when
> no longer required. Recruitment from this group to specialist train-
> ing was highly selective, just as the Royal Colleges[98] wanted it to be …
> There was … no place to go in the hospital service for those left behind
> who didn't get to the next … notch in specialist training … The only

place left open-ended for the 'can't do' was general practice which at the time had no entry standards. This was the quite deliberate and quite ruthless manpower policy of the Department of Health and specialist medicine.[99]

Irvine's account reinforces the sense that the NHS staffing system was based on the assumption that many trainees would fail to fulfil their ambitions but he also indicates that, as I will show later, general practice offered a way of out of the impasse that many found themselves in as a result. In the late 1970s, over 50 per cent of senior house officer posts and 60 per cent of registrar posts[100] were filled by doctors from outside of the UK, as opposed to 16 per cent of consultant posts.[101]

The disregard that the medical establishment held for the type of role fulfilled by many South Asian doctors and the importance to the NHS of their deployment in roles considered peripheral is perhaps best summarised by two letters written by Alan Gilmour, who at the time was the Medical Director of the BMA's Commonwealth Medical Advisory Bureau. The first one was sent to the Conservative MP Victor Goodhew who was supportive of the white minority government in Rhodesia and of the prominent British politician Enoch Powell, who was known for his hostility to immigration.[102] In the letter, Gilmour wrote that the availability of 'cheap labour' in the form of Commonwealth migrants had enabled officials to avoid addressing the need to restructure medical staffing as it had 'helped to perpetuate (and perhaps increase)' the 'serious imbalance of unestablished junior posts offering too few opportunities for advancement'.[103] In the second letter, to Elston Grey-Turner, deputy secretary of the BMA, he writes of overseas doctors who spend many years 'holding registrar posts in Slagthorpe and District', assumedly a disparaging allusion to slagheaps in industrial areas.[104]

As well as often finding themselves confined to junior posts in particular geographical locations, migrant doctors were much more likely to find opportunities in less popular medical specialties. In 1975, the percentages of junior hospital staff born outside of the UK varied from 28.6 per cent in general medicine and 28.1 per cent in cardiology to 81.4 per cent in ophthalmology and 83.6 per cent in geriatrics.[105] In 2001, over 50 per cent of NHS consultants in learning disability who had been appointed between 1964 and 1991 were non-white and overseas trained.[106] The equivalent figure for general medicine was

3 per cent.[107] Overseas-trained consultants were also over-represented in geriatrics, psychiatry and genitourinary medicine.[108] These concentrations essentially reflect professional hierarchies within medical culture: in broad terms, diseases and specialties that involve time-limited and complex interventions in the upper part of the body and dealing with younger patients are afforded a higher status than those that involve chronic conditions and older patients.[109] Racism, which was a significant social force in post-war Britain, also profoundly shaped the development of the NHS and of general practice as Chapter 4 will show.

## The ebbing away of a post-imperial world

### The politics of post-war immigration policy

The freedom of movement that doctors enjoyed in the 1940s and 1950s was restricted in the 1960s and early 1970s, and by the 1980s a new post-imperial context had taken shape.[110] The development of the NHS and the experiences of its migrant workers were part of a wider social context where the movement of non-white migrants to Britain gradually became a significant political issue. In the immediate post-war years, the UK's policy on immigration was in line with its tradition of free movement within its Empire and Commonwealth.[111] This approach had been reaffirmed in the British Nationality Act of 1914 at a time when the immigration of migrants classed as 'aliens' was being subjected to new forms of control.[112] It remained the guiding principle of the 1948 British Nationality Act, which gave colonial and Commonwealth citizens the right to travel to the UK, to work there and to settle as permanent residents.[113] It is in this context that the movement of South Asian doctors to work in the NHS first took place. Subcontinental medical degrees were recognised by the GMC and doctors were free to move to the UK. Immigration policies and medical registration policies both gradually took new forms in the post-imperial space that came into existence in the 1960s and 1970s.

Migration from the British Empire and the Commonwealth increased significantly in the late 1940s and 1950s as various sectors of the UK economy suffered from post-war labour shortages.[114] Employers such as British Rail, London Transport, the NHS, northern textile mills and foundries in the Midlands were amongst the main recruiters.[115] In a pattern not dissimilar to that which characterised the development of British medicine, the limited supply of Irish migrants and of Europeans displaced by war led to an increased recourse to Commonwealth citizens.[116] There was from the outset however a tension between the discourse inherited from empire which stressed equality and freedom of movement and the reality of prejudice against non-white workers, be it from trade unions or service users.[117] Evidence of hostility was also present amongst the public at large. 'Colour bars' operated in pubs and clubs; access to housing was restricted. The media gave prominence to so-called 'race riots' in the Notting Hill area of London and in Nottingham—episodes of violence that mainly involved young white men attacking West Indian men.[118] In 1961, a national opinion poll found that just under three-quarters of the British population wanted immigration to be restricted and that their main concern was 'coloured colonial immigrants'.[119]

Politicians played their part in the development of these sentiments[120] not least because being seen to be pro-immigration became an electoral liability. The Labour politician Patrick Gordon Walker who had opposed the 1962 Immigration Act was defeated in the 1964 general election by the conservative Peter Griffiths, some of whose supporters used the slogan 'If you want a nigger neighbour, vote Labour'. Enoch Powell, in his 1968 'rivers of blood' speech that has come to symbolise post-war British anti-immigrant sentiment, later warned that immigration would lead to civil unrest. Both men were marginalised as a result—Griffiths was labelled a 'parliamentary leper' by the Labour Prime Minister Harold Wilson and Powell was dismissed from the Conservative shadow cabinet by the Tory leader Edward Heath. Their views and those of their supporters were nevertheless influential. The sociologists Stephen Small and John Solomos succinctly summarise how issues around immigration and race gradually came to take centre stage in British politics:

> There was a shift in official policy from decrying an open and explicit discussion of race in the debate on immigration, and allowing it to be shaped by the economic needs of the country (as in the 1940s and 1950s); to a consensus on both sides of the political spectrum, and indeed the general white population, that there should be explicit consideration of the race of immigrants, especially those of African-Caribbean, and Indian/Pakistani background, in framing national policy, and that the 'genuine fears' (a proxy for racial prejudice) of the

indigenous white population should be taken into account in deciding how many such immigrants to allow into the country.[121]

This shift is reflected in the evolution of official policy on immigration between the early 1960s and early 1970s. The 1962 Commonwealth Immigrants Act introduced a system of work vouchers for Commonwealth citizens wanting to move to the UK.[122] The 1968 Commonwealth Immigrants Act and the 1971 Immigration Act introduced further restrictions on the entry and settlement in the UK of citizens of Britain and its colonies who could not demonstrate a 'patrial' connection to the UK, for instance through being born in Britain, having parents or grandparents born in Britain or as a result of long-term residency.[123] These laws of course had a greater effect on non-white than white migrants, the latter being more likely to be able to provide such evidence. As a result of these changes, Commonwealth citizens who were not patrials needed permission to enter the UK and no longer had the automatic right to settle if allowed entry for work purposes.[124]

### 'They are not, and have never been, immigrants': the complex status of South Asian doctors

The movement to restrict non-white migration did not immediately affect doctors in the way that it affected other groups in the 1960s and 1970s. This is at least to a degree, as I will show, because they were not necessarily considered to be migrants. It is also because, as I will discuss later on, the British government was initially using the voucher system to recruit doctors whilst also ensuring that other medical graduates could come to the UK without appearing in official immigration statistics. As a result a number of doctors were able to circumnavigate immigration controls.

Even in the late 1980s, the authors of a Commission for Racial Equality report still felt it necessary to underline the fact that 'The relationship between overseas doctors and the NHS is complex. It is no longer temporary, as some overseas doctors themselves and many of the administration of the NHS thought originally.'[125] The movement of doctors was not officially presented at the time as the permanent importation of a workforce. Oscar Gish's 1969 report *Britain and the Immigrant Doctor* stated that 'The bulk of overseas born doctors are considered to be postgraduate students, in Britain only for advanced training.'[126] A blurring of boundaries was possible as a result of the nature of medical training. Occupying junior posts in hospitals forms part of the postgraduate education that doctors gain when specialising in a particular branch of medicine. It was therefore possible to use doctors in the NHS as an extra 'pair of hands' in junior posts whilst presenting this policy as the temporary proffering of educational opportunity.

This explains the development of an official discourse that presented the reliance of the NHS on migrant labour as a form of aid to the Commonwealth, an argument that a group of researchers described in 1981 as 'the traditional justification' for the presence of large numbers of overseas-born staff in the NHS.[127] If the period from the 1950s to the 1960s can in general terms be seen as characterised by what Bill Schwartz has described as the 're-racialisation' of Britain, with a strong rise in anti-immigrant sentiments leading to a political response, this political response was different, or at least delayed, when it came to the NHS.[128] Enoch Powell's 'rivers of blood' speech, for instance, unequivocally excluded doctors from his apocalyptic warnings about the impact of immigration on the UK's social fabric:

> This has nothing to do with the entry of Commonwealth citizens, any more than of aliens, into this country, for the purposes of study or of improving their qualifications, like (for instance) the Commonwealth doctors who, to the advantage of their own countries, have enabled our hospital service to be expanded faster than would have otherwise have been possible. They are not, and have never been, immigrants.[129]

This view of the role of migrant doctors and their place in British society was shared by a number of migrant doctors. In a letter to the *BMJ* in 1969, a Dr A. S. M. M. Haque wrote to point out that foreign doctors should not be referred to as 'immigrants' because most of them returned to their countries of origin after completing their training.[130] Of course, as a former Minister of Health who had presided over the arrival of large numbers of migrant doctors, Powell might simply have been pre-empting charges of hypocrisy. Irrespective of his motivations, and those of other politicians, what is interesting about this notion that doctors were not migrants is that it was a credible position to adopt at the time.

This is not to say that these arguments were universally accepted. In 1963, L. J. Witts, Professor of Clinical Medicine at Oxford University, was quoted in the *Guardian* as saying that 'The number of resident [i.e. junior] posts in our hospitals which are held by foreign doctors is now 40 per cent of the total and the figure is rising ... It would be hypocrisy to pretend that this has happened out of a desire to educate Commonwealth doctors in Western ways'.[131] A government document from the 1960s which discussed an Indian government statement outlining measures to restrict medical migration shows there was official concern at the prospect of any reduction in migratory movement: a handwritten comment reads 'this sounds ominous'.[132] The author of the document expressed the view that if doctors were to be discouraged from leaving India for 'purely employment purposes' the effect on Britain might be 'catastrophic'.[133] The concern about doctors not being allowed to leave solely to take up employment suggests that within the civil service at least there was a clear sense that facilitating the movement of doctors, at least from the UK's perspective, was about ensuring that NHS posts were filled rather than the philanthropic provision of educational opportunities.

The fact that it was possible to argue that doctors were not migrants nevertheless helped governments reconcile two contradictory political aims: their desire to control Commonwealth immigration and the need to ensure that the NHS was able to function normally. It was of course possible for Commonwealth doctors to enter under the voucher scheme introduced in the early 1960s and many of them did: they numbered 938 in 1967.[134] However, official figures related to the numbers of vouchers issued and used give little sense of the scale of the movement of doctors to the UK. An estimated 2,000 overseas doctors came to the UK in 1968 as postgraduate students with the status of temporary visitors.[135] Moreover, by the late 1960s, the government was, as a civil servant in the Home Office admitted, 'Strictly speaking ... concealing the true number of those admitted for employment',[136] having introduced a parallel system of entry certificates for migrant doctors with job offers or who had been given a place on an attachment scheme.[137] These doctors appeared in statistics as 'other persons coming for settlement' rather than as voucher holders.[138] It seems likely that this was a deliberate ploy to maintain a flow of significant numbers of Commonwealth doctors while creating the impression that immigration was being controlled. A restricted Home Office circular drew attention to the fact that 'Despite the changes described ... the position must be maintained that all doctors must apply for vouchers.'[139] It also reassured readers who were being asked to partake in this deception that 'The form E.D. 431 has been deliberately designed to look like a voucher.'[140] Whilst the new immigration laws clearly did not make it easier for doctors to migrate, substantial numbers of South Asian doctors continued to arrive and take on jobs in the NHS.

*Changes to medical regulations*

Up to the 1970s, many South Asian medical degrees were recognised by the GMC and, once settled in the UK, doctors were free to become general practitioners. By the 1980s, however, the free movement of the 1940s and 1950s and the political accommodations of the 1960s had given way to a much more restrictive environment. The GMC ceased to recognise Sri Lankan, Pakistani and Indian qualifications in 1971, 1972 and 1975 respectively.[141] Pakistan leaving the Commonwealth was one factor behind this change and the GMC also expressed the view that it no longer felt able to vouch for the quality of the degrees delivered by subcontinental medical schools.[142] The (post-) imperial system of mutual recognition of degrees between Britain and the Indian subcontinent was replaced by a requirement to sit a test to demonstrate professional aptitude. The Temporary Registration Assessment Board of the GMC (TRAB, subsequently renamed Professional and Linguistic Assessment Board, PLAB) presided over examinations from 1975.[143] Doctors who successfully passed this examination initially obtained temporary registration, giving them access to hospital work that would be carried out under supervision, but they did not have full registration and therefore could not enter general practice. The Medical Act 1978 replaced temporary registration with limited registration which could lead to full registration after a period of five years in the UK.[144] Full registration could also be gained by sitting the exams of non-university organisations whose qualifications were recognised in the UK.[145] From the 1980s, doctors with full registration who wanted to become GPs would have to undergo a period of vocational training which would focus on the specific skills needed for general practice. In addition to this, new regulations introduced in 1985 stated that migrant doctors would have to prove that the post they were interested in could not be filled by a UK-based doctor. Exceptions were made for those wanting to undertake training in hospitals but their stay would be limited to four years unless they were able to obtain a work permit for a limited period.[146]

One of the principal drivers of this change was the voicing of concerns amongst the British medical profession concerning the quality of the care provided by South Asian doctors. Aneez Esmail's analysis of the correspondence columns of the *BMJ* between 1961 and 1975 revealed that this was a common subject of discussion and he noted that much of what was written would be 'considered offensive and racist if it was published today'.[147] The main issues raised concerned language problems and standards of education.[148] The views of a section of the medical profession were amplified by the media. The *Daily Mail* reported in 1973 that a delegate at the BMA conference, Dr Edward Lewis had suggested that anyone calling their local hospital and asking to speak to the casualty officer could expect to hear the words 'I spikka da no English.'[149]

In fact, the first study to focus on the language skills of migrant doctors estimated that fewer than 13 per cent had 'more than a slight linguistic handicap'.[150] It also found that it was mostly recent arrivals who experienced difficulties.[151] As for the quality of overseas qualifications, in 1969, Walter Pyke-Lees the registrar of the GMC was recorded in the minutes of a meeting at the Department of Health as having defended the standards applied to overseas medical schools before recognition of their degrees was granted, saying that the 'inspection teams were most meticulous' and had 'exacting standards'.[152] This is not to say that there was no evidence of any problems at all: according to a 1967 Memorandum by the Ministry of Health, a third of migrant doctors taking part in a new attachment scheme had been found to be 'deficient in either clinical competence or command of English.'[153] There was certainly however a lack of any conclusive evidence that demonstrated that there was a severe problem that demanded a dramatic shift in policy. This did not prevent the Committee of Inquiry into the Regulation of the Medical Profession from concluding in its 1975 report that 'there are substantial numbers of overseas doctors whose skill and the care they offer to patients fall below that generally acceptable in this country.'[154]

The withdrawal of recognition from South Asian medical colleges whose degrees continued to be recognised and the introduction of professional tests swiftly followed the publication of these conclusions. The government had already indicated that it was open to such moves in 1969 when the Labour Secretary of State for Health and Social Security Richard Crossman met the secretary of the BMA Derek Stevenson and stated that he had discussed issues around professional competence, language and registration with the Chief Medical Officer and the President of the GMC.[155] These changes were however not retrospective. Doctors who had qualified before subcontinental degrees ceased to be recognised could still obtain full registration and become GPs.[156] The impact of the migration of South Asian doctors on general practice therefore continued to be felt into the 1970s and 1980s.

The legacy of the British Empire thus shaped the context of British immigration policy and medical regulation. Its influence can also be detected in the motivations and views of South Asian doctors who came to Britain.

## Notes

1 S. Dadabhoy ('The next generation, the problematic children: A personal story', in Coker (ed.) *Racism in Medicine*, pp. 60–1) for instance compares the National Health Service to a 'sepoy army' — i.e. an organisation, like colonial armies in India, run by white people but dependent on non-white foot soldiers. Esmail ('Asian doctors', p. 830) argues that there are common points between imperial recourse to indentured labour and NHS reliance on overseas doctors. Ali for her part concluded that the NHS, as an institution that recruited from former colonies to meet its staffing needs, was 'one of the last bastions of Empire' (L. Ali, 'West Indian Nurses and the National Health Service in Britain 1950–1968' (Master of Arts by Dissertation, University of York, 2001), p. 110).

2 However, for a discussion of the relevance of a post-colonial approach to the context of the NHS in relation to the treatment of patients see R. Bivins, 'Coming "home" to (post) colonial medicine: Treating tropical bodies in post-war Britain, *Social History of Medicine*, 26:1 (2013) '. Bivins further explores the interactions between the development of the NHS, imperial legacies and migrant patients in *Contagious Communities*.

3 However, see Jones & Snow, *Against the Odds*, pp. 6–22.

4 E. W. Said, *Culture and Imperialism* (London: Vintage Books, 1994), pp. xxii–xxiii.

5 Bivins, 'Coming "home"'.

6  See E. Consterdine, 'Community versus Commonwealth: Reappraising the 1971 Immigration Act', *Immigrants and Minorities*, 35:1 (2017).

7  The term 'race' is used with quotation marks in order to enable its discussion as social reality whilst highlighting that it has no biological basis.

8  Jeffery, 'Recognizing India's doctors: The institutionalisation of medical dependency, 1918–39', *Modern Asian Studies*, 13:2 (1979), pp. 302–3.

9  Jeffery, 'Recognizing India's doctors', p. 303.

10  Ibid.

11  R. O. B. Wijesekera, 'Scientific research in a small developing nation – Sri Lanka', *Economic Review* (June 1976), p. 9.

12  R. Jeffery, *The Politics of Health in India* (Berkeley, Los Angeles, London: University of California Press, 1988), p. 86.

13  M. Harrison, 'Science and the British Empire', *Isis*, 96:1 (2005), p. 60; P. Chakrabarti, *Medicine and Empire 1600–1960* (Basingstoke & New York: Palgrave Macmillan, 2013); M. Gorman, 'Introduction of western science into colonial India: Role of the Calcutta Medical College', *Proceedings of the American Philosophical Society*, 132:3 (1988).

14  Jeffery, 'Recognising India's doctors', p. 316; A. Kumar, *Medicine and the Raj: British Medical Policy in India 1835–1911* (New Delhi, Thousand Oaks, London: Sage Publications, 1998).

15  Jeffery, 'Recognising India's doctors', pp. 301–2.

16  'Indian medical degrees: The General Medical Council and Indian qualifications', *BMJ* (15 March, 1930), p. 508.

17  Ibid.

18  T. J. Johnson & M. Caygill, 'The British Medical Association and its overseas branches: A short history', *The Journal of Imperial and Commonwealth History*, 1:3 (1973), p. 310.

19  Johnson & Caygill, 'The British Medical Association', pp. 308 & 310.

20  Gorman, 'Introduction of western science', p. 293; Ramanna, *Western Medicine and Public Health in Colonial Bombay 1845–1894* (London: Sangam Books, 2002), p. 19.

21  Gorman, 'Introduction of western science', p. 293; M. Ramanna, *Western Medicine*, p. 19; Lahiri, *Indians in Britain*, pp. 5, 7 & 30.

22  Lahiri, *Indians in Britain*, pp. 5–7.

23  Lahiri, *Indians in Britain*, p. 34.

24  Gorman, 'Introduction of western science', p. 290.

25  Jeffery, 'Medical dependency', p. 323.

26 Jeffery, 'Medical dependency', p. 325.

27 Kondapi, *Indians Overseas*, p. 360.

28 A more precise picture of the presence of South Asian GPs in Britain in the 1940s could potentially be produced through a more detailed investigation. This would involve for instance a trawl of medical registers and medical directories. However, South Asian names were at times anglicised and female doctors changed their names on marriage so the result would be imprecise. Research at a local level in surviving papers of medical bodies or newspapers could also be fruitful as could archival research in the Indian subcontinent. Such a task would clearly represent a major undertaking and attempting to identify South Asian doctors who were in Britain before the NHS was established was not one of the main aims of this study.

29 R. Boomla interviews with author, 5 December 2008 & 16 September 2009.

30 Museum of London, London, 92.180, R. Boomla & D. Boomla, interviewed by Rory O'Connell, 20 November 1992.

31 R. Boomla interview with author, 16 September 2009.

32 British Library Sound Archive, London (henceforth BLSA), 'Oral History of General Practice 1936–1952', C648/28/01–06, S. Kutar interviewed by M. Bevan, 1993.

33 Ibid.

34 Sir Netar Mallick interview with author, 23 June 2010; anonymous interview with author; Ajeet Gulati interview with author, 24 May 2011; Jangu Banatvala interview with author, 9 July 2015.

35 Chowdhary, *I Made my Home*, pp. 30–1 & 63.

36 'Living in Barking', *Eastside Community Heritage Newsletter* (September 2010).

37 Chowdhary, *I Made my Home*, p. 61.

38 Visram, *Asians in Britain*, p. 283.

39 Visram, *Asians in Britain*, pp. 286–8.

40 Visram, *Asians in Britain*, pp. 283–4.

41 J. M. Simpson, 'Gulati, Harbans Lall (1896?–1967)', *Oxford Dictionary of National Biography* [online] (Oxford: Oxford University Press, 2012). Accessed 1 July 2012 at: www.oxforddnb.com/index/73/101073274/.

42 S. Creighton, 'Harbans Lal (l) Gulati', Unpublished talk (no date).

43 C. Moreton, 'The dark family secret that drove Ben Kingsley to success', the *Daily Mail* (2012). Accessed 3 May 2012 at: www.dailymail.co.uk/home/moslive/article-1277638/Ben-Kingsley-The-dark-family-secret-drove-success.html.

44 'Immigrants' leader dies in road crash', the *Guardian* (13 November 1979), p. 4.

45 'Indian doctor sent to penal servitude', *The Times* (4 April 1925), p. 9.

46 R. Davenport-Hines, 'Ruxton, Buck (1899–1936)', *Oxford Dictionary of National Biography* [online] (Oxford: Oxford University Press, 2004). Accessed 1 July 2017 at: www.oxforddnb.com/index/73/101073638/.

47 'Lieutenant-Colonel S. S. Vazifdar MRCP, MRCS, IMS (Ret.)', *BMJ* (1971, 3:5776), p. 711.

48 'A. I. Toorawa', *BMJ* (1989, 298:6667), p. 181.

49 'Dorothy M. Satur, BA, MMSA, FRCSED, FRCOG', BMJ (1981, 282:6278), p. 1805.

50 'A. I. Toorawa', *BMJ* (1989, 298:6667), p. 181.

51 'S. K. Sen, MB, BS, DTM', *BMJ* (1974, 3:5926), pp. 354–5.

52 'K. C. Sarkar, MB, MRCS, LRCP, MRCGP', *BMJ* (1982, 285:6352), p. 1435.

53 'H. V. Sankarayya', *BMJ* (1989, 298:6681), p. 1175.

54 'D. Saklatvala, MRCS, LRCP', *BMJ* (1981, 282:6278), p. 1805.

55 'Y. N. Lal, MB, CHB', *BMJ* (1970, 3:5723), p. 651.

56 'K. Kumar, MB, BS', *BMJ* (1981, 283:6288), pp. 444–5.

57 'A. W. Khan, MB, BS, FRCSEd', *BMJ* (1977, 1:6077), p. 1669

58 'H. K.Fozdar, MB, BS', *BMJ* (1975, 3:5980), p. 440.

59 'K. C. Bhattacharyya, MB, MRCS, LRCP, LMSSA', *BMJ* (1982, 285:6341), p. 569.

60 'J. Bhageerutty, LRCP&SED, LRFPSGLAS', *BMJ* (1976, 1:6004), p. 289.

61 'K. A. Anklesaria, MRCS, LRCP', *BMJ* (1970, 1:5689), pp. 179–80.

62 'A. B. Gunasekara, MRCS, LRCP', *BMJ* (1971, 1:5745), p. 408.

63 Lahiri, *Indians in Britain*, p. 61.

64 R. Boomla interviews with author.

65 Lahiri, *Indians in Britain*, pp. 61–2.

66 Sir N. Mallick interview with author; A. Gulati interview with author.

67 Lahiri, *Indians in Britain*, p. 52.

68 C. Muthu, 'Indian doctors and vacant appointments', *The Lancet* (1915, 2:4799), pp. 415–16; Lahiri, *Indians in Britain*, p. 61.

69 Simpson et al., 'Writing migrants'.

70 BMA, Central Medical War Committee, Aliens Committee, meeting of Tuesday 10 December 1946.

71  Hansard, HC Deb, vol. 450 cc71–2W, Alien Doctors (Registration), 29 April 1948. Accessed 15 April 2017 at: http://hansard.mill-banksystems.com/written_answers/1948/apr/29/alien-doctors-registration#S5CV0450P0_19480429_CWA_45.

72  'Work of Foreign doctors: Position in Britain regularised', *The Times* (6 December 1947), p. 2.

73  Weindling, 'Modernisation'; Weindling, 'Introduction'.

74  Simpson et al., 'Writing migrants', p. 392.

75  'London has world "school for doctors"', the *Guardian* (29 December 1946), p. 7.

76  BMA, Empire Medical Advisory Bureau and International Medical Visitors Bureau, Committee of Management, 23 September 1948.

77  BMA, Empire Medical Advisory Bureau and International Medical Visitors Bureau, Committee of Management, 24 April 1952, Report of the Empire Medical Advisory Bureau for the Year Ending 31 December 1951.

78  Webster, *Health Services*, Vol. I, p. 309.

79  Ibid.

80  Ibid.

81  Webster, *Health Services*, Vol. II, p. 283.

82  UK National Archives (henceforth: National Archives), MH 149/1003, note of 21 February 1968.

83  Simpson et al., 'Writing migrants', p. 392.

84  Smith, *Overseas Doctors*, p. 1.

85  Smith, *Overseas Doctors*, p. 210.

86  P. R. L. Mohan, 'Asian doctors in England: Their professional experiences and social life (A case study in Sandwell)' (Master of Social Sciences thesis, University of Birmingham, 1979), p. 27.

87  Report of the Committee of Inquiry into the regulation of the medical profession [Merrison report] (London: HMSO, 1975), p. 54.

88  Simpson et al., 'Writing migrants', p. 392.

89  Ryan, 'Who do you think you are?', p. 417.

90  Jones & Snow, *Against the Odds*, p. 10. See also: A. Kramer, *Many Rivers to Cross: The History of the Caribbean Contribution to the NHS* (London: TSO, 2006).

91  Department of Employment, *The role of immigrants in the labour market: Project report by the unit for manpower studies* (London: Department of Employment, 1976), p. 138.

92  L. Doyal, F. Gee, G. Hunt, J. Mellor, I. Pennell, Migrant workers in the National Health Service: Report of a preliminary survey (Polytechnic of North London: Department of Sociology, 1980), pp. 22–3.

93  J. M. Simpson, 'Diagnosing a flight from care: Medical migration and "dirty work" in the NHS', Policy papers, *History and Policy*, 2014 [online]. Accessed 1 July 2017 at: www.historyandpolicy.org/policy-papers/papers/diagnosing-a-flight-from-care-medical-migration-and-dirty-work-in-the-nhs; Simpson et al., 'Providing "special" types of labour'.

94  Simpson et al., 'Providing "special" types of labour'.

95  J. R. Butler (in collaboration with J. M. Bevan & R. C. Taylor), *Family Doctors and Public Policy* (London: Routledge and Kegan Paul, 1973), p. 111.

96  'Dependence on overseas doctors', *The Times* (31 August 1966), p. 9.

97  Sayeed, *Takdir*, pp. 193–4.

98  Professional bodies in specialised fields of medicine.

99  Sir Donald Irvine interview with author.

100  These are both junior positions in hospitals.

101  Doyal et al., 'Your Life in their hands', p. 57.

102  A. Roth, 'Sir Victor Goodhew: Tory apologist for the Rhodesian regime of UDI leader Ian Smith', the *Guardian*, 26 October 2006. Accessed 27 October 2016 at: www.theguardian.com/news/2006/oct/27/guardianobituaries.zimbabwe; 'Sir Victor Goodhew', The *Telegraph*, 21 October 2006. Accessed 27 October 2016 at: www.telegraph.co.uk/news/obituaries/1531969/Sir-Victor-Goodhew.html.

103  BMA, 'Problems of overseas doctors in UK re employment', A. Gilmour to V. Goodhew, 9 February 1970.

104  BMA, 'Problems of overseas doctors in UK re employment', A. Gilmour to Dr Grey-Turner, 15 September 1970.

105  Raghuram et al., 'Ethnic clustering', p. 290.

106  M. J. Goldacre, J. M. Davidson, T. W. Lambert, 'Country of training and ethnic origin of UK doctors: Database and survey studies', *BMJ*, 2004, doi: 10.1136/bmj.38202.364271.BE.

107  Goldacre et al., 'Country of training and ethnic origin'.

108  Ibid.

109  Simpson et al., 'Providing "special" types of labour', p. 209.

110  Consterdine, 'Community versus Commonwealth'.

111  Holmes, *John Bull's Island*, p. 309.

112  Ibid.

113  Holmes, *John Bull's Island*, p. 257; S. Small & J. Solomos, 'Race, immigration and politics in Britain: Changing policy agendas and conceptual paradigms 1940s–2000s', *International Journal of Comparative Sociology*, 47 (2006), p. 242.

114   Small & Solomos, 'Race, immigration and politics', p. 239; Jones & Snow, *Against the Odds*, pp. 14–15.

115   Small & Solomos, 'Immigration and politics', p. 242; J. Solomos, *Race and Racism in Britain* (Basingstoke & New York: Palgrave Macmillan, 2003).

116   Small & Solomos, 'Immigration and politics', p. 239.

117   Ibid.; Jones & Snow, *Against the Odds*, pp. 14–15.

118   Small & Solomos, 'Immigration and Politics', p. 242.

119   Small & Solomos, 'Immigration and Politics' p. 243.

120   Solomos, *Race and Racism*, p. 57.

121   Small & Solomos, 'Immigration and politics', p. 238.

122   Holmes, *John Bull's Island*, p. 260.

123   Solomos, *Race and Racism*, pp. 60–3; C. Kyriakides & S. Virdee, 'Migrant labour, racism and the British National Health Service', *Ethnicity and Health*, 8:4 (2003), p. 292.

124   Solomos, *Race and Racism*, p. 63.

125   M. Anwar & A. Ali, *Overseas Doctors: Experiences and Expectations* (London: Commission for Racial Equality, 1987), p. 72.

126   Gish, *Britain and the Immigrant Doctor*, p. 5.

127   Doyal et al., 'Your life in their hands', p. 54.

128   B. Schwartz, '"The only white man in there": The re-racialisation of England, 1956–1968', *Race and Class*, 38:1 (1996).

129   E. Powell, Speech to the Conservative association in Birmingham on 20 April 1968 ['rivers of blood' speech]. Accessed 8 December 2012 at: www.telegraph.co.uk/comment/3643826/Enoch-Powells-Rivers-of-Blood-speech.html).

130   A. S. M. M. Haque, '"Immigrant" doctors', Correspondence, *BMJ* (1969, 1:5647), p. 848.

131   'Immigrants keep health service going', the *Guardian* (8 June 1963), p. 10.

132   National Archives, MH149/352, Ministry of Health Note, 8 March 1965.

133   Ibid.

134   Gish, 'Britain and the immigrant doctor', p. 3.

135   BMA, 'Problems of overseas doctors in UK re employment', Note of a discussion on overseas doctors in the National Health Service, 2 March 1969.

136   National Archives, FCO 50/283, Home Office Letter, 12 June 1969.

137   Ibid.

138  Ibid.
139  National Archives, FCO 50/283, Home Office Circular, Revision of the voucher scheme, March 1968.
140  Ibid.
141  Smith, *Overseas Doctors*, pp. 11–12.
142  Ibid.; Kyriakides & Virdee, 'Migrant labour', pp. 393–4.
143  Smith, *Overseas Doctors*, p. 12; I. C. McManus & R. Wakeford, 'PLAB and UK graduates' performance on MRCP (UK) and MRCGP examination: data linkage study', *BMJ*, 348 (2014).
144  Smith, *Overseas Doctors*, p. 13.
145  For instance the Society of Apothecaries of London, the English Conjoint Board and the Scottish Triple Qualification which were criticised for offering a 'back door entry into medicine'. See: R. Wakeford, 'LMSSA: A back door entry into medicine?', *BMJ*, 294 (1987), pp. 890–1. See also: D. Barker, 'Ruling on Pakistani doctors to be raised by High Commission', the *Guardian* (29 July 1972), p. 4.
146  M. McCormack, 'ODA demands stay-away protest in permit row', *Doctor* (4 April 1985), p. 1.
147  Esmail, 'Asian doctors', p. 830.
148  Ibid.; Smith, *Overseas Doctors*, p. 2.
149  'Doctors who "no spikka da English"', the *Daily Mail* (9 June 1973), p. 15.
150  Smith, *Overseas Doctors*, p. 28.
151  Ibid.
152  BMA, Problems of overseas doctors in UK re employment, Minutes of a meeting held at Alexander Fleming House, 27 May 1969.
153  National Archives, MH149/1003, Cabinet Official Committee on Commonwealth Immigration, Memorandum by the Ministry of Health, Doctors and the voucher scheme.
154  Report of the Committee of Enquiry into the regulation of the medical profession, p. 60.
155  BMA, Problems of overseas doctors re employment, Note of meeting between representatives of the BMA and the Department of Health and Social Security, 20 March 1969.
156  Smith, *Overseas Doctors*, p. 12.

# Part II

# The colonial legacy, racism and the staffing of surgeries

# 3

# The empire of the mind and medical migration

It is important, in order to understand how the NHS and British general practice were able to draw on the labour of South Asian doctors, to appreciate, as was shown in the previous chapter, how British immigration and medical registration policies remained defined by imperial legacies for much of this period. It is also crucial to appreciate that these legacies continued to shape medicine in the Indian subcontinent and the thought processes of doctors—as is apparent in their oral history interviews and in documents that they shared with me.

Naturally, post-imperial dynamics were not the only influences on doctors' decisions to migrate. Participants cite the increasing ease of access to air travel[1] as well as dissatisfaction with career options and the medical system in Pakistan,[2] Sri Lanka[3] and India.[4] One informant openly recognised that she hoped to earn more money in Britain than in India, a factor that may also have been important to others even if they chose not to explicitly state this.[5] Medical journals from the time provide further evidence that many South Asian doctors were indeed dissatisfied with their working conditions and salaries and that few Indian doctors wanted to work in rural parts of India.[6] A letter to *The Lancet* in 1967 signed by an anonymous Pakistani doctor stated that:

> Many doctors in my position find it painful to see that, on returning to their countries, the 'brain drain' [sic] find it impossible to practice the Western, more scientific medicine, because of not only lack of adequate scientific facilities or having to deal with a majority of rural and illiterate population but also other reasons peculiar to each country. Surely it is time now to take action to prevent increase in the number of socially, professionally, and even economically frustrated doctors who, having learnt to be 'the engineer', do not want to be 'the plumber' once again.[7]

The fact that doctors could earn higher salaries in the NHS and that air travel made the prospect of taking on work abroad less daunting cannot however on its own explain why such large numbers of South Asian doctors came to Britain. Drawing on interviews with doctors, I will show in this chapter that a key contributor to the large-scale migration of South Asian doctors was the fact that South Asian medical systems continued to work along post-imperial lines rather than being radically redefined. British medicine remained a model to be emulated and South Asian medicine continued to situate itself in relation to medicine in Britain. Those responsible for healthcare systems and medical training on the subcontinent continued to internalise the values of the imperial power, in the way that Frantz Fanon described in *Peau noire, masques blancs* (black skin, white masks): 'A people that has been colonised—by which I mean a people that has developed an inferiority complex … situates itself in relation to the language of the civilising nation, that is of the metropolitan culture.'[8]

This was a political choice made by South Asian governments and medical professionals, rather than an unavoidable development. It is perfectly possible to imagine that post-independence South Asian countries would have radically restructured their systems of medical education, ensuring that they were more closely aligned with the needs of their local populations. The fact that politicians chose to not do this created a situation where doctors developed aspirations that as the anonymous letter to *The Lancet* made clear were more readily met in medical systems in the Global North than in the Global South. If India, and/or Pakistan had decided to prioritise the training of practitioners with basic medical skills who were to be deployed in rural areas and limit the number of doctors trained according to western norms, the history of the NHS would have taken a very different form. As it was, in a post-imperial British context where doctors were until the 1970s relatively free to migrate, they were being educated in settings that remained wedded to British approaches. South Asian medical schools trained 'engineers' more suited to working in better-funded healthcare systems in the Global North rather than 'plumbers' who might be content to work within the constraints of South Asian healthcare provision.

In the post-imperial environment of British medicine in the period from the 1940s to the 1980s, the NHS offered jobs in an

expanding and developing healthcare system and freedom of movement for doctors willing to take them on. In this respect, the UK
was different from the other main importers of medical labour at the
time. In the early 1970s, the WHO estimated that at least 140,000
physicians were based in countries other than those of which they
were nationals or in which they had trained.[9] Three countries were
home to over three quarters of these doctors: the USA (with around
68,000 migrant doctors in 1972, the UK (which had around 21,000
overseas doctors in 1970) and Canada (with an estimated 9,000
international medical graduates in 1971).[10] West Germany and
Australia were also important recipient countries with 6,000 and
4,000 migrant physicians respectively in 1971.[11] For South Asian
doctors thinking of migrating, Germany was not an obvious destination for linguistic reasons. Of the remaining main importers of
medical labour, until the 1960s, the USA and Canada had restrictive immigration laws that made it harder for South Asian migrants
to gain entry and from the 1950s, the USA required migrants to sit
the Educational Council for Foreign Medical Graduates (ECFMG)
examination.[12] In Australia, the medical profession vociferously
opposed political efforts to attract greater numbers of overseas doctors in the 1950s, although more liberal policies were adopted in
the 1960s in a number of states/territories, as was the case in the
USA and Canada.[13] By the 1970s, however, efforts were already
beginning to be made in the USA, Canada and the UK to contain
the flow of migrant doctors.[14] Britain therefore offered a particularly welcoming environment in that from the 1940s to the 1970s,
when subcontinental degrees ceased to be recognised and tests for
doctors wanting to work in the NHS were introduced, it essentially
offered freedom of movement to South Asian-trained doctors and
jobs in an organisation that was, and remains, one of the world's
main employers. It was therefore a logical destination for South
Asian doctors who found themselves on the global medical labour
market.

It is important to emphasise that much of this context was contin-
gent. South Asian medical schools and the South Asian medical profession in general could have chosen not to continue to attach great
importance to the issue of whether degrees were recognised by the

GMC or not. Similarly, policy-makers could have intervened more forcefully to ensure that medical graduates remained in their country of origin. Attempts were made by South Asian governments to prevent doctors from leaving or to encourage them to return but their impact on the broader picture of medical migration was limited.[15]

If South Asian doctors were in a position to move to Britain when dissatisfied with the opportunities they were presented with, it was because they had received an education that continued to see British medicine as a model, because they spoke English and because until the 1970s their degrees were recognised in the UK. All of these factors are connected to the British presence in South Asia. Moreover, issues such as salaries and conditions took on particular importance because doctors who had been educated in a westernised medical system aspired to a particular social status and developed a particular sense of their role through their education. Again, it is not inconceivable that new post-independence governments could have recruited and trained professionals who would have been happy to work in rural areas for the salaries that were on offer in South Asia. More could have been done to challenge the dependency on the UK when it came to the provision of medical training. It is interesting to note, for instance, that as late at 1963, sixteen years after partition, the vice-rector of the Moscow Friendship University claimed that only a small number of Indian students were enrolled in courses in his university because their country did not recognise medical qualifications granted in the Soviet Union.[16]

The interviews carried out with doctors for this project provide evidence of a sense of continuity with imperial traditions, which contributed to the movement of doctors. As a number of studies have shown, the migration of doctors to Britain is the product of a complex array of factors. The geographers Vaughan Robinson and Malcolm Carey have made the case for the need to see this movement as underpinned by colonial ties, traditions of migration and 'Izzet'.[17] This latter notion can be likened to social status and in the context of the history of Indian medicine is not unconnected to imperial legacies: travelling to Britain and obtaining degrees has been and continues to be seen as desirable and prestigious. This chapter builds on Robinson and Carey's insight that the migration of doctors requires to be contextualised socially, culturally and historically.[18] It should not be seen solely as the movement of skilled professionals in search of better salaries.[19] As they put it:

> Although migrants move to 'better themselves', they also make choices based on factors such as the kind of novels they read as children or 'taken for granted' familial obligations rooted in the everyday life of their culture.[20]

This echoes the findings of a study of Asian doctors in England conducted in the 1970s which found that reasons for migrating were not only linked to financial or professional considerations.[21] Its author, P. R. L. Mohan, noted for instance that many doctors' wives were 'fascinated by the idea of the cold weather and the snow falls, the beautiful scenery depicted in English movies'.[22] As David Smith noted in his study of overseas doctors in the NHS published in 1980, a common language as well as shared hospital systems and approaches to medicine made Indian doctors 'naturally' think of Britain as a country in which to train.[23] Doctors were moving within a shared intellectual and social space where common values prevailed, a 'socio-cognitive community' where migration was seen as vital to career progression.[24] Formal imperial domination had come to an end in Pakistan and India in 1947 and in Sri Lanka (then Ceylon) in 1948 but is it important to pay attention to what Andrew Porter has termed the 'empires in the mind': the diffusion of ideas and ways of thinking which continued to mould societies and cultures following the dismantling of the formal empire.[25] The legacy of empire can be detected in doctors' accounts of their medical training and careers in medicine as well as when they discuss their personal backgrounds.

The vast majority of the forty South Asian GPs interviewed for this project talked about their medical education in terms that point to them having been educated in an environment that remained defined by imperial dynamics. The role of the wider cultural influences to which they were subjected however varied much more from one individual to the next. By studying medicine, trainee doctors came into contact with a culture that remained, to a great extent, British. In some cases, this reinforced prior personal experiences, but not always. All of the doctors who took part in this research came from middle-class backgrounds, with parents who were doctors, teachers, artists, administrators, professionals, business people, politicians/political activists and/

or landowners. This should not necessarily be taken as synonymous with affluence in the context of the Indian subcontinent just after independence, but some of the South Asian doctors who became GPs in the NHS were part of a section of society that was strongly shaped by the British presence be it through education, employment or opposition to British rule.

## The continuation of 'medical dependency'

Even if GPs who migrated in the 1960s and 1970s (as did the majority of those who took part in my research) came from newly independent countries, they were trained in a context that was not fundamentally remodelled by independence. Medicine remained shaped by decades of imperial rule and those who had prospered under British rule and often studied and worked in the metropole were in positions of influence. The lingering effect of the movement of South Asian doctors prior to the establishment of the NHS is in evidence in doctors' memories of their training. Independence was not described as marking a rupture from imperial days:

> The medical education curriculum was actually based on University of Dundee at the time … When I got in it was only … 9 years after independence of India so the British influence on the education was still very, very marked. *Why Dundee in particular?* Well, I … understand that couple of our professors, the Professor of Surgery and Professor of … Medicine actually came from that University and I … have absolutely no doubt that they had some sort of influence on what was taught to students.[26]
>
> Most of the education is just like English education in medical schools here … Most of the teachers who were teaching us they were all English-trained professors … The curriculum was … exactly the same like Oxford and Cambridge level. They used to call Andhra Pradesh … where I came from is … like Cambridge and Madras is like Oxford, both they used to adopt the same system of teaching.[27]
>
> It's a very strange experience if you study medicine in India … My mother tongue is Bengali, teachers were mostly Bengali, the textbooks are all written in English by … well-known teachers like Price's textbook of

medicine, Bailey and Love's surgery and all that and these teachers, they all had their postgraduate diplomas from either Edinburgh or London so naturally ... they took that kind of teaching with them when they ... went back to Calcutta and so yes ... the influence was quite a bit ... from their experience in the UK ... when I came here and ... studied a bit in Edinburgh, I found it was very much like what we had in Calcutta.[28]

What is striking in these narratives is the sense of the dominant nature of British medical culture, described as embedded in the minds of lecturers, in textbooks, in the curriculum and in professional identities. L. R. M. Kamal links the education dispensed in his former school in Dhaka to the curriculum in Dundee. Raman N. Rao recalls that Andhra Medical College identified with Cambridge whilst Madras looked to Oxford. In the view of those trained in them, post-independence South Asian medical schools continued to model themselves on the former imperial power and produce doctors steeped in the culture of British medicine.

This does not necessarily mean that there were not by then significant differences between medicine in Britain and South Asia and between different medical schools in India, Pakistan, Bangladesh and Sri Lanka. When it comes to understanding the forces that shaped doctors' professional trajectories, what is important is that they perceived themselves to be part of an inter-connected system. Raj Chandran's choice of words regarding the British royal colleges—bodies responsible for defining standards in specific fields of medicine—when describing his options as a young doctor in Ceylon (present-day Sri Lanka), wanting to become a consultant, is similarly indicative of the perpetuation of an imperial mindset where medicine persisted in looking to London:

> There was a shortage of obstetricians in Sri Lanka and I was told that if you became obstetrician you could become a consultant soon ... Now Sri Lanka at that time ... now we are talking about ... 1960s ... was still under the rule of the ... royal colleges in England. So whatever you wanted to do ... whether you wanted to be a physician, surgeon, obstetrician, or whatever, you had to pass the royal college examinations of London.[29]

The UK educational system thus appears in doctors' recollections as the ultimate reference point for medicine on the Indian subcontinent, rather than being, say, a useful resource for access to information on modern medicine that could be drawn upon as and when necessary. The South Asian doctors who shaped general practice in Britain are therefore not just those who settled and worked as GPs, but also those who had migrated earlier, returned and helped to build South Asian medical systems. These doctors, who are mentioned in the accounts of South Asian GPs, contributed to the survival of a shared British–South Asian medical space after the formal empire came to an end.

In the immediate post-independence context in which the doctors who came to Britain in the 1960s and 1970s were trained, they recalled being left in no doubt that British qualifications continued to be seen as the standard to aspire to:

> All [the teachers] were Indians … But they had studied FRCS, MRCP. They were all been abroad to England and came back as lecturers, readers and professors. They all talked about, during their teaching, a little hint about 'When I was in England' every now and then, everyone said they wanted to show off as well … 'I was in England, I did this … '. And this, subconsciously hits you, that once you qualify you will like to go as well. You know … they never said you should go … but subconsciously … they used to … you can say … brag that they have been to England, done their fellowship, FRCS was a big thing, Fellow of the Royal College of Surgeons and MRCP, Member of the Royal College of Physicians, is a big thing at that time.[30]

Professional legitimacy in doctors' accounts therefore appeared as closely connected to the former colonial power and the qualifications that it dispensed. When they discuss the choices they were faced with as medical students and the environment in which they found themselves doctors portray migration for the purpose of study as a logical step for an ambitious physician to take rather than an option to be considered amongst others:

> I thought at that time that you had to get a postgraduate diploma or a degree from England to be anybody in Indian subcontinent.[31]
> You have to come to Britain to get … further education degrees so that you can enhance your position in Bangladesh.[32]

Migration is thus at times described not as a choice but, up to a point, as a professional necessity: young doctors 'had to' obtain a qualification in Britain if they wanted to be successful. Ruban Prasad's description of his thought processes as a young doctor at the beginning of his career highlights the lack of difference in his mind between the pre-war imperial context that the surgeon he was working with experienced and his own decision to move. When asked about the migration of doctors under the Raj, he spontaneously compared their decisions to his own:

> The professor with whom ... I used to work was extremely eminent surgeon, not only in that state but whole of North East India and he had done his fellowship ... of Royal College of Surgeons from this country, I think it was 1936–37. *Was it quite common for people to have studied overseas at the time?* ... It was almost like a compulsion to tell you very frankly and that was the reason which attracted me to come here. It was like that if you want to succeed in your life ... if you are doing surgery you should have fellowship of the Royal College of Surgeons ... or if you want to do medicine, you perhaps go for Royal College of Physicians, or ... similar thing like Royal College of Obstetricians and Gynaecologists or ... anything like that.[33]

This tendency to think of a trip to Britain as a compulsory part of a medical education is vital to understanding why the South Asian doctors who subsequently became GPs left their countries of origin. Whilst participants were recalling events that occurred decades prior to the interviews, similar answers were given by migrant doctors interviewed for a study published in 1980. David Smith reported that 91 per cent of doctors from the Indian subcontinent he surveyed had moved to Britain chiefly to further their medical training.[34] On the surface this might appear to be a purely professional response but it is difficult to separate such perspectives from the cultural legacy of the British Empire. Naturally, when responding to a survey or answering questions in an oral history interview, people may or may not be revealing their true motivations for moving to Britain. A study of Asian doctors conducted in Sandwell, in the English Midlands, in the 1970s for instance listed being able to meet western women and the possibility of drinking alcohol amongst the attractions of life in Britain.[35] It is not particularly surprising that these factors were not mentioned in oral history interviews conducted with older people. If they had, they would in any case have served to further support the argument being made: they are additional examples of how former colonial subjects could be mesmerised by the metropolitan culture.

The perpetuation of the notion that British postgraduate training was the ideal way in which to crown a medical education undoubtedly contributed to creating the impression that it was in a way, in Ruban Prasad's words, practically compulsory to migrate; a sense that this was the logical course of action to take for a young doctor wanting to succeed professionally. The decisions of South Asian medical students who travelled to Britain in order to undertake postgraduate training, both before and after independence, should be understood in the context of these attitudes. British medicine continued to be seen as a beacon of progress, as part of the 'shining garden' described by the nineteenth-century poet Mirza Asadullah Khan Ghalib:

> Look at the Sahibs of England
> Look at the style and practice of these,
> See what Laws and Rules they have made for all to see
> What none ever saw, they have produced
> Science and skills grew at the hands of these skilled ones ...
> ... Go to London, for in that shining garden
> The city is bright in the night, without candles ... .[36]

## Migration as a 'natural' process: the merging of South Asian and British contexts

Interviews with doctors show that the cultural legacy of empire in the context of South Asian medicine went beyond purely seeing Britain as a 'shining garden'. When doctors discussed their medical education, they did not simply present it as a model to be emulated. Entering medical school in South Asia could also act as a bridge towards British culture. Those teaching in medical schools contributed to the creation of a post-imperial space by talking about life in Britain and presenting their experience of living there and familiarity with British ways of being as something to aspire to. One doctor, for instance, recalled being influenced by a senior colleague who had worked in England:

> My last boss ... under whom I did my MD ... has stayed long in England and he was talking about England and talking about how the people behave, and how's the people, good people ... and I learned lot from him about background of England ... so he was one of the greatest architect of my future in England.[37]

The use of the term 'architect' is intriguing, being suggestive once more of wider social forces that contributed to doctors' decisions to migrate. It was perhaps to be expected that perceptions of Britain might feature prominently when doctors who eventually settled there remembered their youth. What was less predictable was that Britain would appear as a familiar presence in South Asian medical schools:

> They [the teachers at medical school] also mentioned many things about England when they were here, so they were fellows of royal colleges or they were members of various royal colleges and at that time foreign education was very important and they all had qualifications from abroad. *What more can you tell me about what they were saying about Britain at the time?* ... They used to talk about anchovy sauce and we didn't know what anchovies were and we didn't know what the sauce was ... but they used to enjoy telling us and they used to tell us that they enjoyed every minute in England when they did post graduation.[38]

These discourses imply a process of acculturation: in-depth understanding of British medicine and culture was the preserve of an elite that presented it as an ideal to aspire to. The mention of anchovy sauce served as a means of reinforcing the status of medical school lecturers. It may be coincidental that 'gentleman's relish' is a spread made with anchovies but the message that these doctors were able to move amongst the British middle classes was unambiguous. Prem Latha Pathak's description of how her medical college was perceived and how a professor advised her to relate to patients is also redolent of a post-imperial environment:

> Lady Hardinge college ... it was only for women ... and it was one of the very, very posh colleges. If ever you mention, both here, because there were the examiners and in olden days, in the Raj times, [they] used to go from here [Britain]. So everybody knew. Even in this country, in England they knew Lady Hardinge. If you said 'Oh I'm a Hardonian' ... people just ... thought ... highly of you ... When I was in the third year I saw this lady with cancer ... The patient was crying plus the family was crying ... they were saying it was advanced ... As a third year student ... As soon as I saw people crying I rushed in to the professor and said you know ... the family is crying so much ... please, please can you do anything ... so he said to me 'Look here Miss Gupta ... you are not doing allopathy or homeopathy ... or sympathy, we have to do ... the medicine'.[39]

South Asian medical culture appears in these accounts as continuing to be defined by the encounter with the British Empire, not just in terms of its content but also the type of understanding of medicine that it presented to students. It is depicted as shaped by western notions of the rational, scientifically-minded doctor rather than being defined by new post-imperial values sensitive to the needs of Indian patients and open to learning from other traditions of healing or even managing death. It is possible that even in a women-only college, there was a gendered dimension to this exchange, with a senior male doctor taking an opportunity to express his disdain of an emotional response to patient suffering and put forward a patriarchal 'rational' approach. The professor's distance from the realities of patient suffering might not be untypical of medics of his generation; it does speak, though, of an absence of a revolution in medical care in newly independent India.

The way that South Asian GPs who worked in the NHS describe the experience of becoming a doctor in South Asia suggests that they were left in no doubt as to the value of an education obtained in the metropole. It also led them to develop a certain sense of how a doctor should speak and indeed appear. One participant, Shiv Pande, remembers being told that a surgeon should have a 'lion's heart', a 'lady's touch' and 'an eagle's eyes'.[40] Satya Chatterjee offered a variation on this theme in his memoirs. On starting life as a medical student he recalled being advised to acquire 'the heart of a lion, the hands of a woman and the patience of Jove'.[41] The question of whether these expressions are accurately remembered fifty years on or not is ultimately of secondary importance. They indicate a merging of British and Indian contexts in the minds of those who studied in the subcontinent at the time. This description is so typical of the British approach to surgery that virtually the same words are spoken by the archetype of the 'old school' consultant, Sir Lancelot Spratt in the 1950s film *Doctor in the House*. According to the fictional character a successful surgeon required 'The eye of a hawk, the heart of a lion and the hands of a lady'.[42] Lions are naturally also symbolically associated with England. The reference to Jove, i.e. the Roman god Jupiter, further connects this phrase to notions of a traditional gentleman's education, shaped by familiarity with antiquity.

The boundaries between South Asia and Britain remained blurred post-independence. There is nothing in Raman N. Rao's graduation photograph that unambiguously identifies him as a newly qualified doctor from an Indian medical college. It simply shows him in the traditional attire of a British student receiving their degree (see Figure 2). Similarly, Hira Lal Kapur's certificate of registration with the Rajasthan Medical Council from 1968 looks remarkably similar in appearance to his certificate of registration from the GMC in 1970.[43] There appears to have been little political will to create a distinctive medical identity that represented a radical departure from the past. Another interviewee provided a striking example of this blurring of boundaries between Indian

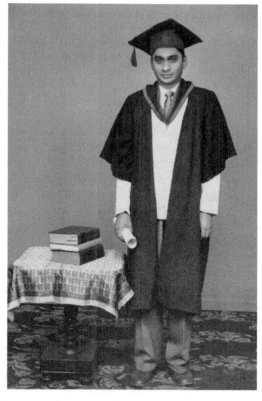

**Figure 2**  Raman N. Rao on his graduation from Andhra Medical College.

and English contexts and of how students might aspire to be a certain 'kind of person' as a result:

> [In] those days the Medical School in Amritsar was one of the best in the country and all the teachers who were initially in Lahore, the Hindus and the Sikhs, they came to Amritsar. So we had the advantage of very experienced professors … who not only taught medicine but also how to speak good, clear English and how to dress properly as a doctor, lots of things … *Can you tell me more about your teachers at medical school and the sort of things they would teach you and talk to you about?* … For example, Professor of surgery, Dr Anand … he must be about 6'3" tall, a Sikh … wearing a turban, and we used to have … surgery class, general surgery—about seven o'clock in the morning. And in winter Amritsar can be very, very cold. As much as it is here in England—and slightly foggy. And Dr Anand used to come in the theatre, anatomy lecture theatre, to tell us about surgery. And always sort of pin-striped suit and the collar—starched white collar … we were quite impressed by … the way he dressed and the way he spoke. His English was impeccable … He was also Hunterian professor at the Royal College of Surgeons in London. So that was the kind of person who taught us surgery.[44]

The medical education that South Asian GPs received was therefore one that exposed them to British methods, British textbooks and British-trained doctors who maintained close links with the former metropole. It encouraged them to perceive British medicine and even ways of speaking and dressing as models. Given this context, it is unsurprising that movement between the Indian sub-continent and Britain continued to be seen as unremarkable, and as something to be encouraged, as illustrated by Syed Ahmad Ali Gilani's description of a UK GMC visit to Nishtar Medical College in Multan, in present-day Pakistan. The reference to a senior British doctor inviting a young Pakistani colleague to come and see him in England 'when you come down', implies that the post-imperial trajectory from Pakistan to England was still seen as being part of the natural order of things:

> I remember the General Medical Council's delegation came to look at the college in order to recognise it for the purpose of registration in this country … that was in '58 and the people who came … that included Professor Ian Aird … and Professor Charles Wells … and the registrar of the General Medical Council … Professor Charles Wells happened to

say 'Gosh, look at your medical college, all this beautiful stonework ... '
He said 'Have you been to England?' I said 'No, sir'. He said 'Oh well, if
you go to Oxford or Cambridge, probably you will think these hospitals
are like cottage hospitals ... as compared with this medical college but I
tell you the work which is done there is very, very good ... So he encouraged me, in a way, that I should go to England for further education ...
Professor Ian Aird ... his textbook was called bible for surgeons ...
he was very kind ... In fact he gave me his card ... saying 'When you
come down, come and see me'.[45]

Those who had studied in Britain naturally had a vested interest in
emphasising the value of the trajectory they followed. In some cases
at least their familiarity with British culture would appear to have been
used as a mechanism to assert superiority and cultivate a mystique.
This would help to explain the apparently obscure reference to anchovy
sauce in the context of a South Asian medical education and Dr Anand's
cultivation of the image of a British gentleman. Whether these discourses and behaviours as described by interviewees were anchored in
a genuine belief in the value of being educated in the British system, or
were a means of justifying personal choices and maintaining prestige is
naturally debatable. S. A. A. Gilani who trained in the 1950s in Pakistan
thus provided an alternative view of the experience of the previous generation of South Asian doctors in Britain:

They always admired it you see, I didn't come across anybody who
would say 'Oh, I have had a bad experience'. Except for one, I remember,
he was a consultant in Ear, Nose [and] Throat ... and he said 'Dr, you
know, when you go there, you can become very depressed. You know,
I took exam in ENT and I failed. And I had no support and I was so
depressed that I went to the Westminster Bridge and jumped into the
Thames to drown myself (laughs). And a police officer ... jumped into it
and he saved me. You see I could have been dead you know ... You have
got to be prepared for bouts of depression ... there is not enough support ...' So that was the only time ... I thought 'Well ...' ... But on the
whole ... the other specialists who have been here, they always praised
it, whether they praised it because they wanted to be recognised, that
they have done something very good ... so they wanted to further their
careers or whether they actually had ... that kind of exposure ...[46]

Whatever the motivations of those described as vaunting the merits of
the British way of medicine and life, their contribution to the survival of

this particular socio-cognitive space is an important dimension of this history. The existence of these attitudes helps to explain why doctors, when they talked about going to Britain, described their movement as part of a logical progression. The moment of migration does not appear as a rupture or as coming at the end of a lengthy period of reflection. Doctors were moving in a post-imperial context where intellectual and cultural values continued to be shared:

> I studied in Dhaka medical college … I qualified in 1961 … It was just standard procedure … and going through the year, class and so on … *At what point in time did you decide to move to the UK?* … Soon after gradu-ation, again influenced by my father, he wanted me to have postgraduate education so that I can be a proper surgeon. *So where did you go in the UK?* My first job in UK was in Scotland, it's a hospital called Greenock Royal Infirmary … From Greenock, I went to Inverness Raigmore Hospital … [47]
>
> During the … years in the medical school, I … decided, I think in the third year that I shall go to England soon after I qualify, for further studies, and this is what I did.[48]
>
> … After graduation, naturally my first aim was to come here and do my post-graduation. *Why do you say 'naturally'?* … It … felt natural in a sense that once you had done your graduation there and I think it was more of a … not peer pressure but peer response as well or peer relation-ship … most of my friends and my colleagues and my classmates you know, we all graduated together and some started coming here and we had an access available in those days and so I thought 'Well, why not?', I should go and do my postgraduation and then decide what I want to do.[49]

The nature of the social and cultural environment that South Asian medicine provided and the ongoing influence of imperial links help to explain that, for a number of young medical graduates, travelling to Britain appeared to be a 'natural' step to take.

### A broader post-imperial legacy and the emergence of a global diaspora

If this was quite clearly the case when it comes to medical culture, the role of the wider cultural influences to which doctors were exposed was harder to gauge. Some participants talked of having little family history of contact with the British or sense of connection to Britain, for others this was an important part of their upbringing which should not be ignored in the context of their decisions to migrate. This could be the product of a certain reticence on the part of participants in the research: some might have felt comfortable discussing the British influences on their medical education but been more reluctant to outline a broader family connection to the former colonial power. It might be a reflection of the fact that the British cultural legacy was more entrenched in medicine than in other domains. It is also the case that the interviews I conducted mainly focused on doctors' lives in medicine.

Nonetheless, the physicians who took part in this research came from middle-class backgrounds. South Asian doctors who became GPs in the NHS were part of a section of society that was shaped by the British presence be it through education, employment or politics. Whilst broader cultural influences were less in evidence in interviews, they undoubtedly played a part in creating and maintaining a connection between Britain and the Indian subcontinent.

For instance, a number of doctors talked of having parents who had served in the British army or who were officials in the colonial administration. Britain could therefore also be a cultural reference point outside of the context of medical education. M. N. I. Talukdar, for example, expressed his pride in the actions of his father, also a doctor, who was involved in British military operations in World War II:

He served at … Burmese front, he was decorated by … his majesty … King George VI, and it was mentioned in the despatch … He was … a field medical officer … *You said you were particularly proud of his work, can you tell me why?* Well basically his achievement which has been recognised by British government … and all my inspiration in the early childhood days came from his activity.[50]

There is a clear link here between medicine in the British Empire, the wider context of the relationship between Britain and India and the 'inspiration' it provided to a South Asian doctor who ended up working as a GP in northern England. Doctors' memories of their upbringing brought forward evidence of well-established links with the rulers of British India and at times revealed that family members had deep-seated affinities with British culture:

> My father ... is the son of a big business magnate. He [the interviewee's grandfather] used to have a lot of ... wholesale business, supplying ... cooking oil ... pulses, other things for the household ... that he used to supply wholesale for all the district ... My father is the son of that ... big business magnate ... He became a magistrate and a social worker, things like that ... *What sort of relationship did your father and your grandfather have with the Raj?* My grandfather ... always like British Raj. Because ... most business people, they like British Raj ... They wanted that type of ... rule to continue in India ... The next generation they sort of slowly changing that view ... saying we must have independence and we can develop more ... My father is in between ... He used to like British Raj: because of British Raj he ... has seen how the railway system is developed, how ... all the provinces fighting with each other all joined together.[51]

Raman N. Rao's account comes across as slightly conflicted—he is keen to highlight the fact that there were changing views about the role of the British Empire amongst the 'next generation'. He clearly conveys, though, that for a middle-class Indian businessman, it may have made sense to want British rule to continue. After all, business circles are known to value stability and certainty.

It would therefore be historically inaccurate to minimise the strength of attachment to the British Empire amongst the middle-class families that produced the vast majority of doctors who worked in the NHS. Rupendra Kumar Majumdar both hesitated and laughed when asked about his father's attitude towards the Raj—laughter apparently act-ing as a means to enable discussion of a subject that was difficult to broach:[52]

> My father was a lawyer, he was a government advocate and public pros-ecutor ... He was a good lawyer and very well known in the district ... My father is very pro to British Raj and British Empire ... *Can you tell me a bit more about that, what do you remember him saying?* Hmm ... (gentle laughter) He always liked British Raj ... he was fascinated with the governor of the Bihar which he used to visit and others ... who used to visit, he never finds any faults of the hierarchy of the British people ... If he goes to anybody's house, he likes to look into the cutlery, where it is made ... if he finds ... .made ... in Sheffield, he enjoyed it [adopts

hugely enthusiastic tone of voice] 'Oh what a lovely ... ' It can't be anything bad. If he finds it's Taiwan manufactured ... (adopts tone indicat-
ing deep disappointment) 'Oh, it's not ... ' ... He used to visit various
places ... in the car ... Morris is very good, Oxford Morris is good, Rolls
Royce is beyond ... (laughs) ... He was a lawyer in the native Rajs and
the kings and zamindars[53] ... they used to have a Rolls Royce and he
used to enjoy with them and take part in their car riding.[54]

At least some of the medical graduates who helped to build the NHS
were therefore the children of people who apparently perceived themselves to be well integrated into the structures of British rule and actively
identified with Britain. To the point of being concerned about the provenance of cutlery. S. A. A. Gilani's memories of his parents' views of
England also offer an insight into how Indians could at times internalise
the values of their colonial rulers, although his father's enthusiasm for
all things British is in marked contrast with his mother's sarcasm:

I remember I used to, as a child, sometimes go to his post office and a
lot of British residents used to come to ... the office for sending money
orders to their families and telegrams and so on ... In a way he was very
anglicized in spite of the fact that he had never been to England. But
since ... England has gone to him, through the British servicemen...
so he ... admired them and appreciated them and in fact it was him
who wanted me to not only learn the local languages which included
Urdu, Persian and Arabic but also English ... He was very happy when
I came here and he was ... very, very satisfied with my progress in this
country and in fact, when I went back on holidays, he encouraged me
to ... go back and ... acquire more knowledge and more skills, that
was his objective ... He had very close friendship with British families,
sometimes it made my mother I think a bit jealous (laughs) ... When
I married an English girl and took her there, I remember ... because my
mother didn't want me to come and live here, she missed me ... and my
father was saying 'Oh it's all right ... you go wherever you are happy' ...
and my mother happened to say 'Oh yes, you always had soft spot for
the English girls' (laughs).[55]

Laughter here possibly serves once more the purpose of defusing tension, of enabling the discussion of attitudes that in a contemporary
context may seem alien.[56] Participants might have found it difficult to
acknowledge that close family members approved of the British presence, worked alongside the representatives of the colonial power and

at times even socialised with them. It is especially relevant to pay attention to these views in a South Asian cultural context as parents, and in
particular fathers were generally described by doctors as having played
an important role in defining their children's career paths. It is telling
that S. A. A. Gilani's account notes that his father was 'very pleased'
with his progress overseas. A successful career in Britain could offer a
means of obtaining the approval of at least one parent whose thinking
had been shaped by contact with the British. Of course his mother's sar-
castic remark also serves as a reminder that others held different views.
Contact with the British who were responsible for running India could
however lead to an identification with British values and a tendency to
perceive anyone or anything associated with them as superior.

In fact, even being actively opposed to British rule did not signify
that parents were not also transmitting positive messages about the
British presence. Urmila Rao reported that her mother, a prominent
follower of Gandhi who was imprisoned for her activism, had no ani-
mosity towards the British and thought that their influence on education in India had been positive.[57] Of course, the possibility that criticism
of Britain was muted as doctors were being interviewed by a white
British researcher cannot be discounted. The laughter that accompanied accounts of parents being pro-British suggests otherwise. The point
made here, in any case, is not that such views were universal but that at
least some doctors' parents held them and that they had a major influence on their children's choices. Ralph Lawrence, a South-African born
South Asian doctor who became a GP in Derbyshire for instance tellingly described his father as an 'old Victorian' who believed that children should be seen and not heard.[58]

The social and cultural influence that is in evidence in GPs' accounts
is therefore not limited to medicine. In a more general sense it is apparent that moving to Britain did not necessarily at the time represent a
move to a fundamentally different post-independence space. One participant recalled receiving a letter from Buckingham Palace and saw this
as a formative moment:

> *At what point did you decide to come to the UK?* ... I was in second or
> third year in medical school ... I had no interest in going to America
> ... I always wanted to ... I used to listen to BBC and also I ... remem-
> ber ... the Queen's inauguration as the Queen ... I listened to all the

commentary which was being made from England and I wrote a letter to the High Commissioner or somebody—I can't remember, I may have written to Her Majesty the Queen of England in London that kind of thing! And after a few months I had a letter from somebody saying I have … been instructed by Her Majesty the Queen to say thank you for your letter … so I had … a lot of interest … in England rather than anywhere else in the world.[59]

Urmila Rao described one of the drivers of her decision to go to Britain as being the influence of the literature of her childhood:

I have always wanted to come to England because I've read many novels … like Thomas Hardy … Brontë sisters novels … So that made me want to come to England more than America like most of my friends … *What sort of image did you have of England through those novels?* … All like cottages, idyllic villages and good living.[60]

Urmila Rao's recollection of her reasons for wanting to come to Britain echo P. R. L. Mohan's finding that doctors' wives were attracted by the British scenery they had seen in films. It also brings to mind the Bengali poet Rabindranath Tagore's account of his (unrealistic) expectations of what he would find on visiting the metropole for the first time:

I had thought that the Island of England was so small and the inhabitants so dedicated to learning that before I arrived here, I expected that the country from one end to the other would echo and re-echo with the lyrical songs of Tennyson; and I had also thought that wherever I might be in this narrow island, I would hear constantly Gladstone's oratory, the explanations of the Vedas by Max Müller, the scientific truth of Tyndall, the profound thoughts of Carlyle and the philosophy of Bain. I was under the impression that wherever I would go I would find the old and young drunk with the pleasure of 'intellectual' enjoyment. But I have been very disappointed in this.[61]

This sense of common destiny and attachment to Britain clearly survived independence with personal and professional identities and reference points appearing in a number of interviews as unconfined by national borders. It undoubtedly contributed to the movement of doctors. Hira Lal Kapur's trajectory, from schoolboy in Kenya to being allocated a place to study medicine in India as a British citizen, qualifying in 1967, being registered as a doctor in Jaipur in 1968, provisionally registered with the GMC in 1968, given permanent registration in 1970 and a job as a GP in north-west England in 1971 is one that is hard to imagine outside of an immediately post-imperial context.[62] The social forces that brought a member of the South Asian Diaspora to India as a British student and subsequently resulted in his move to Britain and entry into general practice are also at play in the way that some doctors talk about their feelings towards Britain when they first started to work in the NHS:

> Yeah, we always felt British ... In Kenya, we always had a British passport ... Whatever ... food was sold here or anything we had it there. So ... for me it was no different. Cadbury's chocolates were Cadbury's chocolates. The chewing gum was the same, you know, so we were used to so many things. Except the weather (laughter), which was very depressing! (laughter)[63]
>
> I think I was absolutely British ... right from the beginning ... I always had this vision you know that there's only one world and I, as a citizen of this world, should be able to go anywhere, anytime and be part of that.[64]

Of course, ironically, commenting on (and complaining about) the weather is another signal of Britishness and thus in this context further serves to emphasise a connection to British culture rather than introduce an element of distance. As for the notion of being a citizen of the world it can be connected to the persistence of imperial identities and the idea that British subjects could travel freely and count on the protection of their government—a notion somewhat grandiosely encapsulated in the phrase 'civis Britannicus sum' ('I am a British citizen') which evoked the Latin 'civis Romanus sum'.[65] It is important however to emphasise that such views were only held by some doctors, with others rejecting any notion of feeling British when they first arrived. A number of other participants did however describe a more nuanced sense of not feeling like an outsider:

> No, I didn't feel British ... I didn't feel anything, I just felt myself ... I didn't put myself whether I was British or Indian or UK or whatsoever ... I was just me.[66]
>
> British? No ... When you say that what exactly you meant? ... *I mean did you feel that you were part of Britain, that you fitted in, did you feel a sense of belonging in Britain when you first arrived, did you feel like an outsider?* No, I didn't feel like an outsider but I didn't become or wanted to become like British.[67]

*Did you feel British when you came to the UK in any way?* (pause) That
is a difficult question. I mean (pause) I ... I didn't feel non-British I
would say in that sense you know ... I had no difficulty integrating with
people and all that but I was an Indian at heart, no doubt.[68]

That an Indian doctor can find it difficult to answer the question of
whether he felt British on arrival in Britain shows how ingrained the
cultural legacy of empire remained during the decades that followed
independence.

Britain thus remained a reference point in medical and to a degree in
wider cultural terms. Raj Chandran's interview offers an example of how
the two could interact with each other. His family's destiny had been closely
tied to the fortunes of the British Empire: his father was a senior administrator working for the British in Malaysia and was awarded an MBE.
Chandran's description of his journey to take up his first medical post
brings to mind Shompa Lahiri's observation that trips to Europe for an
Indian under the Raj fulfilled the function that a Grand Tour of Europe did
for a European: they served to complete a 'gentleman's education'.[69] Once
more, a female figure is described as sceptical towards desires to travel to
the former colonial metropole and settle, hinting that such processes of
acculturation were not universal. In effect, this gives additional weight to
this account. It is not one of uncritical nostalgia:

I left Sri Lanka, I told my mother who was very disappointed because
I was the last of the ... family line ... She knew I will never come
back ... I left Sri Lanka ... on the 20th of December ... it took me
three weeks ... to come to England by plane. That was an experience
because ... I always wanted to see the three ancient civilisations ...
Egyptian civilization, Greek civilization and the Roman civilization ...
I flew to Egypt, stayed there for a week and a half ... and from there
I flew to Greece, to Athens, and spent the week there, going through all
the museums and the ... buildings, and the Parthenon and all that ...
and from there I came to Rome and spent another week in Rome.[70]

This story is one of someone socialised as a middle-class professional,
with an international outlook, shaped by exposure to notions of the
conventional British gentleman's education with its focus on ancient
Greece and Rome.

Through interviews with doctors who formed part of the first generation of migrant South Asian GPs to work in the NHS, this study has

captured something of how empire contributed to the formation of the contemporary middle-class South Asian diaspora. This is not to say that the Indian middle class, which future doctors were born into, was necessarily overwhelmingly dominated by British culture, to the extent that South Asian identities and values became irrelevant. Rather, being born into this middle class under the British Empire and growing up in the immediate aftermath of its demise exposed doctors to different views of the world and could lead to them acquiring a different set of values. Or more accurately perhaps, to reconcile different identities. This was a process that for some doctors began from childhood. Dipak Ray's spontaneous reaction as an older man at being asked to recall his school days 'School? Oh my dear boy! (laughter)' hints at the influence of British (middle-class) culture on his upbringing.[71] He went on to relate that his first experience of education was in a convent: 'I was brought up ... by Irish nun ... "the ship is full of sheep" and all that business ...' after which he was in an English medium school which caused difficulties for him when he later had to continue his education in Bengali.[72] Fiji Biramji Kotwall also started school in a convent before becoming a boarder at the exclusive Bishop Cotton School in the Himalayan city of Simla.[73] His description of the establishment produced another telling merger of British and Indian contexts: 'Simla was the place where most of the viceroys went ... because it is ... cool ... It's at a height of 7,000 feet above sea level ... It's just got the same climate as England.'[74] Rooin Boomla recalled not just going to an English-language school in Bombay but also that 'We were forbidden to speak in our native tongue.'[75]

This is not to say that the encounter with (post-) imperial culture was never problematic. Satya Chatterjee, a specialist chest physician in the North West of England who worked briefly as a GP as a young doctor and later became a leading figure in the ODA, described in his memoirs a trip to Calcutta with his brother and a cousin to buy medical books for his course after he was admitted to medical college.[76] His cousin suggested going for a meal before catching the train back and he decided to have a chicken curry. On his return home, in his words 'all hell broke loose. A Brahmin boy eating chicken and that too in a restaurant—in all probability owned by a Muslim ... It was a taboo of the highest order.'[77] Chatterjee's brother had informed the household of this breach of Hindu vegetarian practice—deemed particularly unacceptable from a member of the highest caste from which priests are drawn.[78] Chatterjee recalls being ordered by his grandfather to go to the river Ganges and rinse his mouth with its holy water 108 times.[79] It is intriguing that his first steps towards medical culture were accompanied by tensions between what he deemed acceptable as an aspiring young doctor and his family's religious values.

As did Raj Chandran's 'disappointed' mother, Chatterjee's strictly observant Hindu grandfather appears here as a representative of an alternative set of South Asian values—founded on family, caste and religion—that doctors drifted away from to embrace a more cosmopolitan sense of being a professional able to move between different worlds. Kumbakonam Srinivasachar Bhanumathi, whose father was a priest, described similar tensions in her family. Her parents died when she was a child and she recalls that her family disagreed about whether or not it was appropriate for her to study medicine in Bangalore:

> I wasn't a very keen person to go into medicine initially, and my eldest sister who had responsibility of bringing us up when my mother died wasn't too keen for me to get into medicine, because those days, her priority was to get me married and … not to have responsibility for me. But … my other sisters are the ones who identified that I really have to be studying, I must be getting somewhere. So then there was a bit of a rift within the family, I was having difficulty in keeping up with the studying for medicine. And at that time I had somebody who was one of my sister's colleagues … in the [independence] movement. And this gentleman was also from our background but he adopted me informally. And he actually more or less took over my care, and he told my sister that she is bright and I am not going to let her suffer just because you want to get her married and settled down and I would like her to complete her medicine.[80]

There could, therefore, be struggles within families but there was also seemingly sufficient social flexibility to allow individuals to move towards developing different identities, to subtly shift towards being members of an international middle class by moving into medicine. At times, they were nudged in this direction by relatives or acquaintances— Chatterjee's cousin who led him to the restaurant 'in all probability owned by a Muslim' or Bhanumathi's sisters who argued that she should continue studying medicine rather than treating marriage as a 'priority'. The legacy of empire contributed to creating the space within which these discussions could happen: the fact that medicine had been open to a significant section of the indigenous population under British rule established a pathway to membership of an international medical culture. This was perhaps facilitated in the case of medical culture because of its status. Even if there could be a tension between traditional South Asian culture and the choice of studying medicine, respect for the views of elders was also, at times, what led doctors to study medicine. A significant number of participants reported becoming doctors because their fathers had decided that that was what they should do. As young people, doctors therefore appear as negotiating a pathway between different values, becoming citizens of what Margret Frenz has described as a 'globalizing' world with a resulting spectrum of social and cultural loyalties.[81]

In this context, however, being middle class from a global cultural perspective does not signify being wealthy in the context of South Asia at the time. K. S. Bhanumathi described herself and most of her contemporaries as coming from a 'poor background' when she discussed her professional options as a doctor and her thoughts about migrating.[82] Financial considerations did not appear as a key driver of decisions to move away from the Indian subcontinent in most doctors' accounts, although this is not particularly surprising. However, it seems unlikely that K. S. Bhanumathi who spoke openly of being attracted by the possibility of earning a better living overseas was unique in having such thoughts. Those doctors who did attempt to build careers in the Indian subcontinent rather than migrate shortly after graduating talk more broadly of their disappointment in the opportunities that were available in their own countries. Sri Venugopal, for instance, professed being more interested in helping deprived rural populations than acquiring material wealth but described his frustration at what he perceived as the excessive control the Indian government exercised over doctors.[83] Anup Kumar Sen described Darjeeling as 'a beautiful place' where 'the tea gardens are alluring' and connected his decision to settle in Britain to his disappointment at not being offered a job there.[84] What these interviews reveal is that doctors had professional and class aspirations that were not limited to national contexts. This could be about money, wanting a sense of professional control or to work in an 'alluring' environment. They are not in this sense radically different from their British counterparts who chose to emigrate rather than work in the NHS. In the post-imperial context of this period, with the freedom of movement that it offered, Britain provided an alternative setting where such aspirations could be met.

This was particularly true as not only were doctors exposed to British culture both generally and more specifically in the context of medicine, their accounts of their early lives also reveal the role played by mobility in their formative years. This could naturally take the form of leaving home to study medicine, but other accounts are also suggestive that movement and uncertainty had for many become a way of life. Raj Chandran's father had taken his family to Malaysia to work for the British there. F. B. Kotwall's father worked for the North Western Railway and in his words 'moved ... from place to place ... when you're in the railway you get transferred very often.'[85] Other doctors described international family trajectories that encompassed movement to South Asia, Africa and Britain, with people basing themselves in different parts of the Empire or former Empire depending on their assessment of their interests.[86] Mobility was frequently a feature of doctors' lives from an early age. Not only because they were in the process of joining an international middle-class culture which involved relocating to study, but because, for a number of them, the imperial legacy was one of the physical mobility of their families, be it within the Raj or the wider British Empire. The experience of having to move because of the partition of India, sometimes in the face of inter-community violence, also appeared vividly in the childhood recollections of some of the doctors I spoke to, raising the intriguing question of the extent of the impact of the events of 1947 on the subsequent decisions of doctors to build lives and careers in Britain.[87]

## Conclusion

The fact that UK borders were relatively open and that the NHS offered salaries that were attractive to South Asian professionals may have been a necessary condition for the movement of doctors. This is not sufficient on its own to explain the scale of post-war medical migration. The 'empire of the mind' continued to exert its influence in medicine and in wider South Asian society allowing the movement of doctors which had begun under British rule to be amplified post-independence. The existence of established flows of doctors and of a post-imperial socio-cognitive community encompassing Britain and South Asian countries provides the context necessary to an understanding of the circumstances surrounding the initial arrival in Britain of the South Asian doctors who subsequently made up a significant part of the NHS's GP workforce. Doctors had been socialised in a middle-class environment under British rule and were as a result equipped to move into British medical culture.

The legacies of empire thus facilitated British access to a pool of doctors who went on to become general practitioners in the NHS. They were not, however, as a rule, directly recruited into general practice. Their initial movement to Great Britain was frequently described as primarily motivated by the desire to gain postgraduate qualifications. In the context of medicine, this involves hospital work. This movement took place on a vast scale and unsurprisingly some doctors decided to stay for personal reasons. The subsequent choices that large numbers of South Asian doctors made to move into general practice and the fact that they were overwhelmingly concentrated in specific areas had a significant structural impact on the way in which general practice developed in the NHS.

## Notes

1  M. S. Kausar interview with author, 26 October 2010.
2  Ibid.
3  Anonymous interview with author.
4  S. Venugopal interview with author, 5 November 2009; two other anonymous interviews with author.
5  K. S. Bhanumathi interview with author, 16 April 2011.
6  B. Senewiratne, 'Emigration of doctors: A problem for the developing and the developed countries. Part I', *BMJ* (1975, 1: 5958), pp. 618–20; T. Richards, 'Impressions of medicine in India: A doctor's lot', *BMJ* (1985, 290), pp. 1276–9.
7  'The brain drain and medical education', *The Lancet* (21 October 1967), p. 890.
8  F. Fanon, *Peau noire, masques blancs* (Paris: Editions du Seuil, 1952) (French), p. 14. Author's translation.
9  Mejia, 'Migration of physicians', p. 208.
10 Ibid.
11 Ibid.

12 J. R. Barnett, 'Foreign medical graduates in New Zealand 1973–79: A test of the "exacerbation hypothesis"', *Social Science and Medicine*, 26:10 (1988), p. 1049; C. B. Keely, 'Effects of the immigration act of 1965 on selected population characteristics of immigrants to the United States', *Demography*, 8:2 (1971); Wright & Mullally, '"Not everyone can be a Gandhi"'.

13 Iredale, 'Luring overseas trained doctors to Australia'; Barnett, 'Foreign medical graduates'; Wright & Mullally, '"Not everyone can be a Gandhi"'.

14 Mejia, 'Migration of physicians', p. 214.

15 Ibid.

16 'Soviet medical degrees "recognition sought"', *Hindustan Times* (8 May 1963), p. 3.

17 V. Robinson & M. Carey, 'Peopling skilled international migration: Indian doctors in the UK', *International Migration*, 38:1 (2000).

18 Robinson & Carey, 'Peopling skilled international migration', p. 95.

19 Ibid.

20 Robinson & Carey, 'Peopling skilled international migration', p. 89.

21 Mohan, 'Asian doctors', p. 105.

22 Ibid.

23 Smith, *Overseas Doctors*, p. 2.

24 J. Bornat, L. Henry, P. Raghuram, 'The making of careers, the making of a discipline: Luck and chance in migrant careers in geriatric medicine', *Journal of Vocational Behavior*, 78 (2011), p. 344.

25 A. Porter, 'Empires in the mind', in P. J. Marshall (ed.), *The Cambridge Illustrated History of the British Empire* (Cambridge: Cambridge University Press, 1996).

26 L. R. M. Kamal interview with author, 8 March 2010.

27 R. N. Rao interview with author, 28 May 2010.

28 A. Chaudhuri interview with author, 30 March 2010.

29 R. Chandran interview with author, 7 March 2011.

30 S. K. Ahuja interview with author, 8 December 2009.

31 L. R. M. Kamal interview with author.

32 M. A. Salam interview with author.

33 R. Prasad interview with author, 20 April 2010.

34 Smith, *Overseas Doctors*, p. 37.

35 Mohan, 'Asian doctors', p. 102.

36 'Preface' to Sayyid Ahmad Khan's edition of the A'in-e Akbari, translation Shamsur Rahman Faruqi, included in R. F. McDermott, L. A.

Gordon, A. T. Embree, F. W. Pritchett, D. Dalton (eds), *Sources of Indian Traditions: Modern India, Pakistan and Bangladesh*, third edition (New York: Columbia University Press, 2014), pp. 95–6.

37  Anonymous interview with author.

38  Anonymous interview with author.

39  P. L. Pathak interview with author, 14 May 2010.

40  S. Pande interview with author, 23 November 2009.

41  Chatterjee, *Yesterdays*, p. 15.

42  *Doctor in the House*, Directed by Ralph Thomas, Group Film Productions Limited, 1954.

43  Personal papers of H. L. Kapur.

44  Anonymous interview with author.

45  S. A. A. Gilani interview with author, 30 June 2010.

46  Ibid.

47  M. N. I. Talukdar interview with author, 1 December 2009.

48  Anonymous interview with author.

49  Anonymous interview with author.

50  M. N. I. Talukdar interview with author.

51  R. N. Rao interview with author.

52  J. M. Simpson & S. J. Snow, 'Why we should try to get the joke: Humor, laughter and healthcare history', *The Oral History Review*, 44:1 (2017).

53  Aristocratic landowners.

54  R. K. Majumdar interview with author.

55  S. A. A. Gilani interview with author, 30 June 2010.

56  Simpson & Snow, 'Why we should try to get the joke'.

57  Urmila Rao interview with author, 28 May 2010.

58  BLSA, C900/03116, Millennium Memory Bank, Ralph Lawrence interviewed by Jan Rogers, 1999.

59  Anonymous interview with author.

60  Urmila Rao interview with author.

61  Quoted in Lahiri, *Indians in Britain*, p. 201.

62  Private papers of H. L. Kapur.

63  P. L. Pathak interview with author.

64  L. R. M. Kamal interview with author.

65  The phrase was used in the House of Commons by the Minister of State for Colonial Affairs as late as 1954 (Consterdine, 'Community versus Commonwealth', p. 3).

66  A. Chaudhuri interview with author.

67  A. K. Sen interview with author.
68  Anonymous interview with author.
69  Lahiri, 'Indians in Britain', p. 34.
70  R. Chandran interview with author.
71  D. Ray interview with author, 5 December 2008.
72  Ibid.
73  Now known as Shimla.
74  F. B. Kotwall interview with author, 11 October 2010.
75  R. Boomla interview with author, 5 December 2008.
76  Chatterjee, *Yesterdays*, pp. 24–6.
77  Chatterjee, *Yesterdays*, p. 25.
78  Ibid.
79  Chatterjee, *Yesterdays*, p. 26. The number 108 is considered to be sacred in Hinduism.
80  K. S. Bhanumathi interview with author.
81  M. Frenz, *Community, Memory and Migration in a Globalizing World: The Goan Experience, c. 1890s–1980* (New Delhi: Oxford University Press, 2014). See in particular pp. 1–5 and 300–2.
82  K. S. Bhanumathi interview with author.
83  S. Venugopal interview with author.
84  A. K. Sen interview with author.
85  F. B. Kotwall interview with author.
86  P. L. Pathak interview with author; H. L. Kapur interview with author, 5 January 2010; Lawrence, *Fire in his Hand*.
87  M. S. Kauser interview with author; S. K. Ahuja interview with author; Bhowmick, *You Can't Climb a Ladder*, pp. 1–11.

# 4

# Discrimination and the development of general practice

The presence of migrant South Asian doctors in the British healthcare system can be linked to the existence of a post-imperial recruitment system in post-war Britain and the lingering effects of the empire of the mind in South Asia. Their movement into general practice, however, requires to be understood in a different way. This chapter and Chapter 5 will show how a discriminatory professional environment limited these doctors' options and how their responses to this context contributed to defining British general practice.

If there was an official strategy aimed at providing additional 'pairs of hands' for British hospitals (albeit one that was presented as involving the provision of training opportunities for temporary migrants), government policy did not extend to bringing doctors to Britain to work in general practice. Some UK government officials were clearly aware of the fact that a number of migrant practitioners were putting down roots and becoming GPs and may well have tacitly approved of this but there was no official programme encouraging the settlement of thousands of South Asian GPs. Nor did most South Asian doctors initially set out to enter general practice. None of the forty South Asian GPs interviewed for this project migrated to take up posts in primary care. Only one had any ambition to become a general practitioner (on his planned return to India) and he stressed that as a result, he was wholly unrepresentative of migrant South Asian doctors in general.[1] His contemporaries mostly entered general practice reluctantly. Participants in this research report spending years working in the NHS before eventually deciding to become GPs. This is consistent with the findings of a survey of overseas doctors conducted in the 1970s which concluded that the vast majority of international medical graduates who became general practitioners could be classed as late entrants into the field with a significant minority having spent more than ten years working in hospitals before opting for primary care.[2] Naturally, there were exceptions to this pattern. Some doctors came directly from the Indian subcontinent to work in specific practices as was mentioned in Chapter 2. The overall picture that I will outline here is however of an unplanned entry of medical migrants into general practice. It was unplanned both by central government and the doctors themselves.

Understanding how these doctors ended up working in specific types of roles involves developing an appreciation of the environment that the NHS provided at the time. Decisions to stay in Britain were made in a professional context which was characterised by racism and what Albert Memmi has termed heterophobia.[3] Discrimination played a key role in the development of the NHS. There is ample evidence that much discrimination was linked to ethnicity. The undoubted existence of racism does not however explain all of the historical dynamics involved when it comes to the history of South Asian doctors in general practice in the NHS. Memmi's distinction between the complementary concepts of racism and heterophobia supports an exploration of the NHS as being historically the product of discrimination based on perceived racial differences but also on difference in a wider sense.[4] Memmi argues for the need to separately consider behaviours that can be linked to a narrow definition of racism as related to perceived biological difference, and those that can be ascribed to the more wide-ranging notion of 'heterophobia'—literally the fear of difference.[5] South Asian migrant doctors could find themselves at a disadvantage because of racism but equally as a result of attitudes toward accent, gender, class, alcohol consumption, nationality, religion and other factors.

Racism was a driver of the development of healthcare but so was, more generally, the tendency of many of those working in the NHS to behave in a heterophobic manner. This had an impact on the career trajectories of those who differed from them and contributed to shaping the form that healthcare provision took. Emphasising the role of difference in a broader sense in the development of medicine also facilitates an engagement with the ways in which migrant doctors can at times be seen to be contributing to making the NHS a racist and heterophobic space through their own thoughts and practices. Although general practice is recognised as being one of the fields of medicine that migrant doctors entered because of racism in the NHS,[6] I will show that racism and heterophobia were also in evidence within the professional culture and practices of the specialty. The existence of this additional layer of discrimination helps to explain the geographical clustering of migrant doctors, which will be described in the next chapter.

I will first outline the evidence that racism and discrimination on the grounds of difference more generally has played a formative role in the development of healthcare in Britain, then explore how South Asian doctors were affected by this context. I conclude by arguing that racism and heterophobia are at the heart of the history of British general practice.

## Discrimination and the NHS workforce

The health policy expert Oscar Gish, describing the position of overseas doctors in the NHS in a 1969 briefing paper for the Institute of Race Relations entitled *Britain and the Immigrant Doctor*, noted that 'the contribution of overseas-born medical graduates to the various medical specialties varies inversely with the attractiveness to British graduates of particular specialties.'[7] This phenomenon might be partially explained by the fact that migrant doctors were outsiders. Patronage networks which were of great importance to hospital careers in the early decades of the NHS naturally tended to work to the disadvantage of migrants who lacked the social and cultural capital and personal contacts of those raised and educated locally.[8] Discrimination within the NHS is not simply about ethnicity: clinicians could be treated differently for instance because of their association with a particular hospital.[9] Overseas doctors could also at times be lacking in familiarity with the modus operandi of British medicine and British society and/or be handicapped when it came to linguistic ability which would have put certain doctors at a disadvantage when competing for posts. It would be disingenuous to simply ignore such issues. It is also clear that widespread discrimination was a major factor in directing non-white doctors towards less popular fields and geographical areas.[10]

At times, discrimination was the product of overt racism, which was undeniably present in the NHS at the time. David Smith's study, *Overseas Doctors in the National Health Service*, published in 1980, showed for instance that 60 per cent of UK/Eire qualified doctors felt that Asian doctors were less competent than British doctors.[11] Informal interviews carried out in hospitals in the course of the same study included an encounter with four members of a district management team who expressed the view that:

> there was considerable prejudice on the part of some consultants against coloured applicants, which went well beyond any ideas about British qualifications being better, or British-qualified doctors having better understanding of the patients, or the fact that an applicant who qualified at a particular medical school might also be known to them.[12]

Moreover, two of the interviewees felt that consultants:

> 'often' took pride in keeping departments white, or—even more—in getting them white when they had been staffed by overseas doctors. They stated unequivocally that some consultants went down lists of candidates for posts, looked at the names, and then said 'There are only two we can shortlist', meaning that there are two whites.[13]

One such consultant, 'Dr Lodge' (not his real name), was also quoted as expressing antagonism towards Asians of whom he claimed that 'As individuals it is fair to say that their sense of values and priorities is quite different.'[14] Evidence for this included the claim that 'they take sick leave unnecessarily and are then seen at the Test match.'[15] These attitudes were directly reflected in his department's recruitment policies:

> Up to two years ago all of the twelve junior doctors in his department had been Asians, whereas now all but one were white and British-qualified. The change had been brought about as a matter of conscious policy by Dr Lodge, and must have involved unlawful discrimination. Dr Lodge was highly satisfied with the results of the change ... [He believed that] the department was happier and more easily run, because staff relations were better and the British doctors were more reliable, punctual, competent and 'honourable'.[16]

Whilst it is hard to estimate how prevalent such attitudes might have been, David Smith's view that they were 'neither rare nor very common'[17] seems a reasonable description, based on interviews with doctors and the evidence that has been sifted through for this project. They were not the preserve of isolated individuals who were only responsible for their own department. Dipak Ray, a member of the GMSC, the national body responsible for matters concerning general practice recalled having to challenge colleagues in the course of professional meetings:

> This guy came up, was cracking jokes about ... OHMS [On Her Majesty's Service]. There's so many bloody foreigners, he said, actually OHMS is 'Only Hindus, Muslims and Sikhs'. He's saying this in a doctors' meeting knowing fully well that at that time thirty percent or thirty-five percent staff came from overseas. So, in the middle of his speech I got up, once I got up there are hushed silence in the room. I said you should be ashamed of yourself, what you have said today. And what hurts me most is that people are laughing in this room ... I'm on the Social Security Advisory Committee ... I'm going to take it up with the Secretary of State ... How people ... like you become chairmen of Health Authorities. There was a huge, huge silence. When I came out of the room, all came to me—the doctors. 'Oh Dipak, we don't agree with him' ... I said 'Why didn't you say something? Why did I have to get up and stop him?'[18]

This account provides further evidence not just that racism existed in the NHS but that those holding racist views felt little need to hide them for much of this period. This applies to consultants such as 'Dr Lodge' and the official that Dipak Ray recalls challenging. This does not mean that all white British doctors were racist. Ray did not describe feeling isolated or unsupported when he spoke up. It seems likely though that this sort of language was employed by at least a significant minority of doctors and formed part of a broader culture of medicine which reflected wider social attitudes of the time rather than distinguishing itself from them.

One white doctor who was a GP during this period and whom I spoke to informally recalled that when walking towards an operating theatre as a trainee medic he could hear from a considerable distance a consultant shouting that he did not want 'a wog' in his operating theatre—the reason for this outburst being that he had been allocated a South Asian doctor to assist with an operation.[19] In the late 1980s another white doctor, in a book on medical politics, wrote that:

> The Royal College of Obstetricians and Gynaecologists includes within its membership examination a question in which candidates are asked to write an essay which will be marked for style and use of English and not for content. White doctors in the specialty sometimes describe this as the 'wog stopper'.[20]

Success rates at professional examinations, supposedly an impartial measure of competence, could therefore be distorted by practices aimed at penalising those marked as different. Not only did these views and practices exist but Dipak Ray's recollection of the incident he described and the fact that racist consultants were working within the NHS also suggests that they were not systematically challenged.

Discrimination on the grounds of ethnicity and national origin was in fact openly practised within the NHS. Explicit bars to entry into particular roles were in place: even as late as the 1970s some posts were advertised as only open to British graduates.[21] In the 1980s, researchers at St George's Medical School in London described how a computer system used to screen students who applied to study there had been programmed in a way that systematically disadvantaged ethnic minority students.[22] David Smith's research showed that 86 per cent of British-trained doctors thought that a non-white overseas-trained graduate would be at a disadvantage when applying for jobs compared to a white British-qualified graduate.[23] Stark evidence of the centrality of discrimination to the professional experiences of ethnic minority doctors was produced in the early 1990s when researchers applied for hospital jobs using comparable CVs purporting to be from doctors, some of whom were given 'traditional British' names while others had 'Asian sounding' names. The candidates presumed to be Asian were significantly less likely to be shortlisted.[24] The fictional CVs were of 'doctors' who had all purportedly trained in Britain, so the study did not reflect any additional disadvantage that might have resulted from having overseas qualifications.

Whilst racism in a narrow sense undoubtedly played a part in blighting the careers of migrant and ethnic minority doctors, the experiences of one of the authors of this study, Aneez Esmail, a British-trained South Asian doctor, also point to the importance of wider issues around difference:

> The results of the pilot study fitted with my own experience of trying for jobs in the mid-eighties. My white peers applied for ten posts, but I must have gone after a hundred in the same time. I found out that the way to get short-listed was to visit the consultants concerned and show myself to be OK. Once, I asked a consultant how he did the short-listing, and he told me about two piles of applications—those with English names and those with foreign ones. Only if there was nobody worthwhile in

the 'English' pile would he look at the 'Foreign' one. He said to me then, 'If you had not come to see me you would not have got an interview.'[25]

As well as providing a further indication of the fact that discrimination on the grounds of ethnicity was indeed being practised, this testimony also highlights the need to engage with the issue of difference in a broader sense: it was possible to be non-white and to still appear 'OK'. In addition to tolerating overt racism, the NHS provided a working environment where difference was not accepted. Racism and heterophobia of course overlapped. This is highlighted by the views of 'Dr Lodge' who was proud to be running an all-white department and claimed that his dislike of graduates from the Indian subcontinent stemmed from their difference: 'I regret that a high proportion of those from India, Pakistan and Bangladesh were different from what we normally expect in medical graduates.'[26]

It would therefore be too simplistic to describe the NHS as operating a form of medical apartheid. Ethnicity intersected with a range of other factors to produce disadvantage. In response to a dissatisfied South Asian doctor who had complained of discrimination, the author of a letter published in the BMJ in 1961 for instance defended the right of a hospital committee to appoint a British doctor ahead of a migrant doctor on the basis that the British doctor 'wishes to do a job as part of a long-term training plan culminating in a life's work in this country' whereas, they claimed, the migrant doctor 'will only spend a year or two here'.[27]

An article published in the BMJ in 1983 provided additional insight into the nature of more general heterophobic attitudes and outlined some of the effects that they could have. Its author, Philip Rhodes, was at the time Professor of Postgraduate Medical Education at the University of Southampton, so hardly a marginal figure within the profession. He argued that:

> There is very little positive prejudice against overseas doctors in the medical profession in Britain, but there is often positive preference in favour of British graduates, largely because their behaviour is understood and is predictable, since it lies within limits that are familiar.[28]

The fact that neither the author nor the journal's editorial team found fault with the logic of this sentence or felt it would be wise to not express such views in public gives us an insight into British medical culture at the time. Naturally, competing against a candidate who benefits from a 'positive preference' essentially equates to being discriminated against. Nevertheless, it was still considered acceptable in medical circles in the early 1980s to explicitly state that migrant doctors could legitimately find themselves at a disadvantage professionally because of cultural differences. It is worth noting that this was happening fifteen years after the adoption of the Race Relations Act, which outlawed discrimination on the grounds of ethnicity. Although what was being advocated in this case in the pages of the *BMJ* was not explicitly discrimination on the grounds of ethnicity, there are significant areas of overlap between national origin (and hence place of qualification), culture and ethnicity. If it was illegal to discriminate on the basis of ethnicity, placing job applicants at a disadvantage because of their place of qualification or their cultural attributes could apparently still be seen as a respectable position to adopt. The solution advocated in the article was not for the culture of medicine to change but for migrant doctors to do their best to fit in. It gave examples of how they could achieve this, including advice related to clothing and appearance:

> For men a grey, dark blue, or black suit raises least hackles in any interview. It is probably wise to avoid brown, especially brown shoes; a sports jacket and trousers that do not match, since they give an air of casualness, as if you do not understand the nature of what is going on underneath the surface as well as on it; and avoid an open necked shirt without a tie or a polo necked jersey. To play safe, hair should be neat and tidy and shirts and ties not too loud … For women, simple dress will make the best impression on conservative consultants who are trying to visualise you working for them in the wards, theatres, and outpatient departments among their patients. If you are from the Indian subcontinent and can bear to discard the sari while you are in Britain, it may be of help to you. It is a most beautiful garment and much admired, but to Western eyes it often seems out of place in the working environment of a hospital … There is of course no proof that the sari is a dust gatherer, nor that it breaches aseptic practice,[29] but you should know that such supposed objections to the sari have been made and are believed by some.[30]

This guidance, apparently well-intentioned in the context of the time, can only be interpreted as a reflection of a broader professional culture within which doctors were expected to appear and to behave in particular ways, typical of those familiar with a dominant white, male, middle-class culture.

Attitudes and practices such as those that have been described had a profound impact on the working lives of migrant and ethnic minority workers. Of the doctors qualified in the Indian subcontinent who were interviewed for the book *Overseas Doctors in the NHS*, which was published in 1980, 23 per cent claimed that they had personally experienced discrimination when applying for hospital jobs.[31] Amongst non-white[32] hospital doctors who had been in Britain since at least 1964, the figure was of over 40 per cent.[33] A 1987 study for the Commission for Racial Equality, which looked at the experiences of overseas doctors and British-trained doctors with comparable qualifications and experience found that in spite of having similar professional backgrounds, the two groups had diverging experiences of work satisfaction and career progress in the NHS with overseas graduates having to make significantly more job applications before obtaining posts.[34] One doctor, quoted in P. R. L. Mohan's study of Asian doctors in Sandwell, reported that:

A lot of discrimination is here. Specially, I wanted to do GP vocational training. I appeared for more than fifty interviews in one year. In all the cases white candidates were only selected. There is a lot of discrimination going on. At some places only black candidates appeared. In that case, they said that nobody was suitable and turned us down.[35]

The repetition of the phrase 'a lot of discrimination' communicates a strong feeling of personal injustice and a sense that racism and heterophobia were unavoidable and commonplace rather than an occasional inconvenience that it might be possible to avoid. This interview also points to the fact that discrimination operated within the context of general practice as well, as is discussed later in this chapter. Another doctor interviewed for Emma Jones and Stephanie Snow's book on black and minority ethnic clinicians in Manchester remembered experiencing 'Tremendous indirect discrimination ... They looked at your face and that was all that they needed to do about your employment and there was nothing that you could do about it.'[36]

Discrimination similarly affected the careers of overseas-born and ethnic minority nurses. Black and minority ethnic nurses were disproportionately represented in unpopular specialisms such as geriatrics and mental health.[37] Again, difference in a wider sense contributed to shaping the careers of migrant workers: being Irish could prove a barrier to progression and the professional status of healthcare professionals could become interwoven with their personal background. Louise Ryan thus identifies Irishness as a barrier to becoming a State Registered Nurse (SRN) as opposed to having a career in enrolled nursing which was seen as less prestigious.[38] Black and minority ethnic nurses had similar experiences of being 'duped', in the words of one research participant, into enrolling for courses leading to the State Enrolled Nurse certificate as opposed to the SRN certificate.[39] Research in the 1980s on undergraduate nurses studying at university in what was then seen as an unconventional route into the profession found that they were treated differently by nurses who had followed a 'conventional' SRN programme—their professional lives were described as being 'dominated by an all-embracing feeling of difference'.[40] As Parvati Raghuram has pointed out, it is also important to reflect on the extent to which the experiences of women migrant workers were at variance with those of men—a subject that has so far received relatively little attention.[41] David Smith noted in *Overseas Doctors in the NHS* that non-white female doctors were substantially less likely than their male counterparts to report having experienced ethnic or racial discrimination, possibly, he felt, because of the impact of gender-based discrimination.[42]

The geographical clustering of South Asian doctors can therefore, through the adoption of a wider framework encompassing both racism and broader questions around difference, be seen as part of a wider process which results in marginalised practitioners being directed towards specific roles. Interviews with South Asian GPs revealed that they were frequently working alongside female doctors, doctors from Scotland or the island of Ireland and doctors of Central European, Middle Eastern or African origin. The deployment of these doctors in the British healthcare system appears to have followed not dissimilar patterns to those of South Asian doctors. Scottish and Irish doctors were relied on to take on positions in general practice in industrial cities that were in many instances subsequently filled by South Asian doctors.[43] The related concepts of racism and heterophobia provide a tool which connects the experiences of South Asian GPs to the historical experiences of other marginalised groups and points to the need for a greater understanding of the impact of discrimination based on difference on the shaping of healthcare provision in Britain. Reflecting on the importance of racism and heterophobia also provides a better way of making sense of the experiences that doctors describe in their interviews.

## Experiencing difference in the NHS

Understanding the trajectories of South Asian GPs involves bearing in mind the fact that racism was prevalent in the NHS but also more generally being attentive to the nature of the obstacles faced by doctors who were viewed as outsiders.[44] If discrimination is seen as based more broadly on difference rather than solely ethnicity, an ability to minimise that difference can contribute to diminishing its effect. Equally, differences other than those of ethnicity, in a system dominated by white English middle-class men, can be seen as being just as important or indeed more relevant. Using the framework of racism and heterophobia for instance helps to incorporate into our analysis of the development of general practice the narratives of doctors who say they were not discriminated against on the basis of ethnicity, even if this did not preclude all forms of discrimination. Thinking of discrimination as being based on difference rather than purely on ethnicity makes it easier to read the following testimonies of doctors who did not perceive themselves as being at a disadvantage in the British medical profession because of their ethnicity:

> I know lots of Asian doctors have been discriminated but maybe the way we were brought up or behaved … we have never been discriminated. If I was ever discriminated, only by the other Asian doctors … because I was a woman … *You … said that you felt that some Asian doctors said they were discriminated against in the UK but you felt that wasn't the case for yourself, why do you think that was?* … I don't know … I think we may be an exception … our background is … we talk well, we are the … generation that read Enid Blyton and you know, went to school and … sang hymns … we had that English sort of background … we went to schools and we were taught by English teachers—not necessarily English … our head teacher was a New Zealander and most of our teachers, Australian, some English.[45]
>
> Discrimination depends on two people, who you are and how you conduct yourself … In that, I feel that language is important … If you

speak the kind of language which is spoken in England then you have no problem.[46]

It is notable, however, that both of the above doctors practised in working-class areas; they might not therefore have been immune to the effects of processes of indirect discrimination on the allocation of roles within general practice. It remains that being South Asian was not an automatic bar to progression. The effects of racism and heterophobia could be perceived to be minimised through evidence of good language skills or an anglicised education. The participant who spoke of her familiarity with the English children's writer Enid Blyton and her exposure to British culture also described how her husband's prowess in a sport associated with the British establishment greatly enhanced his popularity with a consultant and hence his career prospects.[47] A doctor who migrated as a child and was educated in Britain felt that his ability to merge into mainstream culture was an important factor in his not being subjected to some of the pressures that South-Asian trained doctors experienced:

> In terms of promotion, they were always faffing around and not really getting on and many went into general practice because they couldn't get any job in a hospital and all that stuff. I mean (pause) it wasn't (pause) absolutely disgraceful but ... it wasn't good for a lot of their experiences ... And of course the other issue which I found and which I think second generation Asians have found is the language/accent magnifies that problem. The fact that I speak with a [local] accent and we go and have a pint of beer and a game of darts when I was a young boy and ... a young man ... you notice ... a lot of the Asian doctors now speak with English accents ... or regional accents and so on, so it was a mixture of their language issues ... the accent, the brownness, all that was a package which (pause)—medicine wasn't as overt as in some hostile parts of the country but it was there.[48]

The marginalisation of doctors as a result of racism was also perceived as something that could also be overcome through the demonstration of professional skills. One doctor expressed the view that his colleagues were not 'incurably racist'—an intriguing phrase when used by a clinician.[49] It hints at the fact that that there might be different types of racism that may or may not respond to 'treatment' and that racism

understood as racism and heterophobia might be dealt with by under-
mining constructions of difference:

> There was a degree of suspicion. We were seen as not highly qualified,
> had a different accent, so could not be as good as English doctors. We
> were accepted with caution. Once you were seen and spoken to by a
> particular doctor they were more accepting but there was a bias. It was
> not irreversible. Doctors by their skills could surprise people who would
> see that he or she is human as everyone else. But it was left to the doctor
> to persuade.[50]

If doctors could at times overcome 'suspicion' by, for instance, demon-
strating their professional ability or going for a beer, conversely, factors
other than ethnicity could be seen as impeding their progression. The
role of alcohol as a lubricant of British society provides an example of
how this could happen:

> The problem is ... when we came we were not given any introduction or ...
> a foundation course—'How to move in the society' ... I still remember
> when I went to the first dinner [hosted by the President of the Royal
> College of Surgeons], Professor ... who was the President, he was from
> Guy's hospital ... he asked his beautiful daughter 'Come on, take Dr
> Gilani and ... give him some drinks and so on' and she asked me 'What
> would like to drink—shall I bring you sherry or so?' I said 'No thank
> you, I don't drink alcohol' (laughs) ... so she brought me soft drink.
> Nowadays of course soft drink probably is considered alright ... In those
> days, if you didn't drink sherry ... you were funny you see (laughter).[51]

In this particular case, ostracism solely on the grounds of ethnicity
does not appear as a major issue: S. A. A. Gilani had been invited to
attend a prestigious medical function. He recognised however that he
was encountering blockages as a result of his position as an outsider
and that he was not always equipped to deal with social situations: for
instance, how, as a non-drinking Muslim, he should deal with a culture
where alcohol played an important part. Laughter again punctuates his
narrative and acts as a sort of relief mechanism, highlighting the extent
to which his abstinence from alcohol marked him as different. The reference to sherry, a drink more likely to be consumed in gentlemen's
clubs than in working-class pubs, is not innocent. Partaking in a glass of
sherry was akin to signalling membership of a particular social group.
Being teetotal could therefore serve to exclude doctors from important

professional rituals and networks. Hira Lal Kapur's account of his time as a hospital doctor, before becoming a GP, offers another illustration of how these dynamics operated:

> I think when we worked together, there was no problem. There might have been some occasions when we were considered as an outsider. Personally I never experienced it and if there was any time anybody said anything to me—it didn't bother my head ... I couldn't be bothered. There were some other doctors who used to grumble that they are being treated shabbily but then I don't know—they had their own experiences. The only thing I can remember is working in Preston Royal Infirmary [in the north of England], we'd be working together all day and then when we go down for our meal in the evening, all the English doctors would sit on one table for their dinner and all the Asian doctors would sit on another table. And I used to think, 'Why is this happening? I mean, we work during the daytime together, we have a laugh, we have a chat and then ... when it come to the dinner table we are all sitting separately ... ' I can't explain why it happened but it did. *Was that just at mealtimes or did that happen in other situations?* Socialising—I suppose they all had their own way of doing things. Most of them would go out to the pub and drink. I personally don't drink and so I wouldn't be invited to join them because they didn't want to take a chap out for a glass of Coca-Cola, and I never bothered my head going out ... The way I look at it that was a ... positive thing in my favour. I can still remember in Sharoe Green hospital [in Preston] when I worked, at about six o'clock they would all come to me and say 'Look, are you going out this evening?' And I would say 'No'. 'Do you mind looking after my telephone and if there is any call to my ward would you cover it?' I would say 'Yes'. So ... most of the local English boys would run off to the pub for their drink while I'm looking after the hospital ... . And on weekends also I would quite happily stand [in] for them ... I never bothered my head with these things. I was happy working.[52]

The laughter in the first interview can be seen as an acknowledgment of the unease caused at the time by behaviours that deviated from the norm, as a way of dealing with a subject that caused discomfort: the same participant, S. A. A. Gilani, also laughed when describing another doctor's anecdote concerning his suicide attempt when studying in London. The second interview bears witness to the insidious nature of marginalisation on the grounds of difference. Hira Lal Kapur maintained that he had not been discriminated against but his account of his time as a hospital doctor provides an example of how difference could be penalising. Whilst he might have felt contented working and gaining additional expertise, his professional experiences may well have been shaped by a lack of opportunities to build networks in the course of conversations in pubs or over a glass of sherry, to hear about opportunities, to understand some of the unspoken dynamics at play in hospitals and in medicine.

Beliefs regarding the merits of different medical training systems also contributed to hindering doctors' careers. As has been discussed, British graduates could be viewed as superior, which would result in them gaining access to the most prestigious opportunities. This in turn would help them be appointed to the most coveted jobs. This process was described by one research participant. Tellingly, echoing doctors who portrayed racism as being an explicit part of the culture of the NHS, he described this form of discrimination as an openly acknowledged dimension of medical culture at the time:

> People in London told me—my consultant ... and senior registrar— ... your chance of getting a job in a teaching hospital in London is nil. So you will have to go outside of London ... *Why did they think that your chances in London would be nil?* ... Because of the competition. London teaching hospital was the most competitive ... I was given the hint that it would be ... not worthwhile ... *Do you think that was because you were from the Indian subcontinent or was that for another reason?* ... You know people who have been trained in this country they have some advantages. They are the product of the system. But we are not product of the system, we came from outside. So we had some gaps and our education probably was not as high a standard ... than the students who qualified in this country ... It was not ... a preference for white but obviously they had ... better opportunities of learning and gaining experience which obviously we didn't have.[53]

Debating the issue of the 'standards' of medical education in the Indian subcontinent and in the UK would of course be a futile exercise. Aside from the issue of variations in standards from one institution to the next, medicine is a product of its social and cultural context rather than a set of universal rules. South Asian trained doctors might for instance be expected to learn more about tropical diseases which would rarely, if ever, be seen in a British context. Irrespective of the issue of whether standards were lower or higher (some South Asian doctors argue for instance that their training in high-demand hospitals in the Global South has advantages over the more controlled environments of the Global North where it can take longer to build up experience) doctors could undoubtedly be perceived as professionally different and be penalised as a result. This explains how the participant just quoted could claim that there was 'not a preference for whites' whilst asserting that they had 'better opportunities'.

The importance of conceiving of the NHS as being heterophobic and racist rather than purely as racist in the context of understanding the experiences of South Asian GPs is further underlined by the account of the distribution of hospital work given by the participant quoted earlier who believed she was discriminated against on the basis of gender rather than ethnicity:

> I was discriminated by the Pakistani doctors because I was an Asian woman ... They used to alter the rota ... so they could go out in the evenings, 'Oh, you don't need to go out' and that sort of thing, I had to do more nights ... It's historical I think that they discriminate against women ... Pakistani doctors, not so much the Indian doctors. Not all of them ... maybe about thirty per cent of the hospital doctors that I worked with ... again, it's individual people. *So why do you think it's specifically to do with Pakistani doctors?* I really don't know ... must be their cultural background, I suppose ... they consider women as inferior, I think, maybe things they have changed now, I don't know.[54]

Such comments also bear witness to the fact that migrant practitioners played their part in defining the NHS as a heterophobic space—they indicate either the existence of a real problem, a problematic perception on the part of the participant (she was not from Pakistan nor Muslim and may have been prejudiced against Pakistanis or Muslims) or an element of both.[55]

Another female doctor emphasised the importance of the increased distance that she perceived between female South Asian doctors and NHS staff and patients:

> They were not used to ... the culture very much ... especially the females, they were not used to ... mainly it was the ... males who came into that and ... coincidentally for some reason these men, some of the men who came in ... early on also wanted to ... be able to blend with the local community and the way that they could blend with them they

thought perhaps at the time ... it was the materialistic comfort and other comforts. That made them go out with the girl—with the nursing staff, lady nursing staff, I mean with the females and so that built a different rapport with them and so they were able to relate better with them ... than with the ... female South Asian Doctors. It was difficult for us to socially mix with them ... it wasn't easy ... you had to be two or four steps higher than anyone else who was with you to be able to get a job, to make an impression, to proceed. It's for both reasons, cultural as well as being a female.[56]

The extent to which female South Asian doctors had different experiences from male South Asian doctors would be worthy of further enquiry (and it would be worth exploring if the same applied to doctors who were Muslim, had a disability or were marked as different in other ways). Kumbakonam Srinivasachar Bhanumathi's recollections do suggest that at least for some female doctors there was an additional layer of marginalisation which is presented here as the result of a complex blend of social and cultural factors. Given that this study's remit was to look at the role of South Asian GPs as a whole and that only a small number of female doctors were interviewed, it is hard to draw definitive conclusions in this respect, although it seems likely that further research would bring these additional obstacles to the fore. Being discriminated against as a South Asian doctor, and more generally, being perceived as diverging from the norms of the people who were in positions of power could therefore be mutually reinforcing processes. Equally, being able to show allegiance to dominant values, by speaking in a certain way, acquiring a white partner, or drinking beer could play a part in bringing South Asian doctors closer to the mainstream. It is in this sense that the experiences of these doctors within the NHS can be said to be defined by racism and heterophobia which in turn contributed to shaping their careers.

## Discrimination within general practice

This racist and heterophobic context resulted in South Asian doctors being directed towards unpopular fields such as psychiatry, geriatrics and general practice where competition for posts was less fierce. General practice did indeed fulfil this role of offering a medical niche to doctors who faced discrimination. However, it also provided a discriminatory environment. As a result, South Asian doctors were able to enter general practice in significant numbers but often only in specific types of role. The evidence of discrimination within general practice is overwhelming. As was the case with hospital medicine, this was quite openly acknowledged by doctors at the time. Again, a spectrum of attitudes could be observed, ranging from explicit racism defined in the narrow sense of the word to a wider intolerance of difference. In his 1967 book *The Doctors*, the writer Paul Ferris described some of the prejudices that came into play when GPs were recruited to practices:

> [A] senior partner on the South Coast … said it had been terrible to see some of the fellows who applied when he had a vacancy. Each applicant was asked to bring his wife and children and stay for a meal, so that one could see if he was a decent fellow who knew how to hold his knife–'It may be petty but it counts.' One of them was an Irishman, who arrived, with his family, two hours late for Sunday lunch, after driving up from the West Country, and had to be invited to stay the night. 'We had to provide them with toothbrushes and nighties,' said the partner 'and they didn't even bother to write and say thank you.' In these situations, a nicely-spoken young English doctor with a pretty wife, a baby or two and, better still, a big retriever is the ideal candidate. The least ideal is a Southern Irishman or an Indian. All sorts of libellous stories are told about feckless Irish doctors with hip-flasks and bad manners, but besides these dubious objections, there is the question of the Irish Catholic's religious beliefs, which can cause trouble in a practice when the patients want contraceptive advice or appliances. If the *B.M.J.* carries twenty or thirty advertisements for partners, one or two of them will probably specify 'Protestant'. Others will say 'British', in order to keep out the Indians and other foreigners. There are various objections— foreigners are incompetent, the patients wouldn't like it, it wouldn't be fair to the children. A particularly explicit doctor in London, agreeing with a partner in a neighbouring practice, said he felt guilty but stood firm. 'He wouldn't employ me in his practice in India,' he said. 'I'd smell in his practice and he'd smell in mine. I'm sorry, but I don't want that.'[57]

Ferris was a freelance writer and his account may well have given more space to doctors with extreme views. There is undoubtedly a greater readership for stories about cantankerous and racist medics than for dispassionate assessments of the challenges of inner-city general practice. It is notable, however, that he described the latter doctor as being 'particularly explicit' when it came to expressing his views, rather than being at odds with the rest of the profession. Ferris' depiction of a professional culture with a strong sense of middle-class propriety that rejected a range of characteristics gives a sense of how racism and heterophobia could work in general practice. He reports the existence of racism in its most crude shape, with racist and heterophobic stereotypes apparently abundant (there are 'all sorts of libellous' stories about Irish doctors according to Ferris) and at times taking particularly crass forms (as in the reference to a doctor's 'smell'). Religious beliefs are relevant as is class (being familiar with rules concerning the use of cutlery 'counts'). As for gender, female doctors are notably absent from this equation. Women are confined to the role of the 'pretty wife'.

The fact that this type of culture existed within general practice is again not a matter for debate or discussion. GPs admitted quite openly to excluding those that were different at the time. An article published in 1969 in *The Lancet* about the increase in the percentage of overseas doctors recruited to general practice in Essex and Birmingham argued that this phenomenon could only be explained by a lack of supply of local doctors as: 'A doctor tries to choose someone with whom he can agree and one who will, he hopes, please the patients. It is rather likely that he will have a preconception in favour of his own kind.'[58] A passage in the memoirs of the GP Ronald Gibson who worked in the prosperous southern English market town of Winchester also offers an insight into how recruitment into the more desirable types of general practice could operate in ways that disadvantaged outsiders:

> Baffer had had a letter from a Dr Robert Forbes … to say that his son, James, would like to practice in or near Winchester. I thought there was no harm in us seeing him … and he duly arrived for interview. He had been trained at St Mary's (he was an excellent rugger player) but had done his house jobs at Bart's. He also wore an old school tie with which I was familiar … By mutual consent Jimmy Forbes joined the practice.[59]

This brief description contains a wealth of coded information that gives us an indication of the range of factors that could ease a candidate's entry into a position as GP in an affluent area. Having personal contacts was clearly an advantage: the new recruit was able to create a vacancy for himself rather than having to rely on scouring advertisements. Having been trained in the 'right' sort of medical school and hospital (St Mary's and Barts being London teaching hospitals) was an advantage. So was being skilled at a sport that has been described as having a 'semi-religious' status at St Mary's and that was associated with the British upper middle class.[60] The reference to 'rugger' rather than 'rugby' indicates that the sport in question was rugby union rather than rugby league—the latter being more associated with the north of England and the working classes. Rugby union on the other hand was popular in public schools—i.e. in the British context elitist private schools. Their alumni can be recognised by the fact that they wear 'old school ties' which act as a signal of belonging to a particular social realm. The pleasing reassurance of the familiar that comes across in Gibson's account is a reminder that those who could not provide such evidence would have found themselves at a significant disadvantage.

When posts were advertised rather than being filled as a result of informal recommendations, it was common, until the practice was discontinued in the 1970s, for advertisements for GP posts in the *BMJ* to state a preference for British graduates.[61] This practice continued elsewhere as evidenced by the advertisements for GP jobs placed up to the late 1970s in supplements to the medical magazine *Pulse*. Practices in affluent areas frequently stated that British graduates were preferred:

> YOUNG GRADUATE of British university with obstetrics experience required in group practice. Sussex seaside resort with full sporting and social amenities.[62]
> EASTBOURNE/SUSSEX Exceptional opportunity for repl. In coastal town, group pract. of four, full ancil. staff, incl. own pn, highly org/efficiently run pract. with consid. private practice, voc. trnd Br. univ. grad. pref.[63]

It might be possible to argue that the emphasis here was on the vocational training, which was being introduced into general practice at the time as it became recognised as a specialised area of medicine in its own right. Opportunities for traineeships were however also advertised as being reserved for British graduates:

> Trainee vacancy for graduate of British university available 1 March, 1977, in four-man semi-rural practice in pleasant area of Cheshire.[64]

As well as providing evidence that outsiders were discriminated against, these advertisements also give an indication of what practice

characteristics were attractive to the British graduates that they targeted. Being able to work in a practice located in a 'pleasant' area, have
access to private practice and being able to rely on support staff were
seen as positive features. These practices tended to be located in areas
where the concentrations of overseas doctors were the lowest.

Discrimination was therefore openly practised and recognised as
part of medical culture. Advertisements such as those quoted above
were commonplace. It is noteworthy that one advertisement in *Pulse*
started with the words 'Partnership offered to a conscientious doctor of
any nationality'.[65] The fact that the opening was potentially available to
any competent professional could obviously not be taken for granted at
the time. Those who remember living through this period articulate a
sense of a field where difference was a key determinant of professional
trajectories. Has Joshi who worked as a GP in Wales recalled hearing a
lecturer boast about favouring white male candidates in a postgraduate
course run by the Royal College of General Practitioners:

> General practice was even worse … as compared to hospital medicine.
> Because general practice clearly used to … —I know that from experi-
> ence later on—that they used to shortlist people into three piles …
> Asians on one side, women on the other one and white male doctors …
> in the third pile and usually it's white male doctors who got appointed
> to general practice … *Who told you about this method of recruitment and
> these different piles that would be made of applications?* (laughs) Well
> that happened … after I went into general practice and I was trying to
> become a member of the Royal College of GPs … I used to go … to the
> local … half-day release course and one of the guys who was lecturing
> there took pride in telling us all that this is how he recruited partners …
> And he told me that that practice was quite widespread those days. *And
> do you think that it was indeed widespread? Did you … hear from other
> people that this was something that happened?* Yeah. It was very, very com-
> mon … You never, ever got into good practices … You know, the ideal
> practices … didn't even have a look at you.[66]

Irrespective of the literal truth of such an allegation which is not hugely
surprising in the context that has been described (and that was made
by someone who at the time of being interviewed was a vice-chair of
the Royal College of GPs rather than an embittered outsider), it is hard
to escape the sense that general practice in the first four decades of the
NHS was defined by racism and heterophobia in the same way that

medicine in hospitals was. Has Joshi's reference to piles of job applications brings to mind Aneez Esmail's memories of applying for hospital posts. Whether such practices were indeed widespread or not is hard to establish. What is not in doubt is that these recollections give a sense of how migrant and ethnic minority practitioners were made to feel in the British healthcare system and that their marginal status was unambiguously communicated to them.

These discriminatory processes were not necessarily solely targeted at South Asian doctors or their ethnic minority colleagues, as illustrated by the example of the different treatment given to applications made by female candidates. Nor was discrimination only the product of the racist attitudes of white doctors. More generally, heterophobia and the fact that doctors sought out other doctors that they identified with was a factor in determining which jobs were available to whom. One South Asian doctor from the north of England described how this worked in his view in the industrial city where he was based:

> If I be open with you … with LMC [Local Medical Committee] … I will give you one example … At one stage when we had annual dinner, we decided that everybody can give an option where they want to sit, which table … and we found that there were three clear demarcation. Asian doctor wanted to sit with Asian doctors … English doctor make their own English group, Jewish doctor wanted to make their own group … We said look that's not on—I mean high professionals like us—so we mixed it up, I said no, everybody don't have a choice, we will … allocate it, everybody will sit, all the three groups sit in the three tables and that's … how we did it. *And in terms of the practices that doctors ended up working in as GPs, how was it, what was the sort of process whereby Asian doctors ended up working in unpopular areas do you think?* Because like I said … English doctors will pick English doctors. If I give you one example … in [inner-city location in northern city] we had … three group practices … one was English doctor who will not take anybody else … Second, a Jewish practice which will take … only Jewish doctor. And my partner was very fair … and we … were both … ethnic minority … and he accepted me.[67]

Racism and heterophobia should therefore not simply be seen as the product of exclusionary processes driven by white hierarchies in middle-class areas. It is important to recognise not just that discrimination was based on an array of intersecting factors rather than solely being the product of ethnic belonging, but also that exclusionary processes could be at play in less popular areas, and be driven by minorities. The previously mentioned *Pulse* advertisements from the 1970s also list posts described as suitable for graduates of Indian universities or demanding that candidates should have knowledge of 'Hindi or Gujurati', which could have been a way of seeking to discourage non-South Asian candidates.[68] If white British doctors dominated the desirable practices, there is some evidence therefore that less desirable areas could be actively developed into professional 'niches'[69] for doctors belonging to other groups who also behaved in a discriminatory fashion. This is hinted at in the description that one participant gives of how he got his first job:

> *How did you go about finding a job in general practice?* It was … very easy, one of my colleagues working with me in the hospital … one of his best friends was [South Asian doctor working in mining area] and he knew that they are looking for … a partner and he talked to the senior partner … and they agreed with him and they said 'All right, call him for the interview'. I came and met all the partners … they all interviewed me and luckily for me, they offered me the job.[70]

The disadvantages that South Asian doctors faced can thus be seen as partially being the result of racism within the medical profession at the time and more generally of a tendency for those marked as different to be directed towards particular roles.

## Notes

1  S. K. Ahuja interview with author.
2  Smith, *Overseas Doctors*, p. 74.
3  A. Memmi, *Le racisme: Description, définitions, traitement*. Nouvelle édition revue (Paris: Gallimard, 1994) (French), pp. 229–34. The term heterophobia is the author's translation. In the original French, Memmi uses the term 'hétérophobie'.
4  Simpson & Ramsay, 'Manifestations and negotiations of racism'.
5  Memmi, *Le racisme*, p. 234.
6  Esmail, 'Asian doctors'.
7  Gish, *Britain and the Immigrant Doctor*, p. 8.
8  Smith, *Overseas Doctors*, pp. 154–6.

9   For an illustration of some of the tensions that prevailed between doctors and nurses from different British hospitals see 'The recent history of Guy's and St Thomas', 21 June 2011 (Witness seminar). Accessed 8 April 2013 at: www.chstm.manchester.ac.uk/research/projects/guysthomas/.

10  See Esmail, *Asian Doctors*; Jones & Snow, *Against the Odds*; Kyriakides & Virdee, 'Migrant labour'; Coker (ed.), *Racism in Medicine*; Simpson et al., 'Providing "special" types of labour'; Simpson & Ramsay, 'Racism and "heterophobia"'.

11  Smith, *Overseas Doctors*, p. 123.

12  Smith, *Overseas Doctors*, p. 181.

13  Ibid.

14  Smith, *Overseas Doctors*, p. 183.

15  Ibid. The expression 'Test match' is a reference to international cricket—a sport which is hugely popular in the Indian subcontinent.

16  Smith, *Overseas Doctors*, p. 183.

17  Smith, *Overseas Doctors*, p. 184.

18  D. Ray interview with author, 5 December 2008.

19  Personal information.

20  S. Watkins, *Medicine and Labour: The Politics of a Profession* (London: Lawrence and Wishart, 1987), p. 199.

21  Esmail, 'Asian doctors', p. 832.

22  A. Esmail, 'Racial discrimination in medical schools', in Coker (ed.), *Racism in Medicine*, p. 86.

23  Smith, *Overseas Doctors*, p. 128.

24  A. Esmail & S. Everington, 'Racial discrimination against doctors from ethnic minorities', *BMJ*, 306 (1993). In developments that illustrate the sensitivities around these issues and the reluctance of the medical profession to address them, the authors were arrested by the police, having been accused of fraud because of their use of false CVs. They were also pursued by the General Medical Council. See 'Racism in medicine: The mask slips', *Medical World* (1993, 11), pp. 8–9.

25  'Racism in medicine: The mask slips', *Medical World* (1993, 11), p. 8.

26  Smith, *Overseas Doctors*, pp. 183–4. The study gave interviewees fictitious names.

27  K. C. D. Gordon, 'Overseas graduates', *BMJ*, (1962, 1:5276), p. 474.

28  P. Rhodes, 'Some hurdles for the overseas doctor', *BMJ* (1983, 286), pp. 1136–7.

29  i.e. the maintenance of a sterile environment.
30  Rhodes, 'Some hurdles for the overseas doctor', p. 1137.
31  Smith, *Overseas Doctors*, p. 141.
32  Smith used the term 'coloured' which is no longer considered acceptable.
33  Smith, *Overseas Doctors*, p. 141.
34  Anwar & Ali, *Overseas Doctors*, pp. 43 & 52.
35  Mohan, 'Asian doctors', p. 171.
36  Jones & Snow, *Against the Odds*, p. 80.
37  Jones & Snow, *Against the Odds*, p. 57.
38  Ryan, 'Who do you think you are?', p. 427.
39  Jones & Snow, *Against the Odds*, p. 54.
40  K. A. Luker, 'Reading nursing: The burden of being different', *International Journal of Nursing Studies*, 21:1 (1984), p. 1.
41  P. Raghuram, 'Asian women medical migrants in the UK', in A. Agrawal (ed.), *Migrant Women and Work* (New Delhi: SAGE, 2006).
42  Smith, *Overseas Doctors*, p. 143.
43  Collings, 'General practice in England', p. 580; Esmail, 'Asian doctors', p. 834.
44  This section draws on arguments and materials first published in Simpson & Ramsay, 'Racism and "heterophobia"'.
45  Anonymous interview with author.
46  Anonymous interview with author.
47  Anonymous interview with author.
48  Anonymous interview with author.
49  Simpson & Ramsay, 'Racism and "heterophobia"', p. 183.
50  K. Korlipara interview with author, 24 September 2009.
51  S. A. A. Gilani interview with author, 30 June 2010.
52  H. L. Kapur interview with author.
53  Anonymous interview with author.
54  Anonymous interview with author.
55  Simpson & Ramsay, 'Racism and "heterophobia"', p. 181.
56  K. S. Bhanumathi interview with author.
57  Ferris, *The Doctors*, pp. 130–1.
58  D. Cargill, 'Recruitment to general practice in Essex and Birmingham', *The Lancet*, 1:7596 (1969), p. 670.
59  R. Gibson, *The Family Doctor: His Life and History* (London: George Allen & Unwin, 1981), p. 83.

60  J. S. Garner, 'The great experiment: The admission of women students to St Mary's Hospital Medical School, 1916–1925', *Medical History*, 42 (1998), p. 84.
61  Esmail, 'Asian doctors', p. 832.
62  Winthrop classified service, supplement to *Pulse*, 8 May 1971.
63  Free classified service, supplement to *Pulse*, 3 December 1977. The meaning of the abbreviated terms is as follows: repl: replacement; pract: practice; ancil: ancillary; pn: practice nurse; consid: considerable; voc.trnd: vocationally trained; Br. univ. grad.: British university graduate; pref: preferred.
64  Winthrop classified service, supplement to *Pulse*, 22 January 1977.
65  Ibid.
66  H. Joshi interview with author, 27 April 2010.
67  Anonymous interview with author.
68  Free classified service, supplement to *Pulse*, 17 September 1977; Free classified service, supplement to *Pulse*, 1 October 1977.
69  Raghuram et al., 'Ethnic clustering', p. 287.
70  Anonymous interview with author.

# 5

# From 'pairs of hands' to family doctors

The professional options of South Asian doctors who decided to stay in Britain were limited, notably as a result of racism and heterophobia. Discrimination operated both in hospital medicine, resulting in migrant doctors being directed towards general practice, and within general practice itself resulting in outsiders being at a disadvantage when it came to obtaining posts in the more desirable areas. The presence of South Asian doctors in general practice in industrial and inner-city areas is nevertheless partly the product of their agency: they actively decided to remain in Britain and forge careers as GPs even though this was not the type of work that they originally envisaged doing. Doctors' decisions to enter general practice were undoubtedly constrained choices but they were not the only choices they could have made. Doctors used their personal initiative to take on the roles in general practice that were available to them at the time.

The UK government and the medical establishment were (at times concerned) observers of this process rather than its instigators. The entry of a significant number of South Asian doctors into the profession of general practice was not officially orchestrated or even explicitly encouraged by the Department of Health. It was at times resisted by the British medical profession.

This chapter describes what was in effect the accidental acquisition by the NHS of a substantial workforce of South Asian GPs. The individual choices made by thousands of South Asian doctors had a major structural impact on the development of British primary care.

## 'What can you do about it?' South Asian doctors' entry into general practice

The accounts that doctors give of their decisions to become general practitioners suggest that they were the product of their decisions to remain in Britain and the result of a compromise between personal agendas and social and professional constraints. A notable dimension of the interviews I conducted was that the experience of discrimination was described as an acknowledged and explicitly discussed characteristic of the NHS. It was part of the reality of professional life in the NHS at the time. The decision to opt for general practice in this context appears in doctors' accounts as a rational response to the situation they found themselves in. The fact that doctors talk about their experiences in this way adds additional detail to the picture provided by the previous chapter of an institution where discrimination was a pervasive influence and its existence openly admitted. As one GP recalled:

> I got advice from one of the Scottish registrar who used to work and he ... give me advice ... 'Doctor, even you pass MRCOG [Membership of the Royal College of Obstetricians and Gynaecologists] you get a degree but you to become a consultant, you are banging your ... head with the wall. Because you won't be able to get any consultant post in this country ... Even Scottish people find difficulty'. He was senior registrar of mine, working in Birmingham ... He gave me advice, if I would be in your place ... go in GP and as soon as you will become a GP you are near about the level of consultant and consultant also will start respecting you. So I ended up in the GP ... *What did he say exactly about the sort of obstacles that you'd encounter if you pursued a career in*—Yeah, he did tell me when you ... even you pass MRCOG ... even you get senior registrar, there is a criteria to select to become a consultant in this country, in Gynaecology particularly, they always prefer the local people first. After local people is not available then they will look after Irish and Scottish and then, sometime Australian ... . and third category would come after that is the Middle East. And forth would come the Asian.[1]

The racist and heterophobic nature of the NHS is once more in evidence in this account of an exchange between a South Asian and a Scottish doctor, which describes the existence of hierarchies based on geographical origin. Discrimination does not appear here as a hidden, unspoken reality but as one generally acknowledged and openly discussed in the NHS of the time. In some respects, when attempting to make sense of the situation they find themselves in, doctors can be seen to be operating as trained medical professionals might be expected to. They gain an understanding of the nature of the problem they are dealing with and subsequently decide on what the best course of action would be. Entering general practice is thus presented as a rational choice based on doctors' interpretations of the reality they were confronted with. Rather than express offence or surprise at finding himself at a disadvantage, one doctor who became a GP in the 1970s thus expressed gratitude towards his superior, a cardiothoracic surgeon, who told him that discrimination would be an obstacle to his progression. He does hint at a degree of regret that things were not different but quickly returns to a professional, pragmatic perspective:

> When you were given that advice ... do you remember how that was expressed, what were the words that were used, was it expressed quite brutally, was it more subtle? No, I think the advice was good at the time ... basically ... I don't blame for people to have some prejudices ... and some sort of anxiety about overseas graduates—but I must say, that if you have worked hard since early and you are genuine persons ... I think the advice ... what I got was perfectly acceptable, not only acceptable ... it was correct advice.[2]

Interestingly, another of Ruban Prasad's superiors advised him to persist with hospital work as he felt that openings might present themselves as a result of the retirement of doctors who had entered the NHS after World War II. In these narratives, South Asian doctors appear as being at a disadvantage in the hospital system rather than in a position that made it impossible to progress. This disadvantage was however a significant professional impediment. The somewhat matter-of-fact attitude towards the existence of discrimination and its consequences is also reflected in Ralph Lawrence's recollection of how the hospital system was described to him a matter of months after the start of the NHS. Lawrence, who was born in South Africa to South Asian parents decided to stay in Britain after marrying a white British woman. Returning to South Africa was not an option because of the apartheid regime's policy on marriages between people classed as belonging to different 'races'. In an interview in 1999 for the Millennium Memory

Bank project, he recalled the way in which his options in the new NHS were presented to him by his superior:

> I discussed this with my chief who was the orthopaedic surgeon Sir Hugh Griffiths and he was an extremely nice man to work with. And he said ... Look, Ralph, you have got to ... accept that you are a foreigner in this country. And when it comes to appointments, you will always get second choice ... British boys and women are going to get first choice when it comes to an appointment. So you have got to decide whether you want to persist with your career in surgery or whether you want to go into general practice.[3]

Lawrence's interview was naturally shaped by the context in which it was given. It is questionable that a surgeon would have spoken of 'British boys and women' being given preferential treatment at the time rather than pointing out that white, British-born and -trained men would inevitably be the preferred candidates. The practice of discrimination appears once more, not as something that was suspected and hidden but as a known quantity. The fact that doctors describe the obstacles they faced in this way means that their recollections cannot be easily dismissed as mere individual and subjective perceptions. The interviews I conducted convey a common sense of operating in a discriminatory system.

Entry into general practice appeared in this context as a logical step to take for a non-white overseas-trained doctor who wanted to remain in Britain. The choice Lawrence was presented with was between persisting in his attempts to become a surgeon (in spite of the handicap he had of being an outsider likely to be discriminated against) and becoming a GP. At times doctors' narratives suggest an internal struggle between their moral indignation and initial professional aspirations on one hand and a scientific engagement with their professional environment on the other, with a realistic assessment of their prospects winning out. Some residual dissatisfaction can be detected but the agency of doctors is also in evidence when they analyse the situation they find themselves in and conclude that general practice offers them a way out of it—albeit one which might represent a compromise containing unsatisfactory elements. Whilst claims of individual agency are to be expected in oral history interviews, its constrained nature in these stories and the internal struggles that led doctors into general practice are not simply a nostalgic recounting of a personal triumph against adversity. The agency described here is borne of an admission of failure to fulfil professional dreams and of disappointment.

This dimension of doctors' experiences is encapsulated in Muhammad Shafi Kausar's account of how he settled for a career in general practice. He recalled having been promised a post by a professor in a cardiology department only to find that a well-connected local candidate was preferred. His account of his move into general practice echoes and amplifies Ruban Prasad's reluctant acceptance of unpleasant realities. It culminates in his resignation to the fact that rights available in theory might not be accessible in practice:

> When the interview came, he called me for interview and then when I was sitting there, he came with face down and he said: 'Dr Kausar, sorry, the other professor of medicine has recommended strongly his own student, graduate of this university, this school, and we have an obligation to give him preference'. He said: ... 'I can give you a registrar job' ... I said: 'I won't know anything, registrar is a third level and I have to teach him [the other doctor] ... money wise, prestige wise, registrar is a big thing but ... I want to learn the subject.' He said: 'Sorry, I can't help you' ... I came to get my specialisation and go back. But I couldn't ... go into a job where I could get specialisation ... So then I had to find, you know ... a drowning man, catches at every straw ... So I then finally settled in general practice which was not my kettle of fish. But ... afterwards I knew it's the best thing I did. Before that I didn't really ... I came here to become cardiologist ... But could never go there. Wrote to deans, wrote to professors, interviewed, post promised and finally ... 'Sorry sir, my own school boy has come'. So what can you do about it? And I used to accept that because they have to give preference to their own people ... it was not that ... I used to accept it ... Things happen, it's better you accept it, to feel less pinched and less aggrieved ... I knew it was my right but it was not achievable right.[4]

Opting for general practice therefore appears as the 'best thing' for doctors to do within an unsatisfactory environment where their initial aims and ambitions might not be 'achievable', a way of reaching an accommodation with a discriminatory healthcare system within which they had decided to work. When it came to the more prestigious positions in the most competitive fields (such as cardiology), the uncertainties of life as a junior hospital doctor and the difficulties involved in attaining consultant status were to a degree structural problems that faced all doctors. South Asian doctors who had concluded that they wanted to stay in Britain and aspired to stable careers had to contend not only with the lack of career opportunities in the NHS but also with the disadvantage of being an outsider and non-white in a racist and heterophobic environment.

Doctors frequently spoke of their entry into the field as offering a practical way of serving their personal agendas at the time. They had found themselves working as a 'pair of hands' while acquiring specialist training and talked of wanting to settle in Britain. Most South Asian medical migrants initially arrived as young doctors seeking training opportunities. Large numbers of doctors took part in this post-imperial exodus. It is unsurprising that during the time of their stay, some of them formed relationships with British people, developed responsibilities towards growing families or simply found that their circumstances had changed and decided not to return to their countries of origin. They describe being at a stage in their lives when they craved the professional status and personal stability that was in short supply in the hospital system. Decisions to settle in Britain and to become GPs were, as a result, often one and the same. General practice was perceived as a discipline that offered a predictable career path and was described as providing the means for doctors and their families to lead a settled life. The following three accounts give a sense of how the GPs I met spoke of their entry into the profession:

> *At what point did you decide to stay in the UK?* The point that I worked about ten years in hospitals and after that I joined the general practice. By that time, I came to know local nurse, and I was married to her and then as I joined the general practice and I thought this is my way of life ... and I thought it will be very difficult to adjust if I go back to Bangladesh and to start a new life there.[5]
>
> The thing is if I keep on doing the hospital practice then I have to keep on changing the place. And because I had two children and changing place and education and everything was a question. So I thought if I go in general practice at least I will be in one place where I can decide my life and my children's education ... And I will be my own boss. So I decided to go for general practice for that particular reason, family reason.[6]

> I felt children needed stability which would help their education. And I wanted to be top of the ladder. It was only way to fulfil both dreams. I was my own boss in general practice. To be consultant in hospital I had to go through hoops, I felt didn't have the time.[7]

It is worth emphasising that the narratives that doctors develop around their entry into general practice can of course be seen as providing a means of justifying their acceptance of medical 'dirty work'. The fact that they describe subordinating professional ambitions to family priorities may indeed be an accurate reflection of their thought processes at the time. Equally, these narratives could be driven by a need to reflect on a life story in a way that is personally satisfying and demands social respect. If it was not possible for them to climb the professional 'ladder', at least they can be seen here to be successful as providers for their families. Muhammad Shafi Kausar's allusion to drowning and clutching at straws might have allowed a glimpse of a deeper emotional truth that others may have chosen not to put into words. It remains that these stories are indicative of the fact that entering general practice was a 'choice' that doctors made and that certain types of practice provided an entry point into the profession for South Asian doctors who had made this choice, irrespective of what deep-seated factors might have been driving their decisions.

The fact that doctors recall practical aspects of their day-to-day existence and their relevance to their entry into general practice contributes to a sense that decisions to become GPs were pragmatic and attributable ultimately to doctors' agency rather than the result say of NHS recruitment efforts or of shifting professional ambitions. Dipak Ray spoke of the pressure of making ends meet as a junior hospital doctor with a wife who was a teacher and a young son.[8] He described being offered a post as a GP in the Welsh Valleys as a 'godsend'. Urmila Rao spoke of being able to work in the same location as her husband, also a GP, and of being able to look after her children.[9] Similarly Kumbakonam Srinivasachar Bhanumathi remembered finding it difficult to arrange childcare when it came to working nightshifts and weekends.[10] The photographs of Satish Kumar Ahuja and his wife Raj Ahuja as young doctors with their children (Figure 3) and subsequently as GPs (Figure 4) provide an illustration of the personal context that drove these processes.

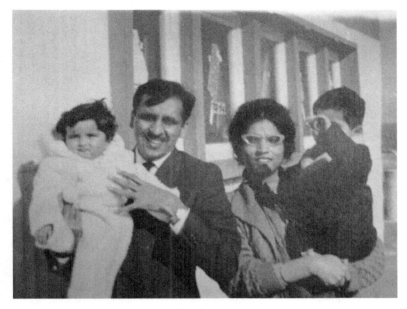

**Figure 3**  Satish Kumar Ahuja (left) and Raj Ahuja as young doctors with their children.

Although it is tempting to see people as migrants from the moment they cross borders, migration is in fact an ongoing process that unfolds over time and is shaped by circumstances. Doctors were not necessarily planning to remain in Britain, they were responding to the social and professional environments that they found and to their changing circumstances. They describe taking opportunities that presented themselves to them. As was the case when it came to the development of geriatrics in the UK, 'luck and chance'[11] played a significant part in the evolution of general practice. One doctor had planned to return to Pakistan to take up a position teaching surgery at King Edward Medical College in Lahore but described how a new law aimed at citizens who had married a foreign national resulted in the job offer being withdrawn.[12] Another spoke of planning to go to the USA but being offered a position in general practice through a professional contact.[13]

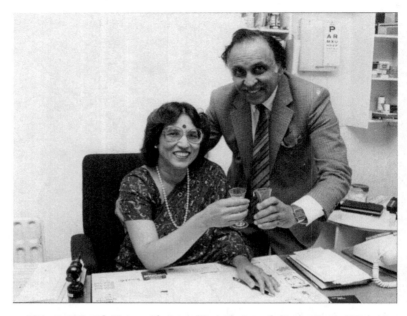

**Figure 4**  Satish Kumar Ahuja and Raj Ahuja at their practice in Wigan.

The combined effect of these individual decisions to become a GP had a considerable impact on the development of the NHS.

### 'If there was an open area you can open your surgery': identifying professional opportunities

If the prospect of becoming a GP offered a means of avoiding discrimination within the hospital system, racism and heterophobia within general practice remained an obstacle to be negotiated. Entering general practice was a constrained choice made because of the lack of other career options. There was also however a lack of options within the field itself and doctors described making a second successive constrained choice to enter a particular type of general practice. One female doctor spoke of setting up her own single-handed practice as a response to the experience of being interviewed for jobs in established surgeries. Her account draws additional attention to the gendered nature of doctors' experiences and the need to see the NHS as both racist and heterophobic. In her view, the difficulties she encountered were the product of institutional sexism rather than resulting from her ethnicity:

> They said I had the right qualification, I've got this, I've got everything right but they looked at me and they said to me: 'Oh, you look very young, your husband … he's a consultant here, a … busy job' and like that they are saying to me 'You are very young and you could still have a family' … They said: … 'You are the right candidate' but unfortunately they didn't give me the job and I was so disappointed … I said: 'Oh my God, wherever I go they'll all be saying to you: "You look young, you're still going to have a family"' and there was no way of convincing … them … I read … that if there was an open area [i.e. where doctors were free to set up new practices] you can open your surgery so I decided to go that way.[14]

The narrative presented here is one of a doctor taking action as a result of structural constraints. General practice was therefore, in one sense, one of the limited options available to South Asian doctors, but also an opportunity to be one's 'own boss' and to occupy a prominent position in particular communities. The 'choice' to go into general practice can therefore be seen as an entrepreneurial act. It appears more explicitly as such in Sri Venugopal's description of his entry into general practice in Birmingham:

> Aston is inner-city, deprived, it's mostly Irish and African families who went there. At the time, immigration from the Indian subcontinent was growing and a lot of Indian families were coming in, living next to each other. Also, Kenyan Asians were coming in: there was a lot of opportunities, a lot of new patients. It was a tough and deprived area but I wanted to work there.[15]

Oral history interviews where participants describe being in control of their destiny and shaping their lives through their actions should clearly be treated with caution. Who would not want to recall their life in such terms? This is arguably particularly the case in situations where people have faced discrimination. It is conceivable that doctors overemphasised the extent to which they were able to influence their professional trajectories at the time. What appears beyond doubt is that ultimately, they were able to reconcile themselves to careers in general practice and actively chose to enter the field.

The opening of a surgery was a constrained choice actively made by South Asian doctors rather than a career option that was purposefully presented to them in a coordinated fashion by the British government or the NHS administration. The 'open areas' mentioned by P. L. Pathak are a reference to what were known as 'under-doctored' areas where there were no administrative obstacles to opening up practices[16] as a consequence of the long-established trends that led to an unequal distribution of GPs in Great Britain.[17] This offered South Asian doctors a way into the profession that could be embraced as an opportunity. By definition, these opportunities were available in areas that were unpopular with British medical graduates. Sri Venugopal described opening a surgery in Aston, in inner-city Birmingham, while Dr P. L. Pathak found a niche in general practice in Rusholme, in inner-city Manchester (Figure 5). When she was asked to pose for a photograph after the interview she gave for the project, she chose to stand in front of

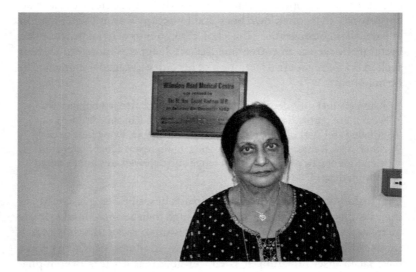

**Figure 5**  Self-staged portrait of Dr P. L. Pathak at her practice in Rusholme, inner-city Manchester.

a plaque commemorating the opening of her practice, adding to a sense that she saw herself as an actor of the development of healthcare, rather than simply filling a particular professional role.

The gaps in British healthcare provision thus gave migrant South Asian doctors a space in which they had at least some scope to create their own professional trajectory and lay claim to agency. In his memoirs, the Leicester GP Akram Sayeed gives a description of becoming a GP that bears witness to the professional reluctance of other doctors to make it easy for their South Asian colleagues to enter general practice and the resulting creation of a professional opportunity by a doctor reliant on his own judgement and professional contacts:

> I started looking for a suitable practice to go to as partner. Again, it turned out to be very disquieting; in two interviews I was faced with the first question: 'Why on earth does an overseas doctor want to get into general practice in this country?' ... Consultations with the Asian community leaders ... helped me to make the decision. I would start a completely fresh practice on the eastern side of Leicester.[18]

Sayeed had earlier described how his initial move into general practice had been prompted by the desire of members of the local South Asian community to be able to draw upon the services of a South Asian practitioner and the availability of work in a practice staffed by a Central European doctor:

> One Friday in early February, after the Juma—the Friday midday prayer—one Pakistani gentleman took me to the Leicester Executive Council Office [an administrative body responsible for local general practice]. Some members of the Pakistani and Indian community were requesting me repeatedly to enter into general practice as there was not an Asian doctor in the city, and the sizeable Asian community was finding it quite difficult to manage. As requested, I left my details ... The following Monday morning I received a telephone call from one Dr Ludwig, a Polish doctor with a dual practice in the West End and St Nicholas Circle. His senior partner had died suddenly on the previous Saturday ... I found myself in the shoes of the late Dr Myers.[19]

Akram Sayeed's account of trying to launch a career in general practice is typical of the experiences of South Asian doctors who wanted to become GPs in the NHS. There were two main ways into the profession. As qualified doctors, they could, at the time, simply choose to establish their own practice and count on being able to build up a patient list. The other way into the profession was to find work in an established practice where racism and heterophobia were not insurmountable obstacles. This also generally involved being located in industrial areas with high proportions of working-class patients. When it came to posts in these parts of Britain, other South Asian doctors could play a role in facilitating the entry of South Asian colleagues into general practice, as Sri Venugopal recalled:

> The locum I did was for the late Dr Saidi from India. He had been in UK from the late forties. He was an elderly gentleman, a well-respected doctor in that area. He was going for 2 months and it was difficult to get a locum to do continuous cover. I had holidays, it was convenient, I said I would do it. He was very good, like an elder brother to me. But he was also a teacher and it was him who introduced me to general practice.[20]

Once one South Asian doctor had succeeded in getting established in a particular area, they could then offer support to others. Burgeoning networks of South Asian doctors were undoubtedly a factor when it came to obtaining positions in general practice and this was the case even before the inception of the NHS.[21] The accounts of South Asian GPs however provide a much more general sense that the pressures of providing a service in industrial and working-class areas and the difficulties involved in finding doctors willing to staff particular surgeries meant that opportunities were available to South Asian GPs if they wanted to take them up. Shiv Pande's account of becoming a GP suggests that he was offered work as a result of the 'plight' of the single-handed doctor and his entrepreneurial assessment of where work was likely to be available, rather than because of ethnic solidarity:

> After doing the … training, when I finished, I felt that: 'Who will be needing me as a locum?'. In a group practice they will be covering each other so they won't need me. So I rung a few single-handed doctors that if you need me I'm available. And it so happened that Dr Paes in Liverpool … I rung him on Friday and unfortunately he had a … heart attack that evening. And see, that is the plight of a single-handed doctor: when he was being taken by an ambulance, he was telling his wife— he was a Goanese doctor married to a Welsh lady—and he was telling her 'Dilys, Dr Pande's number is there on my desk and he is available, give him a ring'. And it so happened that … my mother had come … so

we had gone to Isle of Man for weekend visit. She started ringing from Friday evening till Sunday evening, must have rung twenty times and on Sunday evening at about six o'clock when I picked the phone up, she was the happiest person ... because she had no doctor to look after ... Dr Paes' patients.[22]

It is notable that whereas doctors found it difficult to progress in prestigious hospital specialties, accounts of going into general practice point to the intensity of the need for doctors in particular parts of the country and to the pressure that practitioners who were already in a post were under. Both Akram Sayeed and Shiv Pande recall very short periods of time elapsing between expressing an interest in a role and being offered it. One talks of his predecessor dying suddenly, the other of the doctor he had spoken to being taken seriously ill. Akram Sayeed writes of being approached by the local South Asian community who were, he says, 'finding it quite difficult to manage'. Shiv Pande's memories provide an insight into the pressures on primary care provision in industrial cities such as Liverpool in the 1970s. His story of how an ill doctor's wife repeatedly called his number over a period of days as there was nobody else available to deal with patients signals that such opportunities were available to South Asian doctors at least in part because nobody else was competing against them. It is also notable that the doctor who had suffered a heart attack was himself from the Indian subcontinent.

One of the telling characteristics of South Asian doctors' accounts of their entry into general practice was the extent to which it involved encounters with female doctors, Scottish doctors, doctors from Northern Ireland and Eire, Central European doctors, African doctors as well as other South Asian doctors who had found themselves working in less desirable areas. The contrast with attempts to progress in hospital hierarchies dominated by white male consultants was marked. Even before the inception of the NHS, a substantial number of practices had been dependent on migrant and otherwise marginalised practitioners. A study of general practice in the London borough of Camden in the 1960s concluded that:

The predominant picture is of ageing, single-handed doctors, many of them trained in Central European or Mediterranean countries, working in isolation from inadequate premises and by-passed by many of the innovations in the delivery of medical care. Many of the features of practice in the Borough appeared characteristic of metropolitan general practice.[23]

It seems reasonable to assume that a non-negligible proportion of these Camden-based practitioners who were described as 'ageing' in the 1960s had been working in Britain when the NHS was set up. Little is known about these doctors' work in general practice or how they came to occupy such roles. One interview conducted for an oral history of general practice from the 1930s to the 1950s does however point to parallels with the subsequent experiences of South Asian doctors. Margarete Tuteur Samuel came to Britain from Germany in the 1930s. She was initially minded to pursue a career in psychiatry but recalled being told by a psychiatrist that as 'A Jewish person with your accent, coming from Germany, you'll never make a career here'.[24]

Once more, the importance that we can attach to this memory lies not in any belief in its literal truth (although there is no particular reason to believe it to be inaccurate either). What it does signal is that British medicine's history of making migrant doctors feel like outsiders is a long one. Margarete Tuteur Samuel's reaction was to enter general practice, which she saw as offering her an obvious opportunity to define a professional role for herself: 'I thought, I'm going in a Jewish district and I'm going to work with Jewish women and children. That's what I did.'[25] She subsequently had a career in general practice and reported that three quarters of her patients were Jewish.[26] Her testimony serves to connect the history of South Asian GPs to longer trends in British medicine, characterised by the devolution of certain aspects of care to incomers.

Hira Lal Kapur's first job in general practice was in the coastal resort of Morecambe in the North West of England where he worked alongside a female doctor from Glasgow of East European ancestry.[27] Rupendra Kumar Majumdar recalled being offered a job in the Welsh Valleys by a Central European doctor who did not know him without being interviewed for the position, which is once more suggestive of a lack of competition for these posts:

> I did ... twenty to twenty-four [applications] to the various places, within a week, I received an ... answer that ... says the practice is yours if you come and join ... I just told my wife that it's very strange, he hasn't

seen me, he doesn't know me and he is … offering the practice. And he says that we will work as a father and son.[28]

This recourse to language from the realm of the personal and private highlights the fact that the destinies of different generations of migrant doctors and other marginalised professionals became intertwined through their confinement to specific social and medical roles. A moving illustration of this process is provided by F. B. Kotwall, a Parsee doctor who worked in the small town of Spennymoor in the industrial north-east of England. He spoke of his sense of connection through religion to his older partner, a practising Jew who had migrated from Central Europe:

> Dr Brauer was German, of Jewish origin … What I found enchanting was that when the Jewish festival came round, he used to pray in the same way as the Parsees pray … rocking the body back and forward with a book in his hand. He was very good to me. He had to flee Germany because he was Jewish and he had to come to the UK in 1938–39. He was first put in a … camp because he was German, they then released him when they realised he was not a threat and he came into general practice.[29]

A working-class town therefore provided a professional environment for marginalised doctors of different generations and different backgrounds throughout the first forty years of the NHS.

Even though South Asian doctors were moving into general practice in areas that local graduates did not consider desirable, this development was not met with universal approval by the government or the medical profession—as already indicated by doctors' accounts of attending job interviews. Two of the GPs interviewed for this project described strong resistance to their entry into general practice as single-handed practitioners in the areas they worked in and one reported only being given the right to open his practice after appealing to central government.[30] The movement of South Asian doctors into general practice appears as primarily driven by their agency rather than by the agendas of central government or bodies representing the medical profession.

Notes of discussions between the Department of Health and Social Security (DHSS), the GMC and the BMA in the late 1960s reveal these organisations to have been observers rather than orchestrators of the movement of South Asian doctors into general practice, with figures showing an increase in the numbers of overseas-trained GPs being circulated and analysed.[31] Officials discussed the potential lowering of the status of general practice amongst British graduates as a result of migrant doctors entering the profession without undergoing vocational training[32] and the fact that white doctors might feel obliged to hire an unsuitably qualified overseas doctor because of fears of being challenged under the Race Relations Act.[33] BMA notes of a meeting with the DHSS and the GMC in May 1969 suggest official concern rather than any sense that an increased reliance on migrant doctors was a deliberately engineered solution to staffing shortages in general practice:

> It was apparent that, apart from restricted areas which already had their full complement of general practitioners, there was no legal authority to preclude doctors from overseas who were fully recognised with the General Medical Council from filling a vacancy in a designated area or from putting up their plates and practising single-handed ... In the case of those who set up in single-handed practice, reliance must be placed upon the discretion of the public in registering with a doctor who might not be fully conversant with the manners and the customs of this country.[34]

If South Asian doctors were helping to address shortages in the staffing of general practice at the time, this was the result of their willingness to open practices and to take on 'special' jobs rather than the consequence of a deliberate policy aimed at directing them towards areas of high need.

It is questionable naturally that when doctors described becoming GPs decades after the event, they were giving an entirely accurate description of their thought processes at the time. What their interviews do however reveal is that although they shared white British-born and -trained doctors' reluctance to become GPs, they found ways of reaching an accommodation with what was in most cases a professional and personal compromise. Of course, it is also possible that the UK government found it politically convenient to tolerate the large-scale movement of South Asian doctors into general practice without feeling the need to share this perspective explicitly with representatives of the medical profession. Civil servants were certainly aware from the 1960s that certain parts of Britain had become dependent on overseas-trained

GPs.[35] Governments also had the power to do something about the absence of 'legal authority' preventing doctors from moving into general practice. They did not and might have been content to allow this to happen. It remains that the constrained agency of South Asian doctors seeking to build careers in general practice was the main driver behind the staffing of hundreds of GP surgeries between the late 1940s and the early 1980s.

## The structural impact of South Asian medical migration on British primary care

The function fulfilled by South Asian doctors in the early years of the NHS is therefore one of meeting not just the recruitment needs of British general practice in general but more specifically those of general practice in the areas where it was hardest to recruit. It was noteworthy that the vast majority of interviews carried out with doctors revealed that their main practice area was in a deprived inner-city area, a (former) industrial town or a coalfield community. The four exceptions to this pattern amongst interviewees were three doctors who benefited from the patronage of colleagues who helped them find work in practices based in more desirable areas and a fourth doctor who went to work at the surgery her husband was based in.[36] The fact that South Asian doctors were becoming GPs masked the recruitment problems that were affecting the field.

Moreover, it is conceivable that general practice would have continued to function without these doctors had they been evenly distributed throughout the system. It is their over-representation in particular parts of Britain that made them indispensable to the development of general practice. By the 1980s, 16 per cent of the overall GP workforce had been born in the Indian subcontinent. The fact that in some areas South Asian GPs accounted for between a third and half (Table 1) of all general practitioners means that provision would have been very severely affected in their absence. There are therefore two dimensions to the structural impact that the agency of South Asian doctors had on the development of general practice. Because they were being directed towards general practice, they contributed to maintaining overall staffing levels. Because they were also over-represented in industrial and inner-city areas, they were playing an essential role in enabling primary care to continue to exist as a central dimension of the British healthcare system.

## Maintaining the levels of the GP workforce

Although the 1960s have been described as a turning point for British general practice, following the introduction of the Family Doctors' Charter and as a result of moves towards greater invest-ment in primary care, recruitment to the field remained problem-atic. The image of general practice did gradually evolve between the late 1940s and the early 1980s as detailed in Chapter 1 but entering the field was still an unpopular career choice amongst graduates of British medical schools.[37] This was particularly true in less popular areas such as the industrial north of England. In 1961, the *Guardian* newspaper quoted an official of the left-wing Medical Practitioners' Union as saying that 'few people' had applied to take over when established doctors' practices had become available in the North and that local NHS executive councils were sometimes 'at their wits' end to look after their patients' due to a local shortage of doctors (and dentists).[38]

Not only was general practice unpopular with British graduates but the influx of doctors from across the Irish Sea had also slowed by the mid-twentieth century. Medical migrants from Ireland had started to favour the USA as a destination over Great Britain.[39] The number of doctors born in Northern Ireland or the Irish Republic and practising as unrestricted principals in general practice declined from 1,901 in 1968 to 1,294 in 1978.[40] Central European practitioners who had come to Britain in the 1930s and 1940s were for their part reaching retire-ment age by the 1960s and 1970s. The presence of South Asian doctors in the NHS workforce compensated both for the lack of British-born and -trained doctors willing to take on these roles and the decreasing availability of other sources of migrant labour.

The fact that increasing numbers of South Asian doctors were com-ing to Britain and subsequently choosing to become general practition-ers had a considerable impact on overall staffing levels in the NHS. This process gathered pace from the 1960s. A study looking at the recruit-ment of general practitioners in Essex and Birmingham found that the percentage of doctors qualified in India and Pakistan was very small until 1960 and increased markedly afterwards.[41] At a meeting at the

Department of Health and Social Security in 1969, a BMA official noted that he was getting 'a growing volume of enquiries from overseas doctors about the regulations for getting into general practice.'[42]

The rise in the numbers of South Asian hospital doctors after the establishment of the NHS led to increasing numbers of these doctors opting for general practice. Between 1968 and 1975, 78 per cent of the increase in the number of GPs in England and Wales was accounted for by overseas-born doctors.[43] This was largely attributable to the entry of South Asian hospital doctors into general practice. In 1968, overseas doctors accounted for 11.8 per cent of GP principals in Great Britain.[44] By 1975, doctors born outside of the British Isles made up 18.3 per cent of the UK GP population and half of these overseas doctors were born in the Indian subcontinent.[45] By the mid-1970s, the post-imperial movement of South Asian doctors had therefore resulted in the NHS drawing just under a tenth of its GP workforce from India, Pakistan, Bangladesh or Sri Lanka. The annual reports produced by the UK government's Chief Medical Officer in the 1970s provide further details regarding the extent of the impact of South Asian medical migration on NHS general practice. The 1975 report noted that the UK was becoming dependent on doctors from outside the British Isles to staff primary care.[46] The 1979 edition reported that 'only' 25 per cent of those entering general practice for the first time were from overseas—the figure for the previous year had been 31 per cent.[47]

These developments are reflected in figures that show that between 1968 and 1978, the percentage of unrestricted principals in general practice born in Great Britain fell from 79.8 per cent to 76.3 per cent and the proportion of GPs born on the island of Ireland fell from 8.4 per cent to 5.1 per cent.[48] The percentage of doctors born 'elsewhere', in contrast, rose from 11.8 to 18.6 per cent.[49] As has already been noted, a large proportion of the doctors who made up this category were from the Indian subcontinent.

Between 1949 and 1979, the number of doctors in general medical practice in England and Wales increased from 19,200 to 22,100.[50] The difference between the two figures roughly equates to the increase in the number of South Asian doctors working in general practice during this period. One observer estimated that at least 1,000 Indian doctors were working in the UK in the early 1950s.[51] Even if we accept this figure (as previously noted it appears rather high) and assume that nearly all of these doctors were GPs, their numbers rose by at least 3,000 over the following four decades: by the late 1980s, over 4,300 GPs working in the NHS were born in India, Pakistan, Bangladesh or Sri Lanka.[52] The influx of these doctors into general practice resulted in doctors' average patient list sizes remaining stable between 1958 and 1977, rising slightly from 2,234 to 2,275.[53]

Medical migration was instrumental in ensuring that the NHS was able to maintain staffing levels as the UK population rose. In 1971, *The Times* noted that for the first time since 1958 the number of GP principals had increased at a faster rate than the number of patients, mainly because significant numbers of foreign-born doctors were becoming GPs.[54]

### Delivering Bevan's vision in primary care settings

The overall figures do not however truly do justice to the importance of South Asian doctors to the staffing of general practice. Their movement into general practice was principally an influx into the parts of Britain that experienced the highest levels of medical need: industrial towns and inner-cities. Although there is no detailed statistical evidence of the concentration of South Asian[55] doctors in these parts of Britain up to the 1980s, as Table 1 shows, in the early 1990s a third of practitioners in the (post-) industrial cities of Manchester and Sunderland and over 50 per cent in working-class parts of Greater London (Barking and Havering) and the industrial Midlands (Walsall) had been trained as doctors in the Indian subcontinent. The figures for the more rural and traditionally portrayed as picturesque areas such as Somerset and Devon were 0.87 per cent and 1.29 per cent respectively. The more working-class and the more urban or industrialised an area, the more likely it was to be reliant on South Asian GPs. Admittedly, these statistics do not relate directly to the first forty years of the NHS but it is simply not credible to believe that doctors would have suddenly moved en masse to these parts of Britain in the late 1980s or early 1990s, particularly as the authors of the article these figures are drawn from noted that most of these doctors were approaching retirement age.[56] Moreover, official government figures from the 1970s confirm that this pattern was already established well before (see Table 2). They show that 2,106 doctors born in India, Pakistan, Sri Lanka and Bangladesh were working as

**Table 1** South Asian-trained GPs in different areas of England and Wales in 1992.*

| Family health services authority | Percentage of general practitioners who qualified in South Asia |
| --- | --- |
| Barking and Havering | 56.50 |
| Walsall | 51.59 |
| Wales 5 | 43.90 |
| City and East London | 42.25 |
| Salford | 37.50 |
| Sunderland | 31.85 |
| Manchester | 30.00 |
| Birmingham | 29.79 |
| Kensington, Chelsea and Westminster | 10.59 |
| Northumberland | 8.18 |
| Wales 4 | 3.42 |
| Devon | 1.29 |
| Somerset | 0.87 |
| Cornwall and the Isles of Scilly | 0.75 |

* Adapted from D. H. Taylor Jr and A. Esmail, 'Retrospective analysis of census data on general practitioners who qualified in South Asia: Who will replace them as they retire?', *BMJ*, 1999 (318), pp. 307–8.

unrestricted principals in the NHS at the time.[57] Although they provide a less precise picture of the deployment of South Asian doctors, only showing regions, the tendency for South Asian doctors to cluster in industrial areas is already pronounced. Large numbers of physicians had established themselves in industrial regions such as the North-West and the West Midlands. The figures for Greater London (Thames) show that they were present in greater numbers in the eastern regions, which were traditionally more working-class. As the data from the 1990s showed, concentrations of South Asian doctors in less industrialised areas, such as Wessex or the South-West, were lower.

There is ample additional evidence that overseas doctors tended to be over-represented in areas of high demand that were unpopular with locally-born and -trained doctors. Earlier research in the 1960s and 1970s had already shown that locations such as Birmingham and

**Table 2** Distribution of South Asian GPs in England and Wales in 1974.*

| Regional Health Authority | Number of unrestricted GP principals born in India, Pakistan, Sri Lanka and Bangladesh |
|---|---|
| Northern | 99 |
| Yorkshire | 136 |
| Trent | 208 |
| East Anglia | 25 |
| NW Thames | 167 |
| NE Thames | 294 |
| SE Thames | 188 |
| SW Thames | 96 |
| Wessex | 39 |
| Oxford | 54 |
| South Western | 35 |
| West Midlands | 312 |
| Mersey | 64 |
| North Western | 259 |
| Wales | 130 |

* General Medical Services—England and Wales, 1 October 1974. Number of unrestricted principals: analysis by Regional Health Authority and country of birth, ACE J 32-2 Primary care in inner cities 1977–1981 ACE J 32-3 Symposium on problems of care in inner cities 1980, File 20/2, Archives of the Royal College of General Practitioners.

Barking and Havering had high concentrations of South Asian GPs and that migrant doctors were more likely to be found working in conurbations.[58] The survey of migrant medics conducted for David Smith's *Overseas Doctors in the NHS* found that 3 per cent of overseas doctors working as GPs were based in the Wessex and South Western Regional Health Authorities as opposed to 22 per cent who were in the Oxford and West Midlands areas.[59]

The highest concentration of South Asian GPs noted by Taylor and Esmail in the 1990s was in Barking and Havering. Findings from a study published in 1979 showed that 45 per cent of doctors in general practice in this working-class area of Greater London in 1975 were already from

outside of the UK: three times the then national average.[60] The percentage was poised to increase as 100 per cent of trainees as well as
70 per cent of recruits into general practice in 1976/77 had graduated
outside of the UK and the Republic of Ireland.[61] The researchers make
it clear that it was principally South Asian doctors who were moving
into general practice in an area where there was an established pattern
of dependency on migrant doctors:

> There have been two waves of immigrant doctors into the Region—
> one from Europe in the pre-war period and the more recent flow of
> Commonwealth doctors mainly from India and Pakistan. The European
> doctors are now at the end of their working life, having graduated—in
> many instances—more than 40 years ago.[62]

Another study conducted in Essex and Birmingham found that by the
mid-1960s, 15.8 per cent of recruits in the former and 26.8 per cent
in the latter had qualified in Asia or in the Middle East—with most of
these doctors having been trained in India or Pakistan.[63] An additional
significant group of migrant doctors was in evidence in these areas,
namely the Irish who made up 12.2 per cent of recruits in Birmingham
and 7.5 per cent in Essex at the same time.[64]

In the late 1970s, the GMSC and some Family Practitioner
Committees (local bodies with responsibility for primary care which
replaced Executive Councils in the early 1970s) were concerned about
future recruitment in areas which were unpopular with local graduates
as 'the entry of doctors of overseas origin willing to go to these areas
cannot be expected to continue at the same rate as in recent years', providing further evidence of the increasing dependency of British general
practice on overseas doctors.[65]

The fact that the Chief Medical Officer's report for 1979 found that
the number of patients living in under-doctored areas had fallen by over
one million[66] is therefore in great part attributable to the decisions of
South Asian doctors to enter general practice and to the fact that their
options in the field were limited to work in areas likely to be under-
doctored. The professional and personal choices of doctors from the
Indian subcontinent were supporting the provision of services and
serving to avoid the need for the type of policy response which would
have been necessary to attract indigenous graduates or indeed one
which would have led to the development of a different type of primary

care provision. The relationship between British general practice and South Asian doctors was one of dependency: the field could not have existed at the time in the form that it took without their labour.

## Conclusion

Britain's ability to rely on an overseas supply of doctors drawn to a great extent from the Indian subcontinent was instrumental in shaping the provision of primary care at a local and national level in the first four decades of the NHS. In the second reading of the NHS Bill before the House of Commons in 1946, Aneurin Bevan stated that the first reason that justified the establishment of the NHS was the need to deal with the 'evil' that was the link between money and the provision of medical services.[67] Although in absolute terms the numbers of South Asian doctors may be relatively small, due to their extreme concentration in particular parts of the country and the nature of the role of general practitioners, their presence was hugely significant in enabling the NHS to provide care to the sections of British society that had historically found it difficult to access treatment because of concerns around cost.

The availability of a workforce acquired as a result of post-imperial dynamics and its subsequent deployment as a result of the agency of doctors operating in a racist and heterophobic environment were fundamental characteristics of the history of general practice. If it can be argued that without racism there would be no specialism of geriatrics,[68] the same can be said of general practice provision between the 1940s and the 1980s in inner cities, working-class towns and mining communities without racism and heterophobia, allied to the willingness of South Asian doctors to take on medical 'dirty work'.

Unlike two other fields which were also heavily dependent on migrant doctors, psychiatry and geriatrics, which involve care for specific patient groups, general practice placed South Asian doctors in roles where they were in contact with a substantial proportion of the general population. In 1967, Paul Ferris estimated that GPs saw close to a million people a week, which was roughly equivalent to one-sixtieth of the UK population.[69] The movement of South Asian doctors into the specialty had a profound effect on the day-to-day functioning of the British healthcare system and its long-term development.

## Notes

1  N. Shah interview with author, 7 June 2010.
2  R. Prasad interview with author.
3  BLSA, C900/03116, Millennium Memory Bank, R. Lawrence interviewed by J. Rogers, 1999.
4  M. S. Kausar interview with author.
5  M. A. Khaled interview with author, 2 April 2010.
6  Anonymous interview with author.
7  M. N. I. Talukdar interview with author.
8  D. Ray interview with author, 5 December 2008.
9  U. Rao interview with author.
10  K. S. Bhanumathi interview with author.
11  Bornat et al., 'The making of careers', pp. 342–50.
12  S. A. A. Gilani interview with author, 30 June 2010.
13  K. Korlipara interview with author.
14  P. L. Pathak interview with author.
15  S. Venugopal interview with author.
16  BMA, Problems of overseas doctors in UK re employment, Report of a meeting with representatives of the Department of Health and Social Security, General Medical Council and British Medical Association, 27 May 1969.
17  Webster, *Political History*, p. 57; Hann & Gravelle, 'Maldistribution', pp. 894–8.
18  Sayeed, *Taqdir*, p. 122.
19  Sayeed, *Taqdir*, p. 164.
20  S. Venugopal interview with author.
21  R. Boomla interview with author, 16 September 2009; BLSA, C648/28/01–05, Oral history of general practice 1936–1952, S. Kutar interviewed by M. Bevan, 1993.
22  S. Pande interview with author, 23 November 2009.
23  V. W. Sidel, M. Jefferys, P. J. Mansfield, 'General practice in the London borough of Camden: Report of an enquiry in 1968', *Journal of the Royal College of General Practitioners*, 22 (Suppl.3) (1972), p. 1.
24  BLSA, C648/62/01–03, 'Oral History of General Practice 1936–1952', Margarete Tuteur Samuel interviewed by Michael Bevan, 1993.
25  Ibid.
26  Ibid.

27  H. L. Kapur interview with author.
28  R. K. Majumdar interview with author.
29  F. B. Kotwall interview with author.
30  M. S. Kausar interview with author; anonymous interview with author.
31  BMA, Problems of overseas doctors in UK re employment, Report of a meeting with representatives of the Department of Health and Social Security, General Medical Council and British Medical Association, 27 May 1969; BMA, Problems of overseas doctors in UK re employment, Note of a meeting between representatives of the Department of Health and the British Medical Association, 22 October 1969.
32  BMA, Problems of overseas doctors in UK re employment, Note of a meeting between representatives of the Department of Health and the British Medical Association, 22 October 1969.
33  Ibid.
34  BMA, Problems of overseas doctors in UK re employment, Report of a meeting with representatives of the Department of Health and Social Security, General Medical Council and British Medical Association, 27 May 1969.
35  National Archives, MH149/352, Ministry of Health, Note 8 September 1965.
36  Anonymous interview with author; K. Korlipara interview with author; A. Chaudhuri interview with author; K. S. Bhanumathi interview with author.
37  Berridge, *Health and Society*, p. 42.
38  'North fails to draw enough doctors: Shortage of dentists, too', the *Guardian* (11 September 1961), p. 16.
39  Gish, 'The Irish case', p. 675; G. Jones, '"A mysterious discrimination": Irish medical emigration to the United States in the 1950s', in Monnais & Wright, *Doctors Beyond Borders*.
40  BMA, Executive Committee of Council 1978–79, Report of a working party on medical manpower, staffing and training requirements, 9 May 1979.
41  Cargill, 'Recruitment to general practice'.
42  BMA, E/2541/9, Record of a Meeting held at Alexander Fleming House on 27 May 1969.
43  Department of Employment, *The role of immigrants in the labour market*, pp. 58–9.

44  BMA, Minutes of Executive Committee of Council 1978–79, Report of a working party on medical manpower, staffing and training requirements, Distribution of Overseas Doctors in Great Britain, 9 May 1979.

45  Department of Employment, *The Role of Immigrants in the Labour market*, p. 58.

46  Department of Health and Social Security, *On the state of public health: the annual report of the Chief Medical Officer of the Department of Health and Social Security for the year 1975*, p. 55.

47  Department of Health and Social Security, *On the state of public health: the annual report of the Chief Medical Officer of the Department of Health and Social Security for the year 1979*, p. 112.

48  BMA, Executive Committee of Council 1978–79, Report of a working party on medical manpower, staffing and training requirements, 9 May 1979.

49  Ibid.

50  Webster, *Health Services*, Vol. II, p. 828.

51  Kondapi, *Indians Overseas*, p. 360.

52  Gill, 'General practitioners', pp. 107 & 111.

53  BMA, Executive Committee of Council 1978–79, Report of a working party on medical manpower, staffing and training requirements, 9 May 1979.

54  J. Roper, 'Influx of foreign doctors kept lists of patients down in 1970 but hospitals were busier', *The Times* (5 August 1971), p. 4.

55  Naturally, doctors who qualified in South Asia were not necessarily South Asian but the overwhelming majority of them were.

56  Taylor & Esmail, 'Retrospective analysis', p. 306.

57  As previously mentioned, figures which only count unrestricted principals in general practice do not account for all GPs.

58  R. F. L. Logan, J. A. Roberts, P. Stockton, 'General practice – The immigrant doctor in N.E.T.R.H.A.', *Medicos*, 4:1 (1979), pp. 3–5; Cargill, 'Recruitment to general practice', p. 669; Smith, *Overseas Doctors*, p. 211.

59  Smith, *Overseas Doctors*, p. 211.

60  Logan et al., 'The immigrant doctor', p. 3.

61  Ibid.

62  Ibid.

63  Cargill, 'Recruitment to general practice', p. 669.

64  Ibid.

65  RCGP, ACE J 32-2, Primary care in inner cities 1977–1981, Primary health care in conurbations: general medical practice, December 1977.

66  Department of Health and Social Security, *On the state of public health: the annual report of the Chief Medical Officer of the Department of Health and Social Security for the year 1979*, p. 112.

67  Hansard, vol. 422, cc. 43–142, HC Deb, 30 April 1946, accessed 24 May 2013 at: http://hansard.millbanksystems.com/commons/1946/apr/30/national-health-service-bill#S5cv0422PO-19460430-hoc-7.

68  Raghuram et al., 'Ethnic clustering', p. 295.

69  Ferris, *The Doctors*, p. 119.

# Part III

# Shaping British medicine and British society

# 6

# 'The more you did, the more they depended on you': memories of practice on the periphery

Having described how doctors came to be in Britain, the discrimination that they faced and the processes leading to their geographical clustering, I will now turn my attention to their interactions with their environment and the influence they had on British society and medicine. The present chapter draws on doctors' accounts to explore the nature of general practice in the first forty years of the NHS in the peripheral areas where many medical migrants built careers. If migrant doctors provided labour they also served to perpetuate the existence of what might be termed a medical frontier zone, where practice developed in parallel with mainstream healthcare provision and in ways that politicians and the medical profession had limited influence on. Referring to these areas as peripheral is of course not to say that their status was a natural product of their location (they were not peripheral from the perspective of those who lived in them) but to describe their position within the British healthcare system. Doctors' accounts of their working lives provide insights into their contribution to general practice and into the distinctive nature of medicine as it was practised in such areas.

I start by discussing the relationships between doctors and patients in general and by reflecting on the meaning that can be drawn from the ways in which doctors describe being able to successfully build careers and establish positive relationships with local populations. Migrant practitioners carved out a medical niche for themselves by defining a common cause with patients. The second part of this chapter offers an examination of the nature of the relationship between South Asian doctors and ethnic minority patients. I conclude by outlining the problematic nature of the disengagement of the mainstream of British medicine from large parts of Britain and the resulting dependency of particular populations on migrant doctors who were themselves frequently professionally marginalised.

## Embracing 'dirty work'; finding common ground

If entering general practice was a logical option to pursue for practitioners who found themselves with limited career options within a racist and heterophobic NHS, it also involved encountering an additional potential barrier. A doctor pursuing a career as a GP was ultimately dependent on a degree of patient goodwill. The fact that large concentrations of South Asian doctors built up in major conurbations and in coalfield communities shows that doctors were able to gain acceptance from thousands of people. In light of the points that have been made about British attitudes towards immigration from the 1960s onwards and the hostility towards outsiders that prevailed in British medicine, the fact that thousands of doctors from the Indian subcontinent were able to enjoy successful careers as GPs requires to be explained. It is quite conceivable that patients could have systematically chosen to register with a white British-trained doctor where one was available. Equally, there could have been large-scale patient protests against the fact that significant numbers of British 'family doctors' were non-white and overseas trained.

In fact, the geographical clustering of South Asian doctors generated relatively little hostile reaction, which undoubtedly explains in part why it has received scant attention from historians. As Mica Nava has pointed out, it is important to acknowledge that whilst racism and discrimination were undoubtedly powerful social forces in postwar Britain, there was also a space in which more welcoming attitudes towards migrants and anti-racism could emerge.[1] This chapter offers a reflection, based on their accounts of their experiences, on how practice on the periphery came to be a professional and personal haven for South Asian doctors.

The way in which South Asian doctors talk about their careers suggests that their embracing of medical 'dirty work' in pursuit of a career in the NHS led to them building acceptable and at times fulfilling and satisfying relationships with patients. This type of account might, to an extent, be seen as a natural product of oral history interviews where participants might be tempted to construct positive accounts of their lives.

However, their stories do not ignore difficult episodes of racism and exclusion. Nor do they suggest an unproblematic acceptance. Doctors' descriptions of exchanges with patients on the periphery differ from those of contacts with the medical profession and also hint at the fact they were accepted as professionals filling a specific skills gap rather than as migrants, members of an ethnic minority group or middle-class professionals. Whilst these accounts are clearly subjective, they also offer an insight into what was a social reality: it is hard to imagine that doctors would have been able to function as professionals for periods of decades without at least a degree of acceptance. The overwhelming impression given by doctors is that whilst they may have faced serious obstacles within the medical profession or in wider society, as general practitioners, they were accepted and embraced by the majority of the populations they served.

It is of course conceivable that patient racism is a subject that doctors were reluctant to discuss and that to thrive in general practice doctors had to develop ways of sublimating the presence of racism in society and amongst patients. There is evidence that some doctors faced hostility, which at times manifested as violence. An Asian GP in Coventry was fatally stabbed by a teenager in Coventry in a racially-motivated attack in 1981, although it seems he was targeted as a result of his ethnicity and that the attack was random rather than aimed specifically at a doctor who had settled in the area.[2] In a GMC hearing in 1976, an Indian doctor working in the village of Caistor in Lincolnshire claimed that female patients had made complaints against him as part of a racially-motivated plot to force him out of the area. This explanation seemed credible to the local vicar who appeared as a witness for the doctor and stated that 'I can well see and well appreciate, Caistor being the sort of place that it is, that it could be so', a somewhat equivocal but nevertheless unambiguous indication from an outsider that patient racism could have an impact on migrant medical professionals.[3] Of the doctors interviewed for this book, one reported having received a racially motivated death threat; another was attacked, suffering life-threatening injuries.[4] Both of these incidents took place after the period under examination in this book but this does not imply that similar events were not taking place earlier. It is also possible that if these doctors had been targeted at the beginning rather than towards the end of their careers, they might have chosen to leave their practice area and been harder to locate in the context of this study. One doctor described being attacked in his practice by a drug addict and encountering violence when working in psychiatric departments of hospitals, being called an 'Asian bastard' for refusing to prescribe drugs.[5] Another recalled being 'turfed out', when he went to carry out a home visit, by a patient who said 'I don't want any Pakis here'.[6] Yet another participant related that she had been 'physically thrown out' of a house and faced 'violence, threats when doing visits, physical abuse, mental abuse', although she felt that this could have been the result of a number of factors: her being an Asian woman, having to give patients unwelcome news or social deprivation in the area she was working in at the time.[7] Other participants talk of some patients demanding to see a white doctor at the practice they worked in.[8] The existence of a degree of patient hostility which at times took extreme forms should not be minimised, not least because it may well be a subject doctors preferred not to dwell on in the context of oral history interviews.

Nevertheless, the accounts that doctors give of their relationships with patients contrast markedly with the views that they had of British medicine. If the more desirable hospital roles were seen as out of reach as a result of racism and heterophobia, the social context in which doctors worked as GPs tended to be portrayed as more malleable. This view was not solely the preserve of overseas-trained doctors. One participant apparently tried to second-guess my research agenda and believed I was keen to hear accounts of patient racism. He seemingly strived to identify patterns of racism but struggled to describe his father's experience in the north of England in the early years of the NHS in such terms:

> *What do you remember about his practice and what did he tell you about those early days in general practice?* Surprisingly, he didn't have that many problems ... In one sense, there weren't many Asians in England [in the 1940s]. And if you, I suppose, came from a professional background, and were a doctor, some of the more nasty elements of racism didn't seem to be around. Of course, there were racist comments and all that stuff at times that we all had but ... So, building up his practice was arduous because he started with no patients, but gradually he got to over several thousand patients over many years ... I remember it as quite a contented childhood ... I didn't find anything untoward that was negative ... it was a pleasant time and he built up his practice and worked hard.[9]

What might be dismissed years later as 'racist comments and all that stuff' could of course be corrosive at the time. It is instructive though that even a doctor trying to think of instances of racism in the context of everyday general practice struggled to come up with relevant examples when reflecting on his father's entire career as a practitioner.

Descriptions of relationships with patients have a different quality to those pertaining to the ways in which the British medical profession perceived South Asian doctors. Whilst doctors themselves might be tempted to leave difficult episodes out of interviews, it seems less likely that a doctor's son would express 'surprise' at the fact that his father did not experience grave difficulties and find himself unable to provide instances of problems when he appeared willing to provide them. Similarly, Savitri Chowdhary's account of the relationship between her husband Dharm Sheel Chowdhary (a contemporary of the previous interviewee's father) and his patients in Laindon, near Basildon, in the southern English county of Essex, reads as a world-weary and possibly slightly ironic one rather than an attempt to gloss over any tensions. It projects a sense that her husband was seen primarily as 'a country doctor' rather than as a non-white migrant:

> A country doctor's wife has to accept the fact that her husband is idolised by many of his grateful patients, men, women and even children. He can do nothing wrong, he is the best person on earth to them. You get used to hearing the phrase: 'Oh, he is a darling. He is adorable. He is a real friend besides being a doctor. He has the magic touch. You are lucky to be living with such a wonderful healer.'[10]

Practice in areas in which doctors had settled was therefore perceived as offering an environment where practitioners could first and foremost be seen as professionals. This offers a stark contrast to doctors' descriptions of their experiences as outsiders in the world of medicine.

When it comes to the accounts given by doctors themselves, if they talk at length about the difficulties encountered within the hospital career structure, once they have moved into general practice, the development of relationships with patients is not presented as a major obstacle to be overcome but rather as a gradual and relatively unproblematic process of gaining trust:

> It was just a doctor/patient relationship. In the beginning it was hard to get accepted. In practice when I retired I had 2,200 patients and only

30–40 who are not white—either Pakistan or Caribbean—the rest are local people. I must have got accepted otherwise they would not have stayed for more than one generation. I did not see much difference at all. I was accepted and trusted. There were other doctors there, white doctors, I did not lose patients. *In what way was it difficult to get accepted?* Well you can't blame them—same if a doctor from here sets up a practice in Bangladesh in a village, particularly a man, don't think patients will go and see him and the women will never go. It's similar here. But practising with other partners in early years, gradually, even if people were first not sociable, they get used to it. Human relationships develop after period of time. Many left when I became single practice, but many came as well. I did not take new patients because of workload.[11]

Such accounts cannot realistically be read as simple nostalgia. As mentioned, they contrast with the strong criticisms directed at the culture of medicine. Moreover, doctors did not seek to deny the existence of problems with patients. Nor do they idealise them. Patients are described as having got 'used to' migrant doctors rather than offering an unconditional and warm welcome from the outset.

What doctors describe is in fact what Laura Tabili calls a process of negotiation of inclusion which should invite us to reconsider views of British society as monolithically hostile to incomers.[12] Although Tabili's work on 'natives and newcomers' explores their interactions in the town of South Shields in the North East of England from the mid-nineteenth century to World War II, her conclusions are relevant to understanding how doctors described the development of their relationships with patients, in areas where the population could be overwhelmingly white. For instance, Mohammed Abu Khaled, who was a GP in the Fife coalfields in Scotland, described a relatively straightforward process of gaining acceptance once initial linguistic barriers had been overcome:

As the overseas doctors joined the practice, initially, people did not have any experience of overseas doctors, so I had certain difficulty with the patients and probably in Fife, they had more difficulty to understand me. So definitely, it took a bit time to accept me but when they knew me, they tried to understand me … eventually after a few months I did not have much difficulty … however one or two patients did have some prejudice for overseas doctors but that was very few and I wouldn't say it was any problem and I did not have any abuse or any offensive comment from my patients. When I left the practice, they showed quite respect and sympathy for my service I gave to the community … and the people of Kennoway still have much love and respect for me. So as ethnic doctor in a local community, always will have some problems but it was not a major problem for me in my practice.[13]

It seems therefore that there was more room for negotiated acceptance when it came to relationships with patients, when interviews offered little sense of this being the case in hospital medicine. Ralph Lawrence's memoirs also contrast the attitude of other GPs who were opposed to his arrival as a GP in Derbyshire, and who discouraged patients from joining his practice,[14] with that of the local miners and their families:

There certainly was no racialism amongst the local people who gave me every sign of respect and friendship. One of the first things that I did when I came to the area was to go down a mine to see first-hand the conditions under which many of my patients worked. Our immediate next-door neighbours were miners and we couldn't have wished for better. It was one of them, John Burnham, who took me down the mine and subsequently I became very involved with the St John's Ambulance division of the Derbyshire collieries. I spent many happy years lecturing to them in first aid and judging their local, county and national competitions.[15]

The apparent acceptance of South Asian doctors was not necessarily instantaneous and appears as the product of a process whereby they gradually carved out roles for themselves in local communities. The relationship that Lawrence described can be seen as symptomatic of an objective alliance between doctors seeking a place in Britain and populations in areas where doctors had historically been in short supply. It is possible also that doctors' class status helped them to become integrated into working-class communities.

The central role of migrant doctors in medical provision in areas perceived as peripheral was at times implicitly or explicitly acknowledged by patients, many of whom were from ethnic minority backgrounds themselves but a considerable number of whom were white. Naturally, this would vary from one area to the next. Doctors working in inner-cities could have significant numbers of ethnic minority patients; those working in coalmining villages would be serving a mainly white population. The heterophobia that could be directed towards doctors as immigrants could thus be deflected when they were perceived primarily as medical professionals. One doctor described how the reactions he generated could evolve depending on how likely he was to be perceived primarily as a doctor, a likelihood which varied according to professional and geographical contexts:

> In Wigan, if any Asian person was walking down the road, they will say 'Hello doc, how are you?'. At the time, black, brown people in the town were all in medicine, Indian and Pakistani doctors at the Royal Albert Edward Infirmary. They were well respected. But when I was in London I saw different aspect. In hospital: they knew you as a colleague. Outside, you are a Paki for them. When I went to Liverpool, at the surgery, in the medical profession: you were protected. London is a major international city, they don't have time for anybody. In Liverpool, people have time for others, they will be helpful. But there was lot of resentment: jobs being taken by immigrants ... In ordinary masses there is a love and hate relationship. I was respected as doctor but found it difficult as a brown, coloured man.[16]

Perhaps contrary to expectation, physicians working in areas with very small non-white populations may well have therefore encountered less hostility than those working in areas of greater population diversity as they were primarily identified as medical professionals rather than as migrants or members of an ethnic minority group.[17] Being South Asian in a small community could in fact be seen as an advantage as it had the potential to make it easier to draw on the goodwill associated with doctors' social status:

> The practice was small, almost 100% local population. It was a very small town, there were only 8 GPs in all. Life was very quiet. Everyone there knew I was a doctor: there was one road with shops ... my wife was known as the doctor's wife—she got discounts (laughs). The general rapport with the population was very good. Being Asian, I was more recognisable from that point of view.[18]

When they came to be seen as professionals who were deemed to be playing an important part in the local community, the ethnicity of doctors could be relegated to a secondary consideration for the majority of the populations amongst whom they worked. It does not seem that this acceptance derived purely from class status. Assumedly, most doctors would have been recognisable as middle-class professionals outside of their surgeries. This did not protect them from racist abuse, nor

did their professional status prevent them from encountering difficulties when looking for accommodation.[19] The best explanation for this
is perhaps to be found in the words of one doctor who felt that 'when
they needed help, they did not care who I was'.[20] Sickness and the vul-
nerability it engendered in patients could thus be perceived as serving
to neutralise any sense of resentment towards outsiders. Having gained
acceptance, doctors became embedded in communities that required
their professional skills and they relied on that need for a career, a living
and status.

The lack of historical attention to questions outside the realm of
high policy and professionalisation in twentieth-century general practice makes it difficult to establish how specifically connected to their
ethnicity the experiences of South Asian doctors may have been. Two
surveys examining British doctors' relationships with their patients carried out in the 1960s and 1970s[21] did not convey the degree of enthusiasm about interactions with patients that some participants transmit.
Nor does Paul Ferris' *The Doctors* which captured the views of medical
professionals including GPs in the 1960s.[22] This could, however, simply reflect the contrast between younger doctors talking about patients
they were seeing at the time when they were in demanding full-time
jobs and older medics reminiscing about their patients from the vantage point of retirement or towards the end of their careers. Even though
interviews with white contemporaries might conceivably have yielded
similar views, the fact that doctors do not describe themselves as outsiders is noteworthy. They could quite conceivably have felt confined
to the roles of professionals who were tolerated, rather than integrated.
In fact, many doctors drew on a vocabulary from the realm of the personal and private domains when discussing the relationships they built
up with patients rather than analysing them dispassionately in professional, medical terms.

To a degree, this may well be specific to the experience of migrant
doctors, certainly when it comes to the intensity of feeling expressed.
One interviewee made it explicit that as he had few local networks,
work naturally assumed a more personal dimension:

> I developed some fantastic relationships with my patients. I used to see
> them as friends who were in difficulty and they also saw me as their
> friend. I got to know loads and loads of families … Patients were friends,

they gave advice, we had fantastic times, particularly older patients—I had no family here—I talked to them and they gave me solace, helped me through it, it was absolutely brilliant … It was that type of relationship where you were considered one of them rather than an immigrant doctor who had come and settled in the town.[23]

It is not just the fact that doctors do not report severe difficulties that is telling. That could arguably be ascribed to reticence on the part of the interviewees. The degree of positivity that emerged from some of the discussions about patients was striking. It went well beyond simply communicating that doctors were able to work without being rejected:

*How would you describe your relationship with patients?* It was very good. In some ways a relationship of love in the fullest sense. I think they love me and I love my patients. I would do anything for my patients, no matter what their background, what wealth they have. I would campaign for them, go wherever had to go to achieve for them.[24]

I feel part of the community, being a family doctor I know most of patients in my area and I think of them as part of my practice, and they think of me as a very important member of the family … For me all the patients when they come back, they respect me, I love them and that's the relationship always there.[25]

I'm proud of the way I've given my patients care, I tried my best. I think I would give my life … that's how I feel (laughs). That's the care I have given. I liked my job and my patients.[26]

Love, friendship, doing 'anything', and putting one's life on the line were not words and expressions that might have been expected in the context of GPs describing their work.

The ability of doctors to build this type of relationship is possibly partly ascribable to cultural factors. One doctor claimed to have heard that some patients felt they got better care from South Asian doctors and ascribed this to a superior ability to empathise with older patients because of traditional South Asian attitudes towards elders.[27] Another interviewee spoke of feeling compelled to make himself available to patients at his home as 'It's our old Eastern hospitality, once a person comes to your house you never turn them away, no matter what.'[28]

There is little in the testimony I gathered that is suggestive of a great distance between doctors and patients as a result of social or ethnic difference. Whilst cultural factors undoubtedly shaped doctors' experiences, medical migrants' willingness to embrace medical 'dirty work' that played an important part in patients' lives provides a more compelling general explanatory framework for the nature of the relationships between South Asian doctors and non-South Asian patients. As is the case with other groups of migrants, doctors were doing jobs that involved a workload and conditions that were simply not acceptable to many British graduates and were prepared to take on more work in order to define a professional niche.

The way in which many doctors talk about their relationship with patients suggests a degree of self-actualisation through work. This may result from the fact that this relationship was likely to take on a more personal dimension at the time or from the specific nature of the relationships between doctors and communities in inner cities, mining areas and/or single-handed practices. In this respect, doctors from the Indian subcontinent are possibly more typical of migrants generally rather than South Asians specifically, both in terms of the type of work they took on and the at times difficult circumstances in which they did it. One doctor when asked about his workload responded that it was heavy and that 'they would say too much work, but it's gratifying'.[29] Another felt that as a young GP she was seen as more available to patients:

> Behind the practice, there was an old people's home, I got patients from there through word of mouth … In Sale [in Greater Manchester] initially, many patients were older patients. *Do you have any thoughts on why that was?* Yeah, yeah, they felt I devoted more time to them and if they sent for the visits I was readily doing it.[30]

In Derbyshire, Ralph Lawrence described not having a day off for 'about fifteen years' as other local practices would not allow him to join their out-of-hours roster.[31] Another doctor who worked in the Welsh Valleys, when asked to describe a typical day's work in the 1960s or 1970s spoke of one day merging into the next, space for private pursuits and time being nullified by pressures of work:

> I started surgery at nine. Got up at seven … then getting into car, there is a call, the man is gasping, will you come before surgery, or child is vomiting, please come before surgery. The very words before surgery: before nine o'clock. The patients are waiting, they don't like it either, so you have to go there, sort it out and then go back to the surgery. Receptionist

with a sombre look says 'Why are you late?', 'This happened', 'Oh'. Then
surgery starts, you see 20–24 patients, all of a sudden another 10 joined,
so you should have finished at 11 but it went on and on, half past 11.
Then there is a call, 8 or 9, out of which 1 or 2 is terminally ill, one is
heart failure, and if there is a mental case, better not to say anything.
This takes quite a bit of time, mental or social worker comes, or epilep-
tic patient comes, epilepsy is not controlled, they've got to be admitted,
anyway that's finished at 5. You've got a lunch or whatever it may be, then
start again at 7, night surgery, come back home, there are 2 calls, so you
go there, see the patient, if necessary admit the patient, if not arrange the
district nurse, if not arrange the chemist, out-of-hours chemist ... Then
you go back home, have supper, by this time, two calls came. You've got
to go, see the patient. Then came back, little bit to drink, soda lemonade
or anything, go to bed. After an hour there is a call. So you have to go.'[32]

The final sentence of this extract suggests a feeling of being obliged to
respond to patient demands that may be seen as unreasonable in order
to avoid professional difficulties. The disruption to private lives caused
by the requirement to provide round-the-clock care in areas of high
need was such that several doctors mentioned that their children had
been dissuaded from following them into general practice as a result.[33]
One interviewee quipped in reference to his workload that: 'You come
in as a cause célèbre and end up as a cause macabre'.[34] Although this was
said flippantly and appeared to be a well-rehearsed line from someone
used to public speaking, Dipak Ray's recourse to humour was perhaps
not accidental in this context. It offered a way of alluding to an unpalat-
able truth about the roles of South Asian doctors in high-need communities: 'cause célèbre' as provider of services, 'cause macabre' as a result
of the pressures endured to fulfil such a role. The high workload in the
areas most doctors were based in and their willingness, as migrants, to
shoulder this burden helps to explain how they were able to gain acceptance. One doctor whose practice was in a deprived area of a major city
defined his relationship with his patients as 'give and take' before adding that 'The more you did, the more they depended on you'.[35]
    Perceiving the relationship between South Asian doctors and
patients living in peripheral areas in this way helps to explain contemporary newspaper reports that point to a degree of passion in the
actions of patients defending their doctors, which echoes the words
used by doctors to describe their feelings for their patients. In one case,

a group of patients blocked access to a surgery when a South Asian doctor in west London was denied the opportunity to take over a practice by the Local Health Authority.[36] A member of the patients' action committee was quoted as saying that Mustafa Rahim was 'sympathetic' and 'prepared to turn out at any hour on emergency calls'. A doctor in Lancashire continued to treat patients in a tent in the course of a dispute with the local medical authorities.[37] These reports offer glimpses into the perspectives of patients that add weight to the views expressed by doctors. In the words of Muhammad Noorul Islam Talukdar, who worked in what he described as the 'sleepy hollow' of Bacup, a working-class town in Lancashire:

> There was a lot of deprivation but people were kind to their doctor. Even in rough parts of town, there were no problems walking around in middle of night. It possibly made the bond stronger.[38]

Edal Banatvala was also based in a working-class area. He came to Britain in 1929 and became a GP in the East End of London, in Leyton where he worked until his retirement some forty years later. An anecdote recounted by his son Jangu, who became a professor of clinical virology at St Thomas' Hospital in the British capital, gives a sense of the nature of this bond and of the ways in which doctors' and patients' lives could become enmeshed. It offers an example of how oral history can serve to access truths that lie beyond other forms of historical research. It is the subjective sense of a shared destiny that is important here, irrespective of whether the story is factually accurate or not:

> I do remember a story he told me ... My father used to leave his car at a garage about a mile down the road. He'd cycle back ... The garage was owned by a taxi driver and his—I thought—delightful cockney wife. He liked her too ... And she had two sons. Stanley and I can't remember the other one ... And she said 'My sons, you know, they don't want ... to learn to swim because they've got bad ears' ... And he looked in the ears and he says 'Rubbish, they should learn to swim.' Well they did learn to swim. Thank God. Dunkirk: They made it! (laughter) Right. That sort of thing, you know. That stuck in my mind.[39]

Not only does Jangu Banatvala's father appear as embedded in his local community but as playing his part in a triumph over adversity in the shape of Dunkirk (i.e. the evacuation of allied soldiers from the French port in 1940). The story acts as a metaphor for South Asian doctors' relationships with working-class communities and their contribution to their lives. It is hard to see how it could emerge from a broader context of widespread xenophobic hostility.

## South Asian doctors and ethnic minority patients

The interviews I did in the course of my research took me to the post-industrial cities of Manchester and Glasgow, the former coalmining areas of South Wales, Yorkshire and Fife, and other traditionally industrial and working-class parts of Britain such as the north-east of England and London's East End. A large proportion of the populations that the NHS was primarily established to serve lived in these areas. These are also the locations where South Asian doctors have sought out professional opportunities ever since the NHS was set up. It is unsurprising therefore to find that South Asian doctors played a major role in providing care for migrant and ethnic minority patients, many of whom lived in the areas where South Asian doctors tended to be based. A survey carried out in the West Midlands in 1981 found that two-thirds of South Asians were registered with a GP of South Asian origin, and an additional 10 per cent were registered with a practice where an Asian doctor worked.[40] The same was true of 9 per cent and 15 per cent of white patients and 29 per cent and 9 per cent of those of African-Caribbean origin.[41] To a degree, this was the product of co-location: South Asian doctors were disproportionately concentrated in industrial and inner-city areas and when it came to cities at least this meant that they would find themselves working in areas with higher than average concentrations of ethnic minority patients. However, the relationship between South Asian GPs and South Asian patients took on specific dimensions. In the early 1990s it was estimated for instance that between 40 and 60 per cent of Asians communicated with their GP in a South Asian language.[42] Research conducted in Birmingham and published in 1985 found that significant numbers of South Asian patients expressed a positive preference for a South Asian doctor.[43]

One participant did talk of enjoying the contact with a range of cultures that was a feature of his work in Aston, a multicultural area of Birmingham.[44] Overall, however, doctors' testimony suggests that the relationship between South Asian doctors and non-South Asian ethnic minority patients is probably best defined as being shaped by forces not dissimilar to those that came into play with white patients. Whilst relationships between South Asian doctors and their South Asian patients were different, in ways that will be described, there was little to suggest that the same could be said of the relationship between South Asian doctors and other ethnic minority patients. However, as they were frequently working as GPs in unpopular areas, South Asian doctors could as a result find themselves caring for members of socially marginalised groups such as Gypsies, Roma and Travellers who encountered difficulty in accessing care. Shirin Kutar, a doctor from Bombay who was working as a GP in south-east London from the 1940s along with her husband, provided an insight into the nature of this encounter between marginalised practitioners and patients on the wrong side of the tracks:

> One of the gypsies said to him: 'Doctor, nobody wants us on their list. Will you take my family?'. So he said: 'Where do you live?' He says: 'Lower Abbey Wood, near the railway lines.' In those days, the railway lines didn't have an overhead bridge. A man would come running, open the gate for you, you cross the lines, see the gypsies in their caravan, then again he stands, sees there is no train coming ... and to deliver mothers in that caravan—by the time you finish with the job your back is like this ... so gypsies were our patients.'[45]

Dipak Ray provided an echo of this account, although his recollections relate to South Wales, rather than a working-class London district. Focusing on doctors who were discriminated against and professionally marginalised brings to the fore the history of patient groups in under-served areas:

> The problem was there was stigma about them, it's still there now ... They couldn't get doctors, sometimes it happened ... I think I was the only doctor—there was another doctor who used to take on, from Merthyr [Tydfil], and they were absolutely lovely people ... One child I remember out in the Valleys ... the police called me out and I went with the midwife and the baby ... the woman was 18 years old, no ante-natal care, nothing, I delivered the child, a girl and she said 'What is your name?'. I said 'Dipak Kumar—Dipak'. 'Can I call him Dipak?' she said, I said 'You can't call it Dipak, it's a male name!'. 'I don't care' she said (laughs). Police car took us up, she filled it up with chicken and duck and all that business ... sweet memories ... *Why would other doctors not*

*take them on*? Doctors took them but … they had problems in terms of local doctors who would have them … they could be forced on to doctors by the LMC, there is no problem there, but they don't want to be forced on, that is the point. I can't make any judgment on that … but I got all the Gypsy patients, I don't know what it means. Three families, they were all my patients.[46]

Dipak Ray was apparently reluctant to criticise his colleagues of the time. As he was a highly eloquent anti-racism campaigner, it seems unlikely that he was genuinely unable to think of a reason why these patients ended up being treated by him. The fact that a number of Gypsy, Roma and Traveller patients had to be 'forced on' to other doctors in the Welsh Valleys suggests that they were being shunned by other doctors and it is quite possible that some of these doctors were South Asian given the high concentrations of medical migrants from the Indian subcontinent in the area. One doctor who worked in the Midlands pointed out that although Gypsies, Roma and Travellers consulted at the practice she worked at, some covered significant distances to see her or her (white British, female) colleague although other South Asian doctors were working in the area.[47]

Based on the interviews carried out for this project, the role of doctors from the Indian subcontinent in the treatment of non-South Asian ethnic minority patients would seem to be best perceived as a continuation of their roles of practitioners on the periphery. The provision of medical services and the reciprocal offer of food, the appropriation of a doctor's name for a new-born child and the evocation of this encounter with a patient as a 'sweet memory' all fit with the notions of 'give and take' and of finding common ground which defined relationships between doctors in search of professional roles and patients stigmatised by other professionals.

The relationship between South Asian doctors and South Asian patients at times took different forms. As was discussed in Chapter 2, the entry of South Asian doctors into general practice coincided with a more general increase in immigration from the Indian subcontinent. At least from the mid-1960s, it was apparent that South Asian migrants living in Britain were disproportionately affected by certain conditions such as tuberculosis,[48] diabetes and ischaemic heart disease[49] and more likely to suffer from vitamin D or B12 deficiency.[50] In 1965, *The Lancet* reported that:

> Of the 300,000 people living in Bradford in 1963, about 12,000 were immigrants from Asia. Of the 353 new cases of tuberculosis reported during the year, 203 were in Asians; in other words, 4% of the population accounted for nearly 60% of the cases.[51]

As well as being disproportionally affected by particular conditions, South Asian patients encountered significant obstacles when accessing services as a result of linguistic and literacy barriers: a study of elderly Asians in Leicester published in 1986 found that only 37 per cent of men and 2 per cent of women could speak English and that two-thirds of elderly women were illiterate in all languages.[52] A survey conducted in the mid-1970s concluded that 15 per cent of Asians (7 per cent of men and 27 per cent of women) were 'not at all' able to speak English.[53] The Pakistani Welfare and Information Centre described the situation in Manchester in the 1960s in the following terms:

> Today the number of Pakistanis in Manchester is approximately 7,000. Most of them are illiterate or semi-illiterate. They speak little English, find it difficult to communicate and express their views and problems, and are unable to utilise fully the Welfare Services available in this country. Most of them do now know where to get proper information and guidance, how to get it and how to express their problems; on the other hand the voluntary and statutory bodies and the local authorities find it difficult to understand the problems of the Pakistanis and Indians who speak little or no English at all.[54]

This context is crucial when considering the nature of the relationship between South Asian doctors and South Asian patients at the time. It developed in a health service where patients were disproportionately suffering from ill-health and ill-equipped to access NHS services. The next two chapters will show how doctors from the Indian subcontinent were involved in addressing this agenda at the level of policy and practice at least from the 1970s onwards.

A wider effect of the presence of South Asian doctors can be located at a practice level in the contacts that they had with South Asian patients. I did not interview doctors' patients for this project so can only offer a perspective from one side of this relationship. I am not suggesting that the NHS was able to address all issues concerning ethnic minority health simply because a significant proportion of its medical staff were South Asian. At a very basic level though, South Asian doctors were able to lift some of the barriers to access that patients faced. They for instance attributed some of their professional success to their ability to communicate with patients in South Asian languages:

> If doctor speaks the same language as the patient, patients prefer to go to the same practices. It is quite understandable and person can express their own things in their own language to doctor. I mostly speak Bengali so my patients come from far away ... [55]
>
> Gradually more and more Asian are coming to me because it went to various people that I do my practice in Punjabi, in my local language. Because they can't speak English. I can speak Punjabi and Urdu, their language. That was good for them. Otherwise when a patient would go to the doctors they would bring their sons and daughters to interpret. And they always could not say everything.[56]

If linguistic ability was an important factor, gender also played a role in directing patients towards particular practitioners. In the late 1980s, a study in Bradford found that a majority (62 per cent) of Pakistani women objected to being examined by a male doctor.[57] Two of the female doctors interviewed in the course of this research suggested that their arrival in practices helped to meet a suppressed need amongst the South Asian population in general and in the female South Asian population in particular:

> Because of the cultural issues I think, they didn't know the English language. Lot of the Muslim families they said it will be better to go to the lady doctor. But I had the whole families, even the men. Probably the way I approached them. I had the time, I could talk to them, whatever they wanted to talk about, besides medicine.[58]
>
> When joined the practice ... was on the edge of Asian community. They came to join me like mad—put medical cards through the letterbox even ... *Why was there such a demand from patients?* It was not particularly me—any Asian doctor and specialised in gyne/obs who could speak the languages. I had all the qualities they were looking for.[59]

These interviews suggest once more a confluence of patient need and professional ability and willingness to offer a service. As P. L. Pathak put it, she 'had the time'. It is noteworthy that the second doctor quoted here did not lay claim to any unique talent that served to attract patients. She felt that being South Asian, having South Asian languages and expertise in gynaecology and obstetrics was sufficient. Regardless of how effective individual South Asian doctors might have been in meeting the specific needs of their patients it seems reasonable to conclude that, taken collectively, their presence served to fill a gap at least at a very basic level, namely when it came to the ability to communicate with patients and the availability of a doctor that it was considered culturally acceptable to consult.

These accounts are given additional credibility by two press reports from the 1970s and 1980s which indicate that there was a wider public perception at the time that South Asian doctors could help to address some of the existing gaps in primary care provision. In the mid-1970s the Camden Committee for Community Relations supported the appeal of a Sylheti-speaking Bengali doctor who was seeking permission to practise in the King's Cross area of London.[60] The Medical Practices Committee argued that there were already enough doctors practising locally. *The Times* reported that community relations workers felt that a Sylheti-speaking doctor was needed to overcome the language barrier faced by many patients. Abdul Momen, a support worker with the South Asian community in King's Cross told the newspaper that the problems faced by immigrants were such that some people were 'near to nervous breakdowns' and that a doctor was required 'not only for their ills but as someone they could talk to about personal and family problems'.[61] In the early 1980s, the Buckinghamshire Family Practitioner Committee (FPC) turned down a request from a female South Asian doctor who wanted to open a surgery in High Wycombe.[62] The *Bucks Free Press* reported that the doctor had been told by a relative that there was a need for a practitioner who spoke South Asian languages.[63] Alfred Webley, the chief officer of the local Community Relations Council was quoted as saying that although the town had a male South Asian doctor he did not speak Urdu, which led to 'enormous complications and waste of time'.[64] He added that the female doctor would have been able to 'give special care to Asian women, a section of the community particularly sensitive when it comes to attending a surgery'.[65] More generally, in the context of understanding how important the role of doctors from

the Indian subcontinent was seen to be, it is not uninteresting to note
that the newspaper's headline for this article was 'Asian woman doctor shock' and that the FPC's decision was viewed as controversial.
The proposed arrival of an 'Asian woman doctor' was presented as
being welcome and as a means of addressing many of the healthcare
needs of the local Asian population in ways that would prove beyond
most British-trained graduates:

> An Asian woman doctor had been refused permission to open a surgery
> in High Wycombe. This is despite the fact that the town has one of the
> largest Asian populations in the south of England. According to the
> latest estimates, there are 9,000 Urdu-speakers in the area.[66]

This evidence suggests that doctors from the Indian subcontinent
played an important part in the provision of care to South Asian patients
and that they constituted an important cultural resource for the NHS at
the time. Their impact at this level is comparable to their role in staffing
British general practice at a time of doctor shortages. Their presence
prevented the development of an even greater problem. Sri Venugopal,
a GP in Birmingham, described migrant doctors as having had a 'cushioning' effect when it came to the NHS's ability to respond to the needs
of ethnic minority communities:

> The NHS is very privileged to have lot of these overseas doctors in this
> country who have given this cushioning effect in the inner-city areas,
> otherwise there the NHS system would have failed … the government
> of the day, if the overseas doctors were not there, was not capable of
> providing appropriate service to a multiethnic community. They would
> have been deprived … of … many ways to utilise the NHS system.[67]

Whilst it remains questionable that services were indeed 'appropriate'
even when they were offered by South Asian doctors, the presence of
doctors from the Indian subcontinent did have an effect on the NHS's
capacity to engage effectively with South Asian patients. The roles
played in this respect by South Asian doctors, as alluded to in *The
Times* report on the Bengali community in Kings' Cross, extended to
services that further down the line would be provided by a range of
staff and agencies. One doctor for instance described responding to his
patients' needs for advice and support by 'working as a counsellor'. His

description of his work as a GP suggests a position in the local community that extended well beyond the boundaries of his surgery:

> Asian patients they treated a doctor more or less as a family members. They will tell all the problems—that the son is not doing well at school ... not just ailments. They treated you like a family elder or a church vicar (laughs) so in that way it was a bit different. Sometimes I had to work as a counsellor. In those days we had no trained counsellors attached to practice. *How much time did you spend like this?* Twenty minutes to thirty minutes per consultation. Sometimes, husband and wife would both come and would try to take it as far as possible ... You knew a little bit about the whole family. Asian patients would invite me to weddings. I used to go for an hour or so. That was the difference.[68]

This is not to say of course that the situation described above was ideal; in fact the interviewee hints at it himself when he says he 'had' to work as a counsellor as no trained counsellors were available at the time. Nor is it to say that British-born and -trained GPs did not perform similar functions at the time. However, in the new and developing South Asian communities of post-war Britain, the impact of doctors from the Indian subcontinent extended into areas that would almost certainly have been inaccessible to many other practitioners—if only for linguistic reasons. P. L. Pathak in Rusholme described her role as a female doctor as extending to discussing internal family dynamics in non-clinical settings:

> It was important that I was able to deal with them medically, socially, culturally. I understood all those factors. I got families where mother-in-law and all those things—daughter will make confidences. Mother-in-law says daughter-in-law is rubbish ... have to keep these issues confidential ... Any difficulties I was able to advise: go to social services, do this, do that. I was also involved in so much community work. Some women would meet in this church at the top of Upper Chorlton Road and I used to go and help them. *When did this start?* As soon as I was in the practice. I was able to talk to them about everything, marriages ... they felt comfortable and related to me. Besides medicine I was able to say do this, do that, which was the right path to take.[69]

Doctors were thus working as GPs but at times also talk of incorporating into their work traditional community roles and sometimes even religious functions—one London-based Parsee doctor also being a Zoroastrian priest.[70] The common ground found with white patients is in evidence once more when it comes to South Asian patients. South Asian doctors were well placed to realise that South Asian patients were encountering difficulties in accessing health services and had some advantages when it came to positioning themselves to meet the needs of these patients. They might best be described as a resource that the UK was able to draw upon to meliorate the worst of the effects of the lack of provision for ethnic minorities during the first forty years of the NHS's existence.

## The nature of care on the margins of medicine

The adoption of such roles cannot however be seen as entirely unproblematic. If ethnicity, gender and language could be presented as serving to create a connection between South Asian doctors and South Asian patients there were also barriers between doctors who were mostly urban, male and middle class and patients who tended to originate from rural areas, many of whom were female. What does not seem questionable is the fact that the NHS was not appropriately set up to provide for migrant communities and that South Asian doctors contributed to addressing this state of affairs. If the extent of the 'cushioning effect' is therefore unclear, and doctors' interpretation of this relationship is susceptible to being challenged, there can be little doubt that it existed. The historical role of migrant general practitioners as cultural agents and negotiators of cultural and class differences is, however, little understood. A shared ethnic background could potentially be both of benefit linguistically and a determinant of negative class-based attitudes. Imported social attitudes could also have an impact on care on the periphery. It is therefore important to acknowledge that the cultural diversity of migrant healthcare professionals was a factor in the development of primary healthcare in Britain and reflect on the significance of this fact.

One study from the 1980s suggested for instance that overseas graduates might have different (more negative) attitudes towards patients with HIV/AIDS.[71] There is further evidence from studies conducted beyond the timeframe examined in this study that the influence of migrant doctors can have a range of effects on the nature of care. Research published in 2002[72] found that patients who spoke South

Asian languages were more likely to feel 'enabled' (i.e. able to manage healthcare issues) when consulting a doctor who spoke the same language. An earlier study published in the 1990s had, however, found that Asian doctors tended to have less favourable attitudes towards Asian patients than other doctors, considering that they were more likely to consult for trivial reasons and demand longer consultation times.[73]

Although some doctors might have felt a rapport with South Asian, ethnic minority or working-class patients, others were less than enthusiastic about the arrival in Britain of South Asian migrants from different social backgrounds. Doctors generally describe positive relationships with patients and having a positive impact on the communities in which they lived, but this is, to an extent, to be expected in oral history interviews. Occasional evidence of more problematic behaviours should therefore not be ignored. P. R. L. Mohan's interviews with doctors and their partners carried out in the 1970s revealed that some physicians had strong class prejudices which she assessed as being more pronounced in their relationships with South Asians whereas they were 'very polite to white men doing menial jobs'.[74] At times these views could take extreme forms. Mohan for instance reported that:

> Though most of the Asian General Practitioners depended on Asian working class immigrants for their practice, they only maintained doctor-patient relationship [sic]. Some of the middle class Asians developed a prejudice over the working class immigrants and said, that, 'Enoch Powell's repatriation is the best solution to get rid of those lower class immigrants'.[75]

If patients could, through registering with South Asian doctors, find a useful resource in a system that did not prioritise their needs, they would therefore not necessarily be seen in a particularly sympathetic light. One participant, who recalled his father's views on the increase of immigration from the Indian subcontinent gave a sense of how distant a South Asian GP of the time could feel from other South Asian migrants. It is also interesting to note that the interviewee felt the need to clarify that his family did not endorse Enoch Powell's views on immigration:

> *What view did your father have of changes in terms of migration from the Indian Subcontinent?* They thought on the whole it was disastrous ... Not in the Enoch Powell sense ... they were much more

open about it in their thinking than many other people, they saw a lot of people coming over who weren't educated, being used as work fodder who had no real relationship with the country or concept of it apart from a place where there was work and that they came in too large numbers to really integrate ... They saw the real negative sides of immigration because Blackburn became one of the focal points in the North West. They thought it was very badly handled. It was nothing against people coming, there were always students coming from India, they were always welcome in our house, Indian doctors came who we got to know quite well, mainly for training. When there was a large influx without the educational background to understand they had to assimilate I think they thought this was something which should have been perceived and dealt with much earlier than it was.[76]

Although these views are expressed subtly, there is no mistaking the class perspective that underpins the attitudes described here: 'students ... Indian doctors' were welcome but people who 'weren't educated' were seen as not belonging. Of course, it is precisely such populations that became dependent on migrant doctors. It is naturally difficult to draw any particular conclusions from a son's account of his father's perspective on the growth in post-war South Asian migration years after the events. It should however serve to draw attention to the fact that the delegation of responsibility for the care of South Asian patients to South Asian migrant doctors is not simply to be unquestionably celebrated.

The direct expression of hostility associated with class, ethnic, religious or national origin in oral history interviews carried out in the twenty-first century was predictably rare given the social stigma that is now frequently attached to such views. One doctor working in an area with a large number of ethnic minority patients did nevertheless talk of black (i.e. African or African-Caribbean) patients as 'a bit of rough type' who 'talk rough as well'.[77] Shirin Kutar, who eloquently described how her husband crossed railway lines to treat patients from the Gypsy, Roma and Traveller community, also stated that 'smelly gypsies' were her least favourite type of patient.[78] Whilst their remarks were not targeted directly at patients, one participant stated that: 'Indians are a very criminal-minded nation ... they are the most cruel ... they are very strange people'.[79] Another undermined what started as an ecumenical statement with an expression of Islamophobia which seemed to call for the complicit approval of the interviewer:

> There is only one God, there is some spiritual power who guides the destiny of man, that's what I believe in … You can go to him, through the church or the temple … [sotto voce] I'm not sure about the mosque.[80]

The fact that doctors shared these views naturally raises questions about how this might have affected their professional contacts with Indians or Muslims. Comments about NHS colleagues also bore witness to the fact that migrant practitioners played their part in defining the NHS as a racist and heterophobic space where difference could result in those working for it finding themselves at a disadvantage. As mentioned in Chapter 4, a (non-Pakistani) female doctor complained about the attitudes of some Pakistani doctors towards women, saying that it was due to 'their cultural background, they consider women as inferior'.[81] As previously noted, this suggests either that she was indeed treated differently by these doctors, ethnic stereotyping on the part of the participant or an element of both. The participant who spoke disparagingly of his black patients also engaged in a racist generalisation about black nurses:

> Night nurses in hospitals, they are all black nurses. They are very rough. Very rough, I must tell you. Night nurses, most of them are Black, African or West Indies, they do not know anything. Irish nurses, local nurses and Chinese nurses they are good.[82]

It should be emphasised that these remarks were very isolated in the context of forty in-depth interviews with South Asian GPs. The fact that they were made freely by a not insignificant number of participants and without inhibition in a contemporary context does nevertheless raise questions about how common these views may have been and the extent to which cultural, social and political attitudes imported from the Indian subcontinent may have shaped the care that patients received— for better and for worse. The attitudes towards race, class and disability displayed by some participants may simply be typical of their generation of doctors but their existence requires to be noted. One participant felt that his patients had a 'low mentality' which made his job harder to do and which he attributed to 'the mental IQ of the patient because patients are all poor class'.[83] Another spoke of some of her patients as being 'mentally abnormal or subnormal'.[84] The extent to which such attitudes were prevalent in different groups of practitioners, and the ways in which racism and heterophobia manifested within migrant and ethnic minority groups, would warrant a more detailed investigation.

The fact that certain categories of patients and doctors found themselves marginalised within the context of the NHS also had an effect on the extent to which practitioners were able to access the type of support that they needed to enhance the care they were able to offer their patients. One doctor thus explained how in her view the impact of any 'cushioning effect' she was able to provide was limited because of her poor relationship with those running the healthcare system.[85] It is also clear that the type of workload that doctors took on when working, often single-handed, in deprived communities had an impact on their ability to function effectively as professionals. As M. N. I. Talukdar remarked of his early days in general practice before he moved to a health centre: 'I was on call seven days a week, twenty-four hours. It was unkind and unfair. You can never be fresh if you are doing that kind of work.'[86] Doctors from the Indian subcontinent provided a vital resource for a Health Service that did not prioritise care for certain categories of patients. The fact that they mitigated some of the defects of the system does not mean that it was as a result beyond reproach, nor does it signify that there are only benefits to drawing on the labour of migrant doctors.

## Notes

1 M. Nava, 'Sometimes antagonistic, sometimes ardently sympathetic: Contradictory responses to migrants in postwar Britain', *Ethnicities*, 14:3 (2014).

2 'Doctor dies', the *Guardian* (19 June 1981), p. 25; P. Johnson, 'Skinhead "stabbed Asian to prove himself"', the *Guardian* (27 April 1982), p. 28; P. Johnson, 'Skinhead who stabbed Asian gaoled', the *Guardian* (28 April 1982), p. 3.

3 G. Linscott, 'Women patients "plotted Indian doctor's downfall"', the *Guardian* (9 December 1976), p. 7.

4 K. Korlipara interview with author; anonymous interview with author.

5 N. Shah interview with author.

 6  K. Korlipara interview with author.
 7  K. S. Bhanumathi interview with author.
 8  Anonymous interview with author; M. A. Khaled interview with author.
 9  Anonymous interview with author.
10  Chowdhary, *I Made my Home*, p. 29.
11  Anonymous interview with author.
12  L. Tabili, *Global Migrants, Local Culture: Natives and Newcomers in Provincial England 1841–1939* (London: Palgrave Macmillan, 2011), p. 125.
13  M. A. Khaled interview.
14  Lawrence, *Fire in his Hand*, p. 49.
15  Lawrence, *Fire in his Hand*, p. 53.
16  S. Pande interview with author, 23 November 2009.
17  This was also the impression conveyed by participants in another study of migrant South Asian doctors in England and Wales, with one doctor giving the example of the northern working-class town of Barnsley in the 1960s as a location where the professional identities of migrant doctors came to the fore partly as a result of the fact that the local South Asian population was small. See G. Y. Farooq, 'A study of overseas-trained South Asian doctors in England and Wales' (PhD dissertation, University of Manchester, 2014), p. 231.
18  Anonymous interview with author.
19  Anonymous interview with author; K. S. Bhanumathi interview with author.
20  U. Rao interview with author.
21  A. Cartwright, *Patients and their Doctors: A Study of General Practice* (London: Routledge and Kegan Paul, 1967); A. Cartwright & R. Anderson, *General Practice Revisited: A Second Study of Patients and their Doctors* (London: Tavistock Publications, 1981).
22  Ferris, *The Doctors*.
23  H. Joshi interview with author.
24  L. R. M. Kamal interview with author.
25  Anonymous interview with author.
26  Anonymous interview with author.
27  R. Chandran interview with author.
28  F. B. Kotwall interview with author.
29  M. S. Kauser interview with author.
30  P. L. Pathak interview with author.
31  Lawrence, *Fire in his Hand*, p. 49.

32  R. K. Majumdar interview with author.
33  M. N. I. Talukdar interview with author; S. Pande interview with author, 23 November 2009; R. K. Majumder interview with author.
34  D. Ray interview with author, 19 March 2010.
35  Anonymous interview with author.
36  D. Pallister, 'Loyal patients fight for GP', the *Guardian* (14 September 1977), p. 22.
37  'Barred doctor set up surgery in a tent', the *Daily Telegraph* (3 March 1977), p. 17.
38  M. N. I. Talukdar interview with author.
39  J. Banatvala interview with author, 9 July 2015.
40  M. R. D. Johnson, M. Cross, S. A. Cardew, 'Inner city residents, ethnic minorities and primary health care', *Postgraduate Medical Journal*, 59 (1983), pp. 664–5.
41  Johnson et al., 'Inner city residents', p. 665.
42  Gill, 'General practitioners', p. 108.
43  J. Chanchal, N. Narayan, L. A. Pike, M. E. Clarkson, I. G. Cox, J. Chatterjee, 'Attitudes of Asian patients in Birmingham to general practitioner services', *Journal of the Royal College of General Practitioners*, 35 (1985).
44  S. Venugopal interview with author.
45  BLSA, C648/28/01–06, Oral History of General Practice 1936–1952, S. Kutar interviewed by M. Bevan, 1993.
46  D. Ray interview with author 19 March 2010.
47  Anonymous interview with author.
48  J. Aspin, 'Tuberculosis among Indian immigrants to a Midlands industrial area', *BMJ*, 1:5289 (1962).
49  S. Shaunak, S. R. Lakhani, R. Abraham, J. D. Maxwell, 'Differences among Asian patients', *BMJ*, 293:6555 (1986).
50  Shaunak et al., 'Differences'; P. D. Roberts, H. James, A. Petrie, J. O. Morgan, A. V. Hoffbrand, 'Vitamin B12 status in pregnancy among immigrants to Britain', *BMJ*, 3 (1973).
51  'Health of immigrants', *The Lancet*, 1:7377 (1965), p. 150.
52  L. J. Donaldson, 'Health and social status of elderly Asians: A community survey', *BMJ*, 293 (1986).
53  D. Smith, *The facts of racial disadvantage: A national survey*, PEP, 1976, cited in: Department of Employment, *The role of immigrants in the labour market*, p. 141.

54 Manchester Archives and Local Studies, 301.45 PA19, Pakistani Welfare Trust and Information Centre Manchester, Annual Report 1964–65 (?), p. 3.

55 M. F. Haque interview with author, 16 June 2010.

56 M. S. Kausar interview with author.

57 W. I. U. Ahmad, E. E. M. Kernohan, M. R. Baker, 'Patients' choice of general practitioner: Influence of patients' fluency in English and ethnicity and sex of doctor', *Journal of the Royal College of General Practitioners*, 39 (1989), pp. 153–4.

58 P. L. Pathak interview with author.

59 Anonymous interview with author.

60 'Community workers back appeal by doctor', *The Times* (23 April 1976), p. 2.

61 Ibid.

62 Runnymede Collection at Middlesex University, MDXRT/PC/14/07, J. Pitt, 'Asian woman doctor shock', *Bucks Free Press* (8 February 1983) (no page number).

63 Ibid.

64 Ibid.

65 Ibid.

66 Ibid.

67 S. Venugopal interview with author.

68 Anonymous interview with author.

69 P. L. Pathak interview with author.

70 F. B. Kotwall interview with author.

71 J. A. Shapiro, 'General practitioners' attitudes towards AIDS and their perceived information needs', *BMJ*, 298 (1989) p. 1565.

72 G. K. Freeman, H. Rai, J. J. Walker, J. G. R. Howie, D. J. Heaney, M. Maxwell, 'Non-English speakers consulting with the GP in their own language: A cross-sectional survey', *British Journal of General Practice*, 52 (2002).

73 W. I. U. Ahmad, M. R. Baker, E. E. M. Kernohan, 'General practitioners' perceptions of Asian and non-Asian patients', *Family Practice*, 8:1 (1991).

74 Mohan, 'Asian doctors', p. 174.

75 Mohan, 'Asian doctors', p. 152.

76 Sir N. Mallick interview with author.

77 Anonymous interview with author.

78 BLSA, C648/28/01–06, 'Oral History of General Practice 1936–1952', S. Kutar interviewed by M. Bevan, 1993.

79  Anonymous interview with author.
80  Anonymous interview with author.
81  Anonymous interview with author.
82  Anonymous interview with author.
83  Anonymous interview with author.
84  Anonymous interview with author.
85  Anonymous interview with author.
86  M. N. I. Talukdar interview with author.

# 7

# Beyond the surgery boundaries: doctors' organisations and activist medics

Migrant South Asian GPs, by the very nature of their roles, became embedded in communities. GPs came in contact with a cross-section of the local population at regular intervals, often over long periods of time. They benefited from a great deal of professional autonomy in addition to having substantial amounts of social capital. They were therefore in a position to shape the social and political environment in which they found themselves. Doctors' interviews and archives provide evidence of their agency at a local level. At times, this social and political engagement extended beyond local contexts and resulted in them taking on national roles. South Asian doctors set up voluntary organisations which had an impact on policy and more generally provided a setting in which migrant practitioners could access training and socialise. They also acted to change British medicine in a number of ways.

This chapter describes how migrant doctors became involved in medical politics and in addressing social questions. They added new dimensions to British medical culture by creating groups that catered to their professional ambitions and their social and cultural aspirations as migrants. Of course, not all South Asian medical migrants should be seen as 'activist doctors' who shaped policy; it is entirely possible that such doctors were over-represented in this study as their names were more likely to have left traces in archives. In addition, it could be argued that as people who held strong views that they defended in public they might be expected to be more likely to agree to take part in an interview than contemporaries who kept a lower profile. However, many South Asian doctors clearly had a significant social impact that went beyond their immediate ability to fill a gap in the labour market and provide medical services. Even the actions of an individual GP working in their own practice were significant in the context of the lives of thousands of their patients.

## 'At that time I was a black sheep': local roles beyond the surgery

Not all doctors talked about their roles as incorporating wider social responsibilities and/or political involvement but a significant number of them did. South Asian doctors were, as a result of their social and professional status, able to take action that had a social impact at a local level. This type of involvement is not the sole preserve of South Asian GPs of course.[1] Interviews do however suggest that their personal trajectories and backgrounds and the social problems they encountered in their surgeries led them to have political perspectives that diverged from those of the mainstream of medicine. In a number of cases this directed them towards political activism, which appeared as a natural extension of the fact that they had defined common ground with patients on the periphery. It is also possible that doctors who had been discriminated against and who retained a sense of injustice might have been more likely to become politicised through their contact with social realities in their surgeries. For instance, L. R. M. Kamal who worked in the Yorkshire mining village of Hemsworth spoke of being deeply affected by the impact that the miner's strike of the 1980s had on his patients' health. His account is also coloured by a sense of grievance that positions him as an insider working in an area and identifying with the local residents rather than as a professional retaining his status as an outsider:

> The mining strike in '80s … was horrendous, a period of disgrace to the country. How it was possible to treat one section of the community so badly—I could not believe. There were soup kitchens in Hemsworth and would take bags of potatoes there. I felt so terrible; they were taking up fences to burn them for heat. I remember one patient turning up, he had pneumonia, I had given him antibiotics and told him to take them straight away. I said 'You are going for the medication now aren't you?' At the time the prescription charge was of about £1 but it was a lot of money because there was no social security during the strike. I had done evening surgery, I felt I would go and visit this patient, I had a feeling he may not have got

his medication. I had samples etc ... and took them with me. I was right: there was no heating in house, the chap was wrapped up in his quilt. He had no money to buy antibiotics. I gave him antibiotics, in some ways it was a salve to my conscience for what other people had done to this community. It was a terrible time, there was no justification for it, the eighties was a prosperous time for Britain. How could it happen?[2]

Although L. R. M. Kamal talks of his action being a 'salve to his conscience', doctors' actions on behalf of their patients can also be seen as a way of mounting a challenge to a social order that disadvantaged them as members of a group that faced discrimination. Some doctors reported that they knew they wanted to be politically active before they established themselves as general practitioners. One interviewee said he became a GP because it would give him more scope to be involved in politics;[3] another spoke of deliberately choosing to base himself in a working-class area.[4] South Asian doctors are not unique in this respect: other doctors could equally be motivated by political beliefs. The confrontation with the realities of practice (the Welsh Valleys in the case of Dipak Ray and the Nottinghamshire and Yorkshire coalfields for Raj Chandran and L. R. M. Kamal) could however also be presented as having served to politicise doctors, reinforcing previously held views and acting as a catalyst for social and/or political action.

These interventions are relevant to our understanding of the history of general practice as doctors do not distinguish between their politics and their practice; they see one as informing the other. Dipak Ray talked of being driven to action by witnessing the impact of coalmining on his patients' health:

I was very much involved with the miners ... because of ... the way the dust cases were treated ... which I think was an absolute disgrace ... Some of them had ... the small alveolitis ... small cells are involved in the lungs, clinically it doesn't manifest, x-rays are always misleading. A lot of them were not paid even though they were ... half dead, they ... never had compensation or anything like that.[5]

Although his politics were diametrically opposed to Ray's, Raj Chandran also described his political involvement as being partially grounded in frustrations emerging from the day-to-day running of his practice:

> I also being interested in politics myself ... decided ... I found that a lot of my old age pensioners patients were living in very poor housing conditions and I had to write letters, hundreds of letters to the councils to get them rehoused ... those days they used to have homes for the aged ... and they were in appalling conditions as well. So I thought I would try and get into the council myself to see what I can do. So I stood as an independent candidate for Sutton-in-Ashfield and they elected me ... *In what year was that?* In 1971 ... I thought council was not too ... effective ... out of fifty-two councillors ... fifty-one councillors were Labour and I was the only independent. So I thought I must change the system. And I ... formed the first Conservative Party Association in Sutton-in-Ashfield—against all odds ... I became the chairman ... I was getting a bit ambitious as well and I said right, let me try fighting a general election ... 1982, the party chose me to stand for election as a ... parliamentary candidate [in Preston].[6]

It is important to bear in mind that doctors are professionals and these forays into political activism could arguably be interpreted as motivated by a desire for status. Chandran explicitly recognises that he was 'ambitious' and his desire to effect local change in the Midlands did not prevent him from standing for election as a Member of Parliament in the north west of England.

These accounts are important, however, because they reveal not just that doctors were pushing the boundaries of their medical roles but also that migrant doctors were not, as a group, marginal figures. Involvement at a local level could at times lead doctors to take on national roles as alluded to by Raj Chandran and this will be discussed in the following section of this chapter. The connection between perceived care needs and political context more generally resulted in doctors taking action at a local level, which could be more productively seen as a desire for social change than stemming from a particular fixed political affiliation. Dhani Prem, a GP in the Midlands was elected to Birmingham Council in 1945 as a Labour candidate and served a three-year term.[7] He subsequently became a prominent opponent of local anti-immigrant politics.[8] In 1974, dissatisfied with the Labour party's line on immigration, he stood as a Liberal parliamentary candidate in Coventry South East but was defeated.[9] Harbans Lall Gulati's concern over the poverty he encountered in Battersea in the 1940s led him to start a petition to draw the Minister of Food's attention to the difficulties of older people and those living alone who had to survive on rations in post-war London.[10] He described some of the local residents he encountered as virtually facing starvation. A Conservative member of Battersea Council from 1934 until 1949, he later joined the Labour party and was elected to the London County Council in 1958.[11] Lutfe Rabbi Mustafa Kamal, who worked in a Yorkshire mining village, became an independent councillor on a platform that he described as being 'about Hemsworth':[12]

> I wanted to see social justice, I wanted to see people looking beyond just giving them shelter, they need to be provided with warmth … they needed to be provided with Citizen's Advisory Bureau advice and giving a whole person care, rather than … doing piecemeal things like housing and so on. *Why do you think you had that particular vision of what health-care should be, where do you think that came from?* I don't know, I think … you are born with some ideals aren't you, in life … You probably have to care for the have-nots and I think my being a doctor is part of that.[13]

The idea of caring for the have-nots as being central to the role of the doctor is possibly an example of cultural transfer. L. R. M. Kamal came from a Muslim country[14] where the provision of charity to the poor is considered a religious duty. Naturally, it is also possible that white British-born and -trained doctors would have held similar views and a sense of social responsibility could be ascribed to them. In the absence of an available database of interviews with non-South Asian doctors, it is impossible to be categorical in this respect. Nevertheless, cultural transfer is at times clearly in evidence, even if determining the precise limits of its influence is not an exact science.

The involvement of South Asian doctors in local politics can also be seen as an extension of political views that were at least partly shaped by experiences that can be connected to the background of South Asian doctors. One South Asian-born but British-trained GP described his involvement in council work in a working-class area as a logical consequence of his left-leaning political outlook and of his opinion that the role of local authorities and public health policy was more important to health outcomes than the day-to-day provision of medical treatment.[15] When asked about how he came to hold such views, he spoke of his experiences at university and of his personal hinterland, connecting colonialism with wider questions of social injustice:

> It was when I was at medical school, which is odd because I know universities often can give you a left-wing orientation but generally not medical school, especially in those days. Maybe, as I said, I was never really that excited about medical training and I became friendly with many people outside of medical school. Maybe that influenced me, and just reading, and I know it sounds again superficial, but I began to read the *Guardian*, and I thought, 'Gosh, this is a lot of sense!' ... So ... there was no big moment ... but I began to realise how, for want of a better word, how unfair the colonial set up had been and issues around under-developed countries and so on. So it was much more driven by an international perspective probably originally rather than embedded in English issues either immigrants or otherwise. But then gradually as I got into this ... that's when I decided that I wanted to do more in a working-class community you see.[16]

An even more direct link between colonialism and the history of general practice is provided by Dipak Ray's recounting of his political awakening as a child incarcerated for distributing anti-British literature under the Raj and his activism in Great Britain as a prominent left-wing doctor.[17] In an echo of L. R. M. Kamal's memories of the miners' strike, he recalled being involved in a 'doctors for miners' group which raised funds for those taking industrial action.[18] An election leaflet for the 1974 general election shows that he was a high-profile local figure. He is named as one of the speakers at an eve-of-poll meeting held in support of the sitting Bedwellty MP and future Labour party leader, Neil Kinnock, who also spoke at the gathering.[19]

There was also a close connection between Rooin Boomla's political opposition to British rule in India and his commitment to the NHS before it was established: he described becoming a socialist because he felt like 'a second-class citizen in an imperial design' and being 'in favour of the NHS from the beginning as a socialist.'[20]

If the legacy of empire could shape doctors' opinions, the post-war context of immigration to Britain also influenced the development of their political identities. Margaret Thatcher's views on migrant communities were described by Raj Chandran as being particularly detrimental to the image of the Conservatives amongst South Asian doctors.[21] Enoch Powell's association with the Tories was undoubtedly another polarising factor. At least two South Asian doctors were involved in attempts to debate immigration issues with him.[22] Although the category of 'activist doctor' undoubtedly includes other clinicians, a number of factors, including their location in areas where social problems were more immediately apparent, legacies of empire, and the politics of 'race' in post-war Britain all therefore contributed to politicising South Asian doctors. Evidence of a resulting tendency for them to be more left-leaning than average middle-class professionals is provided by Raj Chandran's account of his attempts to recruit South Asian doctors to the Conservative Medical Society following its establishment in the 1970s, an exercise which he found greatly frustrating, with some of those he approached telling him he was involved with the wrong party.[23] He concluded that they 'probably would have joined the Labour party'.[24]

Not all doctors who can be described to a greater or lesser extent as social and political activists became directly involved in representative democracy. Others did nevertheless perceive the effects of societal change, social policy and social context on patients and saw it as part of their role to act to counter these effects. As doctors, they positioned themselves at times between patients and policy-makers. As already mentioned, GPs had a great deal of autonomy at the time, so it is not particularly surprising to hear one describe his interactions with the local social services as involving him giving out what he described as 'orders':

I had a lot problem when demolition came in, in … 1976 or 1977 when … the area was being demolished and they were trying to move the old patient away from the thing and I had a lot of problem with the social service department because within that six month, I had experience that old people who were used to live in that area for a long time, when they moved, so many people … I can't give a figure but I had a … clinical impression that the old people when they moved … from their own environment they were dying like … quickly than those who were surviving in the same environment. So I was refusing the social services department to move older people unless they get a … right place to go and they are agreeing to go. *What sort of discussions did that lead to with social services?* Oh, ah, so many time, I was adamant and I refused to … let them take the patient away. And one or two patients stayed in … my chosen place for two or three months and then they moved … they died within … three or four week … At that time I was a black sheep with the social service department. I said 'No I won't let you do it. If you want to do it, do it at your own peril. But … against my wish, against my order'.[25]

The use of the expression 'black sheep' is particularly interesting as it underscores the importance of the interviewee's agency: it communicates a sense of trying to achieve something against the will of local authorities. Whilst it would not be uncommon for a professional to present their life story as shaped by their own decisions, this would not necessarily entail being in opposition with the local establishment rather than being integrated into it as a professional. The transmission into a British context of elements of South Asian culture can arguably be located in this defence of older patients which echoes Raj Chandran's concern for badly-housed pensioners. This is naturally debatable but it is possible to read these stories in this way.

The relevance of the cultural background of doctors is clearly in evidence in work that relates more specifically to South Asians living in Britain. Akram Sayeed's concern about racism led him to become one of the founder members of the Leicester Community Relations Commission.[26] M. N. I. Talukdar was part of a similar structure in Lancashire and recalls advising Rossendale Borough Council about Muslim burials.[27] The television programme 'Aap Kaa Hak'[28] presented in Urdu and Hindi was established by a Liverpool GP concerned about social problems faced by the British South Asian community.[29] It was broadcast on Granada TV, which covered the north-west of England. Speaking to the medical magazine *Pulse* in 1983, Shiv Pande said that some South Asian patients were being charged fees as they did not know that healthcare in the UK was free at the point of use.[30] He also reported being approached by patients who asked him for information about non-medical questions, such as how to access support from the Department of Health and Social Security.[31] When I asked him about this programme, he described how his experiences led to the creation of a new public forum in which health, legal and social concerns could be discussed:

> In '79, I was off sick with the 'flu, I was sitting down in the house … I was watching TV and there came an old gentleman, Lord Michael Winstanley … and he presented that you know, 'This is your right', this is how you should be conducting if you have any problem … I thought to myself: 'Here is a gentleman who has to present a programme on rights to the British people who are born in this country, who are educated in this country … If this is the situation then what will be the plight of those people who are not born here?' … We did it with a friend of

mine who was from Pakistan who ... was a barrister ... If there was any
legal problems then he would answer, if there was any medical or social
then I will answer and we started doing the programmes ... We initially
thought that we'll do set of thirteen programmes but we ended up doing
for fourteen years! (laughs) ... *Did you get many questions about health
on the programme?* Oh, yes, we did ... various health issues as well ... I
remember we did about the ... ischemic heart disease, we did about the
diabetes ... all those subjects which are common ... depression in the
... ladies because they were isolated at home.[32]

Another instance of a doctor's background shaping the wider context
of healthcare is provided by a participant's account of how he raised the
issue of the provision of vegetarian food for Hindu patients in hospitals in the context of local medical politics and succeeded in obtaining
its introduction.[33] A doctor in the north of England spoke of visiting
a local food factory to discuss food production and its suitability for
South Asian diets.[34] South Asian doctors described having a degree of
professional freedom and being able to launch initiatives that had a significant impact. Not all of them did of course. Nevertheless, a number
of them described a professional space that intersected with public life
and a social environment where migrant doctors were able to take on
leading roles.

Whilst the ethnicity and geographical origin of doctors was a factor
in shaping their action in a number of instances, individual personal
experience also served to determine the nature of their involvement in
their communities. Doctors became involved in the work of voluntary
organisations dealing with issues in which they took a personal interest
as a direct result of life experiences—be it disability[35] or drug addic-
tion.[36] Social action could also be driven by interests that derived from
medical research, involvement in medical organisations and a wider
concern for public health. Ralph Lawrence described how his involvement in his local division of the BMA of which he became the secretary
in the early 1960s[37] led naturally to other interests:

Things like smoking and smoking-related diseases, this was another
thing that the BMA took a very active part and I supported that very,
very much. I was a founder member of the organisation in Derbyshire
called DASH—Derbyshire Action on Smoking and Health. I ... was
one of the very, very prominent advocates of the abolition or the restric-
tion of smoking, especially amongst young people.[38]

In a number of instances, doctors took on roles that are quite obviously directly connected to their personal background. Elsewhere, the distinction between the influence of ethnic background and geographical origin and that of the nature of the work they were doing is harder to make—reactions to poverty and disagreeing with housing policy and its effect on older people could simply be typical of the attitudes of doctors based in deprived areas. In other instances, factors such as personal experiences would appear to be the main motivation.

A future, broader-based, history of general practice encompassing the involvement of other doctors in these areas would produce a clearer picture. The legacies of empire, debates around 'race' in postwar Great Britain and contact with the everyday concerns of working-class patients were however all factors that were more likely to have an impact on South Asian doctors than on their white counterparts. In a number of instances, South Asian doctors were also involved in work which can be to a greater or lesser extent linked to their social and cultural background. They are not unique in this respect; they form part of a wider group of similarly-motivated doctors whose roles at a local level across the UK have so far attracted little interest from historians of medicine.

## 'I didn't speak English like ... Peter Sellars': entering the national stage

The social and political influence that a number of South Asian doctors managed to exert at a grassroots level was also, as has been alluded to, in evidence in a national context. At times this was through their involvement in collective action by the establishment of new organisations, as the next section of this chapter will show. A number of individual doctors also became prominent GPs. Once more, ascertaining precisely to what extent doctors' origins in the Indian subcontinent served to propel them into certain roles is a difficult exercise. Doctors' accounts do however suggest that one of the legacies of empire in South Asia was the production of anglicised doctors who were culturally well equipped to play prominent parts in British society and medicine. Describing the work of these doctors and highlighting its importance is not to say that indigenous doctors were not engaging with similar issues in similar ways. The important point here is that the influence and prominence that some South Asian doctors attained should be recognised as forming part of the broader picture of the influence of South Asian medical migration to Britain. The impact that South Asian doctors were able to have at a national level on developments within and beyond the field of healthcare can be located in their involvement in medical politics, community relations activism and in the initiation of changes to professional practice.

The ability of individual South Asian doctors to gain representation in mainstream medico-political bodies should not be overstated. According to Bashir Qureshi, as late as 1990, he became the first ethnic minority GP to be nationally elected to the council of the RCGP.[39] A number of doctors had however occupied prominent positions in medical politics prior to that. By the early 1980s, three overseas-qualified South Asian doctors were sitting on the GMSC. M. Hamid Husain was elected to the body which dealt with matters concerning general practice in 1978, having already become secretary of the Rotherham division of the BMA and member of the association's Trent Regional Council.[40] Deb Kumar Bose, a GP in Wolverhampton, had also succeeded in rising through the traditional BMA channels.[41] Dipak Ray had become a member of the GMSC in the early 1970s, having been nominated by the Medical Practitioners' Union.[42]

They were not the first South Asian doctors to occupy senior roles in the BMA. Ralph Lawrence became a senior figure in the organisation, representing the Derby division at the BMA's Annual Representative Meeting for 36 years from 1962 and sitting on the BMA Council from 1972 to 1986 (Figure 6).[43] He was involved in debates on a range of issues which saw him defending surrogate parenthood, demanding a ban on smoking in public places and opposing the lowering of the age of consent for homosexuals.[44] From 1984, Lawrence also chaired a working party of the National Association of Health Authorities looking into black and minority ethnic access to the NHS, argued in favour of patients being able to self-certify sickness, and was active in encouraging the British medical profession to distance itself from the South African apartheid regime.[45] It seems reasonable to suppose that Lawrence's background was a factor

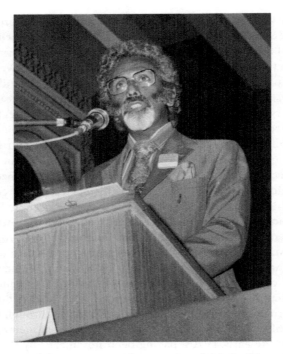

**Figure 6** Ralph Lawrence speaking at a British Medical Association gathering in the 1970s.

in directing him towards some of these particular areas of interest. His involvement in black and minority ethnic health and anti-apartheid politics are the most obvious instances of this. It is also possible that his conservatism on gay rights was the product in part of traditional South Asian socio-cultural attitudes.

The presence in Britain of South Asian GPs capable of successfully negotiating cultural boundaries and playing prominent roles is also arguably an indirect legacy of the British Empire. South Asian doctors were the product of a historical context which exposed them to a greater or lesser extent to the norms of British medicine and British culture. Several of the doctors who took on prominent national roles clearly felt able to 'erase' ethnicity or sidestep stereotypical expectations both within medicine and in wider society:

> I have forgotten what colour I am.[46]
>
> I was chairman of the [political party] locally and we got a letter from some Black voluntary organisation congratulating the ... party locally on ... having a Black chairman. And the look of amazement on the people's face when that was read out was interesting.[47]
>
> I didn't speak English like ... Peter Sellars[48] ... It was quite a bit of an experience for them.[49]

Factors such as accent, education, gender and social background appear to have played a part in determining migrant doctors' ability to prosper in mainstream contexts in the same way that they shaped professional trajectories. If having been brought up in Britain could help to reduce barriers, there are indications that the extent to which adult migrants were anglicised could also influence their ability to be part of national debates. Dipak Ray, self-described as not speaking like Peter Sellars, was an active trade unionist, moving health motions at the annual congress of the Trades Union Congress (TUC) to which he was one of the few non-white delegates.[50] He was a leading anti-racism activist within the trades union movement,[51] wrote for *Tribune*, had a column in the magazine *Doctor*, and in the late 1980s was described in the medical magazine *Pulse* as 'one of the country's most prominent left-wing GPs'.[52] A photograph of him speaking at the TUC Congress in the 1970s (Figure 7) suggests a man in his element and in control of his audience—he is apparently pausing while others around him laugh and smile: he may have just told a joke. His demeanour, along with his relaxed dress sense make him appear as the antithesis of an overawed outsider. He is as much part of the trades union milieu as Ralph Lawrence looks at home as a medical politician addressing other doctors. Ray was also a commissioner of the Commission for Racial Equality as was Raj Chandran. Chandran, whose father worked as an administrator for the British in Malaysia, joined the Conservative Medical Society when it was set up by Shadow Minister for Health Gerard Vaughan and became its secretary.[53]

Ray and Chandran were not the only South Asian doctors playing a leading role in debating issues affecting migrants and ethnic minority groups and influencing policy. M. Hamid Husain was described in

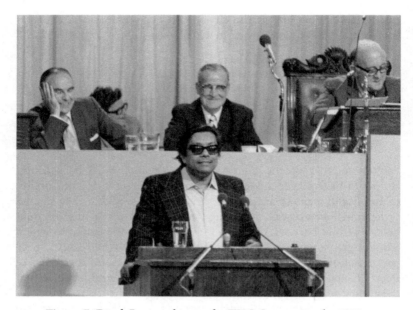

**Figure 7**  Dipak Ray speaking at the TUC Congress in the 1970s.


1983 by the *Guardian* as 'one of the architects' of a BMA plan aimed
at reducing the numbers of migrant doctors coming to the UK which
was being given consideration by the government.[54] Doctors also contributed to the development of organisations established to represent
South Asians in Britain. Akram Sayeed and Dhani Prem became
respectively Chairman and President of the Standing Conference of
Asian Organisations when it came into being in 1970.[55] Sayeed was
also a member of the Community Relations Commission established
following the adoption of the 1968 Race Relations Act. He recounted
having, as a result, acquired a network of medical contacts which he
drew upon when he was involved in setting up the Overseas Doctors'
Association in 1975, providing further evidence that significant numbers of migrant doctors were involved in this agenda.[56]

The involvement of doctors in the politics of 'race' and migration
in post-war Britain is quite obviously connected to their background.
More generally, the ability of South Asian doctors to take part in

national discussions about policy in the first thirty-five years of the NHS can also be linked to a specific historical context which provided some South Asian doctors with social and cultural capital which helped them to become agents of change.

The circumstances surrounding the development of a national network of GP cooperatives as an alternative to recourse to private provision for out-of-hours medical services provides a further illustration of the ability that a number of South Asian doctors had to drive change in policy and practice at a national level. They reinforce the impression that it was most likely to be a certain type of South Asian doctor who could take on such roles. Krishna Korlipara, a GP in Horwich, near Bolton in the north of England, described how dissatisfaction with the service provided by a private company led him to initiate the establishment in 1976 in Bolton of what is recognised as the first GP cooperative in Great Britain:[57]

> I called for a general meeting of all the doctors, you have to remember, this man still in his thirties, calling for a meeting, only in general practice for four years. They all came rather curiously. I spoke extempore about my vision and told them that this is a lifetime's once in a while opportunity, either to pick up the gauntlet and run a service which has never been done before, all collectively owned by all the doctors, no one owning more or less than £1 share but all of us together managing the service to the standards we expect and our patients are entitled to. Is it a dream that we dare have or are we going to be so afraid that we are going to turn our backs?[58]

The language used is again telling and clearly defines the speaker not only as an agent of change but as someone able to embrace the modes of expression of the British establishment—as shown by the reference to speaking 'extempore'.[59] The model which was set up in 1976 in the Bolton area was a success and was later extended to other parts of Great Britain, leading eventually to over two hundred cooperatives being formed, serving a population of thirty million.[60]

If discrimination and marginalisation were a reality, some individual doctors took on prominent roles in medical politics and in wider society. By definition, this involvement was the preserve of a small number of doctors; leading roles can only be taken on by a minority of individuals. Their impact was, however, far from negligible.

The Overseas Doctors' Association and other professional groups

The professional organisations formed by South Asian doctors had a significant impact on the British healthcare system at a national level. A range of professional groups bringing South Asian doctors together were in existence between the 1940s and 1980s, with varying degrees of representativeness and political influence. The ODA, established in 1975,[61] would seem to have been by some distance the most influential in political terms, judging by the number of participants who speak of being involved in its work and the records of contacts with the leaders of the organisation in government archives and in the BMA archives. A number of other associations were also in existence at the time. In the early 1970s, the Pakistan Medical Graduates Association complained that advertisements for GP posts routinely stated that applicants should be graduates of British medical schools and the issue was taken up by the Liberal MP for Rochdale, Cyril Smith.[62] Two letters published in *The Times* in 1975 also suggest that the Indian Medical Association (Great Britain) was seen by the medical establishment as a body that required to be taken seriously and engaged with. A letter from its president M. S. Kataria criticising the media coverage of the withdrawal of GMC registration from Indian medical colleges was published on Thursday 29 May.[63] The following Monday, 2 June, a letter from Henry Yellowlees, the Chief Medical Officer, provided reassurance that the service that Indian doctors had given was 'fully recognised'.[64] By the early 1980s groups representing Bangladeshi and Sri Lankan doctors were also in existence.[65]

There also appears to have been a degree of overlap between the ODA and other groups organised along national lines: at what seems to have been its first meeting with the BMA in 1975, it is described by one of its leaders Akram Sayeed as an 'umbrella organisation' and representatives of the Indian Medical Society, the Indian Medical Association, the Pakistan Medical Society and the Bangladesh Medical Association were also present.[66] A more radical group, the National Association of Ethnic Minority Doctors (NAEMD) emerged in 1983 with an agenda critical of both the ODA and the BMA.[67] The NAEMD announced its intention to approach MPs with a view to bringing a private member's Bill that would modify the UK rules affecting the registration of doctors that had been introduced in the late 1970s.[68] Given that general practice was one of the areas in which South Asian doctors clustered, GPs naturally constituted a significant proportion of the membership of these associations which were involved in the political debates that shaped medicine at the time. Alongside alumni networks, they also performed a social and educational role, which will be examined separately in the third section of this chapter.

The ODA, which came into being in the 1970s as migration (and, gradually, by extension, medical migration) became more politicised and when South Asian doctors were more numerous, appears to have exerted the greatest influence by far. It brought together a significant number of doctors from different countries and had a proactive leadership that was successful in making the organisation's voice heard and efficient when pursuing its objectives. In spite of its apparently inclusive name it was a South Asian-led body: the impetus for its foundation came from South Asian doctors[69] and there is no reference in the writings of its early leaders or in interviews with prominent members to any influential non-South Asian members.[70] Whilst its remit was not specific to general practice a number of its senior figures were GPs. Of the four most prominent founder members, two were general practitioners: Akram Sayeed, a Bangladeshi GP based in Leicester, and Sri Venugopal, an Indian GP from Birmingham.[71] A number of other GPs held senior posts in the years following the establishment of the organisation.[72] The ODA leadership very quickly obtained access to the higher echelons of British parliamentary and medical politics. It was founded on 11 May 1975 at the initiative of a small group of South Asian doctors unhappy at the treatment of migrant doctors in the NHS.[73] An editorial in the first edition of *ODA News* published in October 1976 reported that within a year it had succeeded in gaining recognition from 'the Establishment, and the various august bodies, which control the future of British Medicine, educationally, as well as politically'.[74]

BMA and government archives provide a substantial amount of support for this claim. Within months of the establishment of the organisation, ODA leaders were meeting with cabinet ministers. A letter sent by the ODA to the Labour Secretary of State for Health and Social Security Barbara Castle in September 1975 refers to 'our talk at Dr Rhaman's house on Friday, 5 September 1975'.[75] ODA events were attended by the major figures involved in defining healthcare policy at the time. Both the then Secretary of State for Health and Social Security

David Ennals and his Conservative shadow Patrick Jenkin attended its first annual dinner in 1976.[76]

As appeared to be the case when it came to individual initiatives, the familiarity of South Asian doctors with British culture and identification with it in a post-imperial context could well have contributed to their ability to gain access to the political and medical establishment. One of the main grievances voiced by the ODA following its establishment was that UK-based overseas doctors were being denied the right to practice elsewhere within the European Economic Community while British-trained doctors enjoyed freedom of movement.[77] An editorial in *ODA News* complained that this meant that overseas doctors would not be able to 'treat even their fellow British citizens' in other Common Market countries.[78] Given that it is unlikely that substantial numbers of South Asian doctors would have wanted to move to Hamburg or Bordeaux, the embracing of this cause can only be interpreted as an expression of doctors' strong desire to be fully accepted as equal to other British-based doctors. This, in turn, suggests a strong identification with the culture and values of the former colonial power and a need to be recognised as being part of it.

Shiv Pande, who remembered joining the ODA a few years after it was set up and later became one of its senior members gave a telling description of his conception of politics when he stated in his interview that: 'I am a real committee man. I like to take most people with me'.[79] The description of meetings given by the former Chief Medical Officer, Sir Liam Donaldson also provides evidence that South Asian doctors were particularly apt at engaging the establishment and co-opting its members to further their aims:

> I think the interesting phenomenon ... was ... the extent to which the Asian doctors were organised socially. So they ... would have annual dinners and events ... to which ... they would invite prominent people, so for example the Dean of the Medical School ... and I was in the more junior capacity then but I would be invited to those sorts of functions and events so there ... was a great deal of cohesiveness in ... the professional societies and associations that the Asian doctors formed and they were extremely ... hospitable and keen to get guests from the ... higher echelons of the health service and the medical school ... *Was this the Overseas Doctors' Association you are talking about or is it other organisations as well?* ... Yes, the Overseas Doctor's Association ... I think there

were some more informal groupings than that but I can't remember the detail of it. *And what sort of impact would this have on decision makers, did people talk about it, did it shape their thinking in any way?* Well I think it certainly ... created ... a focus, I think, because it wasn't just the problems of Asian doctors that they would talk about, but ... the problems of ethnic minority health ... so I think it did start to establish that it was an important thing for them to do.[80]

The ODA was led by doctors born under British rule and in some respects its presence in the British medical landscape of the 1970s can be interpreted as an imperial legacy. Its influence also needs to be seen not just in the direct results of its actions but in the changes that it encouraged others to make.

From the 1970s, regular meetings were taking place between government ministers and ODA representatives and a working group was established to bring together the ODA, the Department of Health and Social Security and the Regional Health Authorities with a brief to examine problems facing overseas doctors and explore what action might be taken.[81] The ODA had met with Derek Stevenson and Elston Grey-Turner the Secretary and Deputy Secretary of the BMA as early as June 1975.[82] Discussions eventually led to an agreement in 1976 on the co-option of an ODA representative on the GMSC.[83] South Asian GPs also gained representation on the GMC. By 1984, at least three South Asian GPs (as well as a number of other senior ODA members) had succeeded in being elected: Sunil Chandra Bhattacharya, Sri Venugopal and Krishna Korlipara.[84] The presence of South Asian doctors within the GMC provided an opportunity to attempt to address issues that affected them directly—such as professional discrimination in the context of the treatment of doctors facing complaints.[85] It also meant that they were in a position to offer a GP's perspective on medical regulation. General practitioners had been unable to obtain council membership until the introduction of elections as recommended by the Committee of Inquiry into the Regulation of the Medical Profession in 1975.[86]

As alluded to by Sir Liam Donaldson, as well as defending their own professional interests, South Asian doctors also helped to raise the profile of issues affecting the ethnic minority patients to whom they provided an important service. Sri Venugopal thus recalls using discussions with the DHSS to this effect and encouraging the government to launch a campaign aimed at tackling the high incidence of rickets amongst South Asian children.[87] It can be difficult to gain a sense of the precise nature of the ODA's influence. If Sri Venugopal for instance described a very proactive approach to putting ethnic minority health on the agenda, Akram Sayeed in his memoirs writes that the publication of a report on rickets and anaemia resulted in the Health Minister Gerard Vaughan inviting him to join a committee to look at health problems encountered by South Asians.[88] This, in turn, according to Sayeed, led to the launch of the 'Stop Rickets' campaign.[89]

What is beyond doubt is that the ODA was represented in debates at a national level and was able to have an influence in a number of identifiable areas. The most direct evidence of this was the amendment to the proposed new legislation on medical regulation in the late 1970s to create the category of limited registration. The general secretary of the ODA, S. A. A. Gilani, argued in the *BMJ* in December 1977 for the abolition of the system of temporary registration (which allowed overseas doctors to practice in the UK but could be withdrawn and required renewal[90]) and for migrant doctors to be able to progress to full registration.[91] The following month, Lord Hunt of Fawley put forward two amendments to the Medical Bill in the House of Lords that brought in a system of limited registration and allowed for progress to full registration. He quoted from Gilani's article when moving the amendments and noted that they had the support of the ODA.[92]

The ODA was equally effective in gaining a profile in the mainstream and the medical media. In 1979 the *Guardian* for instance reported its decision to complain to the GMC about the gynaecological examinations that migrant women were subjected to at Heathrow airport, asking for a ruling on the ethics of such practices.[93] In 1985 the magazine *Doctor* devoted its main headline to the news that the ODA was calling for medical migrants to boycott Britain in response to the government's decision to introduce work permits for migrant doctors and restrict postgraduate opportunities.[94] The ODA was considered important enough within the British medical community for arguments over vote-rigging in elections to its leadership positions and its future direction to be considered front page news by *Doctor*, *Pulse* and *Hospital Doctor* in the mid-1980s.[95]

By that time, the ODA was faced with serious internal difficulties and had lost some of the momentum that propelled it into the heart of the

British medical establishment in the 1970s. Some of its leading members had come to think of it as too passive or as being dominated by Indian doctors to the detriment of other nationalities.[96] It was also at times the victim of its own successes in highlighting the mainstream's lack of engagement with overseas doctors. As Steve Watkins observed in 1987:

> The BMA's response [to the ODA] was to emphasise its own role as the representative of all doctors. Overseas doctors who held office in the BMA ... were invited to write articles for BMA publications and for the medical press, and were given prominence in reports of conferences.[97]

Thus, if by 1980, the BMA had decided that it would no longer offer a seat to the ODA on the GMSC, it could by then argue that this was unnecessary as three South Asian doctors who had not been nominated by the ODA were already members. In fact, the BMA was able to rely on a South Asian member of the GMSC to convey this point to the ODA.[98]

By highlighting the issue of discrimination in British medicine, obtaining representation on a range of bodies and raising the national profile of issues surrounding ethnic minority health, the ODA and the GPs who were central to its running were, however, playing a significant part in the development of national policy between the mid-1970s and the early 1980s and thus shaping the context in which general practice developed. The ODA and a number of other associations formed by South Asian doctors also functioned as networks that gave those involved in them access to professional knowledge and social support.

## Establishing new educational and social structures

In addition to medico-political groupings such as the ODA, there were a number of other associations which aimed to bring together graduates of particular sub-continental medical colleges. At least two publications (one run by the ODA) facilitated the exchange of information relevant to migrant doctors. As well as being an instrument of advocacy, the ODA provided professional training for its members and acted as a forum for information sharing and education. South Asian doctors in effect developed a parallel system of professional development. These groupings were also important vectors of professional networking and support.

Ensuring that its members had educational opportunities in British medicine was one of the ODA's priorities from the outset. Its establishment and development can thus be connected to a significant number of doctors' decisions to remain in Britain and their desire to build successful careers rather than be treated as 'pairs of hands'. One of the ten principal demands listed in the first edition of *ODA News* was for 'Full participation in Post graduate training activities'.[99] Although this was not limited to general practice, as one of the principal routes offering migrant doctors a career structure, the developing specialty did feature prominently in the work of the ODA in this area. In 1976, *ODA News* reported that M. S. Swani, secretary of the ODA's West Midlands division, had met with the director of the board of graduate clinical studies of the Birmingham Medical School and the regional adviser in general practice to discuss postgraduate training for overseas doctors.[100] Further evidence that accessing training with a view to entering general practice was amongst the organisation's priorities is provided by the inclusion in the first edition of the magazine *ODA News* of the first part of a guide to passing the Membership of the Royal College of General Practitioners (MRCGP) examination written by the Salford GP S. A. A. Gilani who by then was a trainer in general practice.[101] More generally, the ODA provided South Asian GPs with access to a parallel and informal system of professional development, which brought general practitioners into contact with other doctors who had migrated from the Indian subcontinent. Muhammad Noorul Islam Talukdar, a GP in Bacup in the north of England recalls that this filled a gap in provision by providing training in a form that South Asian doctors were comfortable with:

> There was not a clear idea ... about progression, of ... their educational need. Overseas Doctors' Association started first introducing lot of postgraduate ... lectures. *Can you tell me a bit more about that, about the training aspect?* We used to invite people who we feel will be able to teach us something, for example any medical problem. And we used to invite the consultants of that particular field who possibly had done some work and give us a lecture, some evening, possibly once or twice a month. *Did you not feel that there were other avenues whereby you could access that sort of knowledge?* Each of the local hospital has postgraduate ... medical centre. Unfortunately we felt we needed a forum whereby we can ... be more relaxed and this is the relaxed atmosphere. Postgraduate medical

forum often used to have what they thought we should learn as opposed to what we think we need to learn.[102]

It is not entirely clear what is meant here by South Asian doctors needing to feel 'relaxed'. Did they indeed have specific training needs that could not be addressed satisfactorily through local medical structures or was it simply a case of them having little trust in the wider culture of British medicine? Graduates of South Asian medical schools would undoubtedly have had concerns that their white UK-trained colleagues did not (i.e. understanding the unspoken rules of British medical culture when it came to sitting Royal College examinations). Given the prevalence of racism and heterophobia in British medicine, it would not be surprising if there had been a more widespread distrust and consequently a reluctance to engage with local training provision. Alternatively, the use of the word relaxed might hint at a more fundamental purpose of these structures as a social support network—a dimension I will describe later in this chapter.

Whatever the precise motivations of those who set them up may have been, these new structures clearly played a part in helping migrant doctors develop a sense of belonging in the NHS. As illustrated by the references I have already made to *ODA News*, South Asian doctors found their own ways of disseminating information of relevance to other migrant doctors. Another example of the existence of these parallel systems of professional development and information exchange that had been established by South Asian doctors by the early 1980s is provided by the journal *Medicos* which was launched by S. M. Qureshi, a GP in Nottingham. His testimony serves as a reminder that although South Asian doctors were the most numerous group of overseas doctors working in the NHS, doctors who were nationals of other countries were involved in these organisations and seen as part of their constituency. His aspiration to 'bridge that gap' between 'East and West' highlights its existence at the time and South Asian doctors' agency in attempting to create a professional space for themselves. It is also a subtle reminder of the imperial backdrop to this story; the notion of a divide between East and West (and one that individuals can bridge) being of course an echo of Rudyard Kipling's poem[103] 'The Ballad of East and West':

> *Medicos* journal ... I started in 1975 ... it was just to raise the issues of these ... overseas doctors and the developing countries. We used

to bring some news reviews from most of these countries, for example India, Pakistan ... Nigeria ... Middle Eastern countries. We used to also invite other ... articles ... for general interest. It was not a research sort of a newspaper ... there was a need of a paper just to bring East and West closer ... in medicine ... We thought that we are going to bridge that gap ... We had ... circulation approximately I think about five thousand ... it was quarterly publication and it ran quite nicely for some years until the 2002 ... *Who were your readers?* Mostly readers are the overseas doctors, then all the postgraduate medical centres in England, we used to send them.[104]

Whilst these groups were led by South Asian men, they presented themselves as having an international focus, therefore they should not be seen solely as aiming to bring together doctors from the Indian sub-continent. They also had a remit of engaging with other migrant doctors and the British medical mainstream. They developed a distinct system of educational provision and more generally information exchange.

One of the drivers of these initiatives was the desire of doctors to enhance their professional status (for instance in the case of the advice given with regards to the MRCGP examination or the links with Birmingham Medical School) and careers in the NHS. There was also an overlap between the educational dimension of gatherings and a more general networking function:

We had regular interactive workshops and the meetings ... we had several divisions of the ODA which met regularly. And that enabled ... people to get together to exchange their experiences as well as to be involved in the professional activities, to learn from each other. And they invited the guests, guest speakers from outside the ODA itself ... So it established a forum for dialogue both among themselves within the overseas doctors as well as between the overseas doctors and the native British doctors ... *What ... sort of subjects would have been discussed?* ... Medical subjects like diabetes, the heart disease ... the rheumatology ... and so many other ... topics ... *So would many Asian GPs have attended these workshops do you think?* Oh massively ... There's no doubt at all. I personally have witnessed several hundreds of doctors.[105]

It is of course hard to judge from doctors' interviews the relative import-ance afforded to professional development and socialising at such events. It is likely that this varied across organisations, time periods and depending on the interests of different practitioners. As professionals reminiscing about their working lives some doctors at least may also have been tempted to over-emphasise the importance of the medical dimension of these gatherings. It might make for a more satisfying self-image to talk of spending one's spare time in pursuit of knowledge as opposed to just enjoying a meal and drinks with colleagues. What comes across clearly in recollections though is the sense of belonging derived from membership of organisations like the ODA:

> It was a social event but there will be some … postgraduate … lectures … given by … hospital consultants mostly … And the doctors themselves will choose … what sort of … cardiology, or nephrology or whatever things they are interested into … diabetic management or … chronic respiratory problem, chiropody, all those things … and they'll give a lecture … just like locally, it is the same thing but happens in a different setting … There are maybe two or three hundred GPs … in one place at one time … *You said the ODA and other organisations were also to a certain extent a social network, how did that work, what sort of things happened?* … We are all general practitioners … There will be … topics … small groups will meet together to talk on certain things— how do you cope with this … it is exchange of ideas and experiences … some people were working in Wales, some in England, some in … Scotland … how can they communicate? … There is no … Internet in those days.[106]

The significance of these groups should not be underestimated. They provided important outlets for doctors seeking to build careers and lives in Great Britain, enabling them to access information and form networks. There is little reason to doubt the claim that these meetings were well attended: the ODA was, after all, able to mobilise a sufficiently large membership to obtain representation on the GMC. The overlap between educational and professional exchange and social get-together and the blurring of boundaries between the two seems to have been one of the defining characteristics of such gatherings and was no coincidence. The organisation also saw itself as providing support to its members, seeking, according to its Memorandum of Association, to 'provide a comprehensive counselling and career service.'[107] By the late 1970s, it had established an advisory service with the support of the DHSS.[108] In 1976, *ODA News* was encouraging its readers to create more local divisions 'not only to strengthen the cause of the Overseas doctors but also to perform a social need among Overseas Doctors and their families.'[109]

This social role was also performed by a range of groupings bringing together graduates of South Asian medical colleges. The first reunion of medical graduates from Andhra, Guntur and Rangaraya medical colleges resident in the UK was organised in 1986.[110] The Calcutta Medical College ex-Students' Association in the United Kingdom was also established by the mid-1980s: an obituary in the *BMJ* of K. K. Panja, a GP in the north-west of England who died in 1986, states that he was a founder member.[111] R. P. Shukla who was a GP in Reading was secretary of the Nagpur Medical College Overseas Association when he died in 1983.[112] Alumni organisations were clearly in existence and considered important enough to be mentioned when summing up doctors' lives by the 1980s. Doctors' interviews suggest that such gatherings began earlier. One written account of the creation of the Andhra Medical Graduates Reunion describes meetings of the Indian Students Association giving way to informal gatherings of doctors who had graduated from the same college and then the formal establishment of a network once significant numbers of South Asian doctors had settled in Britain.[113]

The descriptions that doctors give of the function of these organisations is not dissimilar to the way in which they talk about the ODA. They enabled the exchange of information but also facilitated social contact by bringing together British-based doctors who shared a common identity forged in specific medical schools:

> Every ... medical college from India has a reunion every year ... I come from Hyderabad ... We have our own reunion every year ... We all meet. We have two days ... one day we spend for postgraduate lectures. Second day, we have ... dinner and dance and this sort of thing ... Most of the medical college have got reunions in this country. *And how long has that been going on for?* Oh, it's going on for number of years—since at least sixties it's going on ... Basically these are social gatherings, you meet your old friends and enjoy your nostalgia ... But in the same time, one day we always felt that it should be allocated to some ... learning process.[114]

Alumni networks and doctors' organisations played an important social function in helping doctors to adapt to their new lives as well as enabling them to build networks. S. A. A. Gilani described the Pakistan Medical Society as a type of social club, which would bring together doctors and their families for events such as Eid or Pakistan Day.[115] The society would also book well-known musicians and singers.[116] Doctors' cultural and social needs could also be met through groupings that on the surface were not connected to medicine. The development of South Asian organisations in Britain that were apparently purely cultural such as Kannada Balaga could also be in fact driven by doctors seeking to adapt to life away from the Indian subcontinent. They formed a majority of members when the group celebrating the language and culture of the Kannada people of Southern India was established in the 1980s.[117] These voluntary organisations were important to doctors who could suffer from social isolation and professional frustration.[118] A classified ad placed in the *Guardian* in 1969 thus rather poignantly reads 'A YOUNG OVERSEAS DOCTOR recently arrived in London seeks a small social circle'.[119]

These associations are important to the history of the NHS because of the information they allowed doctors to access and the part that they played in their personal lives. The proliferation of networks shows that they were certainly perceived as useful by doctors. Although this was less apparent in interviews, where one might expect participants to be less open about using such groups to further personal agendas, they could also serve to access information essential to careers:

I was a student in medical college in Calcutta and there are lots of other boys and girls from Calcutta Medical College who are here in UK … We set up an organisation [in 1977] … ourselves called Medical College Ex-Student Association UK … We have our annual meet … in July … in various parts of the country … and we have … Friday, Saturday, Sunday … we meet all the other doctors working in different parts of the country and we do get into informal discussions, and … find out the problems … if there be any but the association is not a … pressure group as such, it's just … what you'd call a social gathering … But through … involvement … in that you do get a … lot of information from various other doctors in different parts of the country … and you get to know many things … it's … purely a social gathering … with a bit of scientific things put in. *How important would you say that network was to you over the years?* It helps out in the sense that people do know what's going on … particularly … in the hospital sector … what jobs is going, who is good … what to go for … it helps … networking and helps … anybody who wants to … get a job or … do some research … they get help from each other.[120]

These groupings set up by South Asian doctors undoubtedly served to give their members an advantage when it came to developing their careers and profile. The ODA for instance propelled some of its more high-profile members into prominent positions in British medical politics.

## Conclusion

The fact that large numbers of doctors from the Indian subcontinent settled in Britain in the post-war period led to the emergence of a range of networks which provided access to opportunities for professional development and information exchange as well as social support. They form an important part of the history of British general practice for the role that they played in the professional and personal lives of South Asian GPs. Incorporating these developments into the history of general practice does not result in the production of a complete history of the discipline. Nor does it result in the production of an uncritically celebratory history: drug companies were for instance involved in supporting the development of new organisations.[121] This naturally leaves open the question of what the pharmaceutical industry was able to obtain in exchange for its support. As one interviewee put it: 'Obviously the drug companies would have a speaker on a subject that was to their interest'.[122] What should be clear however is that understanding the development of British general practice involves an appreciation of the fact that its development is multidirectional and contested rather than linear and driven by top-down processes. Migrant doctors played a formative part in its development.

## Notes

1  See Smith et al., 'Speaking for a change'.
2  L. R. M. Kamal interview with author.
3  D. Ray interview with author, 5 December 2008.
4  Anonymous interview with author.
5  D. Ray interview with author, 19 March 2010.
6  R. Chandran interview with author.
7  I. Grosvenor, 'Prem, Dhani Ram (1904–1979)' *Oxford Dictionary of National Biography* [online] (Oxford: Oxford University Press, 2013). Accessed 2 July 2017 at: www.oxforddnb.com/index/103/101103441/.
8  Ibid.

9 Ibid.
10 Simpson, 'Gulati, Harbans Lall'.
11 Ibid.
12 L. R. M. Kamal interview with author.
13 L. R. M. Kamal interview with author.
14 He was born in present-day Bangladesh.
15 Anonymous interview with author.
16 Anonymous interview with author.
17 D. Ray interviews with author, 5 December 2008 & 19 March 2010.
18 D. Ray interview with author, 19 March 2010.
19 Private papers of Dr Dipak Ray.
20 R. Boomla interview with author, 16 September 2009.
21 R. Chandran interview with author.
22 K. Korlipara interview with author; 'Immigrants' leader dies in road crash', the *Guardian* (13 November 1979), p. 4.
23 R. Chandran interview with author.
24 Ibid.
25 Anonymous interview with author.
26 Sayeed, *Taqdir*, pp. 126–9.
27 M. N. I. Talukdar interview with author.
28 The name of the programme is a translation of the title of the English language programme it was based on: 'This is your right'.
29 S. Pande interview with author, 23 November 2009.
30 W. Lloyd, 'TV star breaks down the language barrier', *Pulse* (10 September 1983), p. 28.
31 Ibid.
32 S. Pande interview with author, 23 November 2009.
33 Anonymous interview with author.
34 Anonymous interview with author.
35 R. Boomla interview with author, 16 September 2009.
36 R. Chandran interview with author.
37 BLSA, C900/03116, Millennium Memory Bank, R. Lawrence interviewed by J. Rogers, 1999.
38 Ibid.
39 Personal information: B. Qureshi email to author, 27 January 2011.
40 'Important post for Asian doctor', *West Indian World* (24 August 1978), p. 7; D. Ray & S. Bhattacharya, 'Overseas column: Why ODA must stay on GMSC … and why it is out for now', *Doctor* (4 December 1980), p. 11.

41  Ray & Bhattacharya, 'Overseas column'; A. Chaudhuri, 'Deb Kumar Bose', *BMJ* (1998, 317: 7163), p. 952.
42  D. Ray interview with author, 5 December 2008.
43  Lawrence, *Fire in his Hand*, p. 63.
44  Lawrence, *Fire in his Hand*, p. 64.
45  Lawrence, *Fire in his Hand*, pp. 63 & 66; 'New council member calls for unity', *Pulse* (23 October 1971), p. 3.
46  R. Lawrence, quoted in 'New council member calls for unity', *Pulse* (23 October 1971), p. 3.
47  Anonymous interview with author.
48  This is a reference to the now notorious film *The Millionairess* (A. Asquith, Twentieth Century Fox, 1960) in which a heavily made-up Sellars played the part of an Indian doctor and adopted a caricatural accent.
49  D. Ray interview with author, 5 December 2008.
50  Ibid.
51  'Dipak Ray', *TUC In Touch e-bulletin*, Issue 8 2011/12 (4 May 2012). Accessed 19 November 2015 at: www.tuc.org.uk/about-tuc/touch/touch-e-bulletin-74; D. Ray 2008 interview with author, 5 December 2008.
52  D. Ray interviews with author, 5 December 2008 & 19 March 2010; N. Duncan, 'Breaking the mould of medical politics', *Pulse* (2 January 1988), p. 15.
53  R. Chandran interview with author.
54  A. Veitch, 'Commonwealth doctors in UK may have to go', the *Guardian* (29 December 1983), p. 22.
55  Sayeed, *Taqdir*, p. 160.
56  Sayeed, *Taqdir*, pp. 136–8 & 142.
57  K. Korlipara interview with author; 'CV: Dr Krishna Korlipara', *Pulse* (10 December 2005), p. 56.
58  K. Korlipara interview with author.
59  Meaning literally 'out of the time', i.e. on the spur of the moment, without preparation.
60  K. Korlipara interview with author; 'CV: Dr Krishna Korlipara', *Pulse* (10 December 2005), p. 56.
61  M. I. Akter, 'Overseas Doctors Association in UK', *Medicos* (December 1975), pp. 6–9; 'Why ODA', *ODA News* (1976, 1:1), pp. 1–2; S. Venugopal interview with author.
62  'Job advertisements for doctors "racial"', the *Guardian* (17 February 1973), p. 5.

63  M. S. Kataria, 'Indian doctors in UK', *The Times* (29 May 1975), p. 15.

64  H. Yellowlees, 'Indian doctors in the NHS', *The Times* (2 June 1975), p. 13.

65  M. F. Haque interview with author; anonymous interview with author.

66  BMA, Problems of overseas doctors in UK re employment, Notes of a meeting between representatives of the BMA and representatives of the Overseas Doctors' Association in the UK, 19 June 1975.

67  J. Cousins, 'Ethnic group pledges campaign against limited registration', *Hospital Doctor* (24 November 1983), p. 12.

68  Ibid.

69  Chatterjee, *Yesterdays*, pp. 120–2.

70  Chatterjee, *Yesterdays*; Sayeed, *Taqdir*; K. Korlipara interview with author; S. A. A. Gilani interviews with author; R. Prasad interview with author.

71  Chatterjee, *Yesterdays*, pp. 120–2; S. Venugopal interview with author.

72  K. Korlipara interview with author; M. N. I. Talukdar interview with author; R. Prasad interview with author; S. M. Qureshi interview with author, 20 May 2011.

73  Sayeed, *Taqdir*, p. 194; 'Why ODA?', *ODA News* (1976, 1:1), pp. 1–2.

74  'Why ODA?', *ODA News* (1976, 1:1), pp. 1–2.

75  National Archives, MH 149/1840, Overseas Doctors' Association, Letter to Barbara Castle, 9 September 1975.

76  'News, views and comments', *ODA News* (November–December 1976, 1:2), p. 6.

77  'Editorial: Sad day', *ODA News* (November–December 1976, 1:2), p. 3.

78  Ibid.

79  S. Pande interview with author, 23 November 2009.

80  Sir L. Donaldson interview with author, 9 May 2011.

81  National Archives, MH 149/1840, Briefing Note for S.S. for meeting with ODA, 30 June 1976.

82  BMA, Problems of overseas doctors in UK re employment, Notes of a meeting between representatives of the BMA and representatives of the Overseas Doctors' Association in the UK, 19 June 1975.

83  *ODA News*, 1976 (No title, 1:1), p. 11.

84  D. Fletcher 'Disciplined doctor now on GMC', the *Daily Telegraph* (8 February 1980), p. 3; General Medical Council Archives, Minutes of the General Medical Council, Branch Councils and Committees for the year 1979 with reports of committees etc … , Manchester: 1980 (?);Private papers of Krishna Korlipara, Overseas Doctors' Association, Letter to members, August 1984.

85   S. Venugopal interview with author.
86   S. Harrison & R. McDonald, *The Politics of Healthcare in Britain* (London, Thousand Oaks, New Delhi, Singapore: SAGE Publications, 2008), p. 37; Webster, *Health Services*, Vol. II, p. 706.
87   S. Venugopal interview with author.
88   Sayeed, *Taqdir*, p. 191.
89   Ibid.
90   Smith, *Overseas Doctors*, p. 13.
91   S. A. A. Gilani, 'Reform of the GMC', *BMJ* (1977, 2), p. 1600.
92   Hansard, HL Deb, vol. 388, cols 291–4, Medical Bill, 24 January 1978.
93   M. Philipps, 'Doctors join virgin row', the *Guardian* (15 February 1979), p. 2.
94   M. McCormack, 'ODA demands stay-away protest in permit row', *Doctor* (April 4 1985), p. 1.
95   J. Sims, 'Overseas doctors row on "improper elections"', *Pulse* (1 December 1984), p. 1; 'Ousted boss lashes overseas doctors' leaders', *Hospital Doctor* (9 May 1985), p. 1; M. McCormack 'Ousted leader warns of split in ODA ranks', *Doctor* (9 May 1985), p. 1.
96   'Ousted boss lashes overseas doctors' leaders', *Hospital Doctor* (9 May 1985), p. 1; Sayeed, *Taqdir*, p. 200.
97   Watkins, *Medicine and Labour*, p. 201.
98   Ray & Bhattacharya, 'Overseas column', p. 11.
99   'What the ODA wants to achieve?', *ODA News* (1976, 1:1), p. 10.
100  'West Midlands Division', *ODA News* (1976, 1:2), p. 11.
101  S. A. A. Gilani, 'MRCGP examination', *Supplement to ODA News* (1976, 1:1).
102  M. N. I. Talukdar interview with author.
103  R. Kipling, 'The Ballad of East and West', University of Toronto Libraries, accessed 16 April 2017 at: https://rpo.library.utoronto.ca/poems/ballad-east-and-west.
104  S. M. Qureshi interview with author.
105  K. Korlipara interview with author.
106  Anonymous interview with author.
107  Personal papers of Dr Satya Chatterjee and Mrs Enyd Chatterjee, Memorandum Articles of Association and By-Laws of The Overseas Doctors' Association in the UK Limited, No. of Company: 1396082, Incorporated the 26th day of October, 1978 (Amended on 31st August, 1988).

108 National Archives, BS6/2893, Royal Commission on the NHS, Oral Evidence from the Overseas Doctors' Association; Sayeed, *Taqdir*, p. 199.

109 'New Divisions', *ODA News* (October 1976, 1:1), p. 9.

110 V. A. R. Rao, 'A. M. G. R.: Celebrating the silver jubilee', Andhra Medical Graduates' Reunion (UK) Silver Jubilee Edition: A retrospective. Andhra Medical Graduates' Reunion (UK), 2010, p. 7.

111 'K. K. Panja', *BMJ* (1986: 292), pp. 566–7.

112 'R. P. Shukla', *BMJ* (1983: 286), p. 564.

113 Rao, 'A. M. G. R.: Celebrating the silver jubilee'.

114 S. Venugopal interview with author.

115 S. A. A. Gilani interview with author, 30 June 2010.

116 Ibid.

117 K. S. Bhanumathi interview with author; 'How we started', Kannada Balaga UK. Accessed 23 November 2015 at: www.kannadabalaga.org.uk/How%20we%20Started.aspx#.

118 Mohan, 'Asian doctors', p. 144; S. A. A. Gilani interview with author, 30 June 2010.

119 'Personal', the *Guardian* (6 Sept 1969), p. 4.

120 A. Chaudhuri interview with author.

121 Anonymous interview with author; Chatterjee, *Yesterdays*, p. 123.

122 Anonymous interview with author.

# 8

# Adding to the mosaic of British general practice

The professional and personal lives of South Asian GPs and their social and political activities contributed to defining the nature of British general practice on the periphery and the social and political context in which care was provided between the 1940s and the 1980s. Their presence in Britain also had a significant and more specific impact on the way in which general practice developed as a dimension of healthcare and as a medical specialty. General practice was not a homogenous field where a clearly defined set of practices was implemented by practitioners. GPs working during this era retained a great deal of professional autonomy at a time when their profession was undergoing a profound transformation. During this period, general practice as a discipline consolidated its status as the cornerstone of the NHS. The provision of treatment in primary care settings became increasingly important to governments keen to contain costs. It was at this time that general practice became recognised as a medical specialty and that the College of General Practitioners (later the Royal College of General Practitioners or RCGP) was founded. This chapter explores the relationship between South Asian doctors and what has been termed the 'renaissance'[1] of general practice in the post-war years. Changes in British General practice from the 1960s onwards coincided with the entry into the field of substantial numbers of South Asian doctors. These two historical processes should be seen as interconnected.

This 'renaissance' was not a linear process; it was contested, took on different forms and at times practitioners chose to ignore some of its central elements. Conceiving of general practice as a mosaic facilitates the writing of a history that acknowledges the agency of individual doctors, including South Asian migrants, in the development of general practice. It also serves to highlight the contradictions, tensions and multi-directionality that are characteristic of its development. Many doctors remained sceptical about such developments. The vast majority of them refrained from joining the RCGP. GPs were also mostly technically independent contractors rather than NHS employees. Change could not be entirely imposed from the centre; its effects varied depending on the interests of individual practitioners and the extent to which they supported different initiatives.

The history of general practice from the 1940s to the 1980s is therefore best conceived of as a mosaic—one which South Asian medical migrants helped to create. Professional change in general practice was shaped both by the involvement and marginalisation of South Asian doctors: they contributed to these processes and gave them particular forms but also limited their impact through disengagement from them. It is impossible to generalise when it comes to their effect on the field: some doctors were proactive implementers of new initiatives, others felt disenfranchised. All contributed to making up the professional identity of an atomised field. The interviews conducted with doctors bear witness to the varying individual conceptions of medicine and the array of practices which together made British general practice what it was. It is of course possible, indeed probable, that in a scholarly academic study of South Asian GPs, a disproportionate number of respondents will be those who are more academically minded or politically engaged. The majority of the quotations used in this section are taken from interviews with doctors who were prominent in medical politics and therefore not necessarily representative of the thought processes of South Asian doctors as a whole. This does not mean however that we should underestimate the significance of their role. As ever, it is important to remember that the professional clustering of South Asian doctors means that their involvement in this agenda had a disproportionate impact on the professionalisation of the discipline in specific parts of Britain. If the extent to which their contribution was specific to their social and cultural background and the professional trajectories they followed is debatable and deserving of further investigation, it is certainly apparent that South Asian doctors were involved in the process of change that characterised British general practice between the 1940s and the 1980s.

The nature of the 'renaissance' of general practice was defined in part by the adoption and shaping of its principles by medical migrants.

The large numbers of South Asian doctors and their geographical clustering signify that without the active engagement of many of them the impact of changes that were affecting general practice would have been significantly reduced. Not all migrant doctors were part of the vanguard of the new general practice, but a significant number of them were and others made change possible by engaging with the new culture of general practice. In addition, South Asian doctors, although trained in systems modelled on British approaches to medicine, should also be seen as the product of their social, cultural and professional background.[2] Evidence of this conditioning is apparent in doctors' memories of their work as GPs. The fact that a number of doctors talk of being marginalised by the medical profession and within the NHS should also be integrated into this history and seen as one of its characteristics.

### 'Doc., if you want that, you'll have it': improving practice premises

South Asian doctors report being involved in initiatives to improve the quality of surgeries and playing an active part in shaping a wider trend involving doctors moving to health centres and using government funds to improve premises. The surgeries that many South Asian doctors found themselves based in as a result of the discrimination that they faced were in areas where historically there had been little investment in general practice and the quality of practice premises left much to be desired.[3] This does not mean that these conditions were simply passively accepted by medical migrants. Their recollections at times indicate an element of surprise when confronted with their working environment at the beginning of their careers as GPs and an implicit aspiration to work in different conditions. Satish Ahuja in Wigan provided a reminder that the fact that doctors had moved from the Global South did not necessarily mean they were used to encountering unsatisfactory professional settings:

> When I came to this country I was literally amazed and surprised when I saw the dirty rooms you're in with the dirty chair, wooden chair and you are living in ... big bungalows and mansions. And your place of work is like this. In India, at that time it used to be other way round: you had made a clinic ... nice clinic ... and the house might not be that good but your clinic will be better than your house ... But over the years ...

government realised and ... they started giving notional rent, people started buying, making it up ... and it is for the better of course.[4]

Hasmukh Joshi's description of the conditions in the practice where he went to work in Pontypool in South Wales is striking in its level of detail, suggesting it made a profound impression on him at the time:

> I thought ... when I get there I'm going to find a wonderful modern building. In fact it was nothing but a converted billiard hall. We had one fire, around which all the patients sat. And there were two consulting rooms coming out of that, with one room for the ... office. And all this was just partitioned off ... If the patients were sitting near ... the consulting room they can hear everything that was going on. We had no hot water, no running hot water at all, we only had one toilet that everybody used, we only had one gas ring on which we sterilised the instruments or you know made cup of teas and coffees ... It was very primitive as compared to what it is now ... In winter months ... you dare not go into the toilet. Because the cisterns used to leak ... And there'll be icicles hanging down. You know, it was that [last word accentuated] primitive. And we never had any instruments as well. Surgical instruments, for example ... if you want to do a smear there's no speculi, so you know we used to send them all to the family planning clinic. It was nothing more than just a ... reactive ... service that we used to provide.[5]

Satish Ahuja's memories and those of Hasmukh Joshi go beyond being a simple professional narrative of encountering problems and moving towards a better way of practising medicine. The emotional charge in the physicians' responses to their initial encounter with British general practice in inner-cities and working-class towns is apparent. They do not just remember conditions being poor from the vantage point of the present; they recall being more than disappointed by what they found. These stark descriptions of South Asian doctors' encounters with industrial general practice in post-war Britain illustrate the extent of the under-investment in this part of the NHS following its establishment.

A number of doctors spoke of being actively involved in exploiting the opportunities that were available to build new premises during the 'renaissance' of general practice. As was the case with policy influence and cultural transfer, it is difficult to precisely map the extent to which the contribution they made in this particular respect was distinct in its nature from those of other GPs. To a certain extent, doctors' accounts simply reflect the fact that they were working during a period

of change, which affected the work practices of all GPs. Their involvement in this agenda can also be connected to, for instance, different
expectations of what a surgery may look like or to the embracing of the
new culture of general practice by South Asian doctors frustrated by
their failure to thrive in hospitals that I will describe later in this chapter. It remains noteworthy that South Asian doctors were involved in
improving the facilities available to their patients. The accounts I discuss were of course given many years after the events they describe but
they are supported by other evidence. For instance, Krishna Korlipara
in Bolton in Greater Manchester was responsible for overseeing the
construction of a new medical centre (Figure 8). A report in the local
press in 1981 makes it clear that he was central to the plans and that
it was a major project. A local councillor is quoted as saying that it
was an ambitious scheme and that it could become one of the best
health centres in the region.[6] A letter sent to Hira Lal Kapur by the
Lancashire Executive Council in 1972 regarding the construction of a
health centre in Heysham in the north-west of England requested his
approval of sketch plans.[7] Whilst the degree to which South Asian doctors were driving change might be debatable, the fact that a number of
them were at the centre of this process, particularly in the industrial
and inner-city areas they were concentrated in is beyond doubt. The
mention by one participant of their engagement with local medical
bodies is also indicative of the fact that at least some South Asian GPs
were part of the local medical establishment and enthusiastic agents
of change:

> I keep telling them [the partners] ... NHS is trying to increase people
> who have ... good premises ... at that time the cost rent scheme came.
> Then I used to tell them that we can build our own surgery on the cost
> rent scheme, it won't cost as much ... I had to show some figures and ...
> I have taken them, my senior partners to the Family Practitioners'
> Committee [Family Practitioner Committee] and through them I ...
> got them explained how it works. Then they agreed for it ... It was ...
> a big task to build premises at that time ... it took nearly one and a half
> years ... It worked out very well, the premises is good ... Four doctors
> used to work without any problem. There are separate nurses' rooms,
> separate dressing room ... big reception hall, upstairs there is a doctors'
> meeting room and conference room. It was really purpose built prem-
> ises. *In what year were those premises built?* 1981.[8]

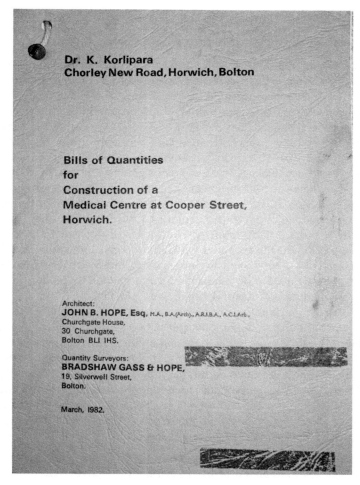

Dr. K. Korlipara
Chorley New Road, Horwich, Bolton

Bills of Quantities
for
Construction of a
Medical Centre at Cooper Street,
Horwich.

Architect:
JOHN B. HOPE, Esq, M.A., B.A.(Arch)., A.R.I.B.A., A.C.I.Arb.,
Churchgate House,
30 Churchgate,
Bolton BL1 1HS.

Quantity Surveyors:
BRADSHAW GASS & HOPE,
19, Silverwell Street,
Bolton.

March, 1982.

**Figure 8** Plans for the building of a health centre in Horwich, near Bolton, under the supervision of Krishna Korlipara.

When I came to my practice, it was very downtrodden practice. It was very cold place and nothing there, and I found that the money's available ... through the LMC to improve it. So I say if I go in ... the LMC then I will have better chance of ... improving my practice. So I joined

the LMC and then I came to know all the ... paraphernalia of LMC how
it works and how it's ... I took the advantage. I was the first practice in
[northern city] to get it on cost rent scheme improvement grant.[9]

It is of course also possible that South Asian doctors were indeed different from their colleagues in this respect and that the discrimination
that they faced when pursuing careers as specialists made them more
determined than other practitioners to participate in the transformation of general practice. It is certainly intriguing to note that in a survey
published in 1980, overseas-trained GPs were found to be more than
twice as likely than their British counterparts to be members or fellows
of a British Royal College (i.e. to have postgraduate qualifications in an
area of medicine outside of general practice).[10] This is, however, hard to
gauge simply on the basis of oral history testimony gathered principally
from one particular group and exploring this question further would
require a more holistic approach to the history of general practice
encompassing the motivations of different groups of practitioners. The
interviews I have conducted do show, though, that South Asian doctors
must be recognised as having been much more than bystanders in the
process of modernisation of British general practice.

It is also important to consider these accounts in the light of the evidence of South Asian doctors' success in becoming embedded in local
communities and influencing social and political developments. If doctors were able to build up surgeries and obtain meetings with ministers, there is little reason to doubt that they could also take centre stage
when it came to developments concerning the buildings they worked
in. Indeed, in some cases, change at a practice level was described as the
result of direct engagement with politicians and senior civil servants of
the type described in the preceding chapter:

First change came in in 1970. At that time ... Secretary of State for
Health was Mr Robinson. I remember writing to him a letter advocating
a health centre and how it will be beneficial for the community. And
that's how we got the very first health centre. At that time, in Bacup
there were three medical practice. One is mine, there was one ... down
the road with two doctors practice and the third one was also a single-
handed practice ... We all moved into the health centre which was first
built in '72 with the exception [of] that last single-handed doctor, he
knew he was retiring, so he never wanted to come into the health centre.
*And what prompted you to write that letter?* It was just feeling that that was

a good thing, having all the primary care under one roof, I felt, would be a good idea.[11]

There is in this description of the evolution of general practice in the working-class Lancashire town of Bacup a sense of possibility, connection to the mainstream and of being able to shape change that is quite striking. It would have been quite conceivable that all of the interviews conducted for this project would have only uncovered stories of migrant doctors working in isolation and contributing to the perpetuation of a more traditional type of general practice. As I have already acknowledged, those who agreed to speak to me were probably more likely than average to be people who were more embedded in the mainstream and believed that they had a positive story to tell. The fact that these doctors describe their experiences in such terms is nonetheless instructive as it emphasises the need to acknowledge the influence that at least some medical migrants were able to have.

Dipak Ray tells a similar story in connection with the construction of a health centre in South Wales where his practice was based. He was a well-known doctor and trade unionist who was used to public speaking and the following extract from his interview reads as a well-rehearsed anecdote. It nevertheless casts light on the extent to which he was integrated into local and national medical politics:

> I was speaking in a rally in … Manchester … Anti-racist rally … I was marching with Barbara Castle and Barbara Castle was then the Minister of Health … She said: 'Do you have a Health Centre?' … 'No'. 'Do you want one?'. I said: 'Yes!' … I came home—a telephone call from the Chief Medical Officer: 'Hey, Dipak, what the hell have you been doing?' (laughs) … 'They want us to come and see you regarding a health centre' … Next day a chap came, within forty-eight hours they started the planning and then the health centre was built in my area.[12]

Not only is Dipak Ray seen here as rubbing shoulders with a senior Labour party figure, he also appears as very close to the Chief Medical Officer for Wales who is described as not only having his home telephone number but as addressing him by his first name and in a jocular fashion. Like Ray, a number of doctors talked about their actions in a way that indicates a sense of being at the centre rather than on the margins of the developments taking place in medicine at the time. The building of new premises, particularly in industrial and inner-city areas of Great Britain was undoubtedly facilitated by their agency. It should of course be recognised that oral history interviews offer people a means to construct a positive narrative around their lives. There would however have been numerous alternative ways of doing this without claiming a stake in the transformation of general practice—doctors could for instance have spoken of seeking solace in the quality of the work they did at a local practice level. Moreover, printed documents, as already mentioned, bear witness to Ray's prominence as a medico-political activist. He does not explicitly claim to have been on close terms with the Chief Medical Officer for Wales but suggests this closeness in an apparently uncalculated way through subtle cues and the recounting of informal language.

Lutfe Rabbi Mustafa Kamal's account of the construction of a new surgery in the Yorkshire mining village of Hemsworth provides an example of how the interweaving of the agendas of governments, initiatives of other doctors and local roles of South Asian doctors played a part in the building of a new practice. His reference to the words used by the architect firmly place the narrator at the helm but whilst this is again unsurprising in the context of an oral history interview, he also tellingly brings into play the gaze of an outsider who viewed South Asian doctors as central to this process:

> The government started investing in ... primary care ... very early on in 1970s. So we took opportunity for that ... There was a doctor in Wakefield, a Dr Elliot (?). He had just made his purpose-built premises on a scheme called cost rent scheme at that time ... We were fired [up] by what he had done ... because he had what at that time was a wonderful surgery ... So I talked to my colleagues. Three of them didn't really want to know because they were ... well into their sixties ... They were not interested ... . But the other partner was ... another Indian colleague ... Dr Sen, the Indian gentleman he was very interested in having a new surgery ... We bought this piece of land and we built this wonderful surgery in 1979 ... We had a wonderful, wonderful, architect who happened to be our patient as well ... We sat down with him and we spent a lot of time with him ... eventually we got the modern surgery ... To be honest, it's still contemporary, even though it was built in 1979 ... I remember saying to him, 'I want to be able to stretch my arms, both my arms and still not touch the walls of the corridor' ... Ian was his name, Ian Massey, Ian said to me 'Doc, if you want that, you'll have it.' ... And that really was the ethos at the time.[13]

L. R. M. Kamal connects his initiative to that of another local doctor, placing it in the broader context of the changing nature of post-war British general practice. By giving voice to the views of the architect contracted to work on the new building he provides a strong sense of the connection of migrant doctors to the 'ethos of the time'. Being recognised by an architect as ultimately responsible for the form that the practice would take was clearly important enough to Kamal for him to recreate the encounter decades later, conjuring up an image of doctor and architect standing together and their associated dialogue. Innovations in general practice were therefore at least in part driven by doctors' perceptions of their necessity and their decisions to become involved in the processes leading to change. In this sense, South Asian doctors can quite literally be described as 'architects of the NHS' as they played an active part in the erection of the buildings which provided the context for the delivery of primary care services.

### 'Hands on' doctors and the development of primary care services

Doctors were also involved in shaping the changing nature of the care provided in surgeries. The emphasis placed on the concept of primary care and on treatment outside of hospital contexts led to the increasing engagement of doctors with other healthcare professionals such as nurses and health visitors.[14] GPs developed areas of specialisation and were more likely to take on roles in specialist units in hospitals in addition to working in their surgeries.[15] For a number of medical migrants, this different conception of the role of the GP resonated with an interventionist narrative that appears in their accounts of their careers as chiming with values associated with South Asian medical education and contexts. Changes to the nature of general practice also offered doctors a means of reconnecting with their initial aspirations to work as specialists in hospitals. Moreover, the influence of the social, cultural and professional background of South Asian doctors on their work as GPs is in evidence when it comes to their work in surgeries around Great Britain. The collective impact of these doctors can be linked to their ethnicity, their medical education on the Indian subcontinent, and their shared experiences of becoming GPs in the NHS after aspiring to become specialists and working for many years in hospitals.

While South Asian doctors were trained in systems which modelled themselves on British medicine,[16] the social and economic environment that medicine on the Indian subcontinent existed in resulted in the emergence of varying forms of medical knowledge. If medicine in the Indian subcontinent looked to Britain, it also took on forms that were particular to local contexts. This had an impact on doctors' approach to medicine. Hasmukh Joshi gave a reflective account of his perception of how approaches to medicine varied between Britain and the Indian subcontinent:

> We were taught mainly clinical medicine in those days because we had issues regarding … investigations particularly … because of the economic problems … you only had … limited number of investigations available to you. So we were taught mainly clinical medicine. You know, try and diagnose patients by just purely on symptoms and science and your examination … so in that respect I think our grounding was much better … looking at somebody, seeing them, and mostly we will arrive at a clinical diagnosis which we will then confirm with some investigations rather than what happens nowadays where they just go for very specialised investigations right from the start … And also … when I qualified … I worked two years there before I came over here and both … the years … I spent in my teaching hospital … I started in surgery … it was a very good grounding again because … the number of patients that we used to see is just unbelievable: I would have something like between sixty-five and sixty-seven admissions every night … and we had to do almost everything ourselves … You were virtually at the coalface with support from your registrar and consultant who rarely came … *Do you feel that gave you a different grounding to the sort of grounding that most British-trained … GPs of your generation would have had?* I would have thought so because I think … we learnt a lot more in that respect. Our theoretical knowledge was much better in some respects as well. However … what I realised when I came here was that the way that they were brought up was slightly different than us in some respects … In our med schools, there was much more emphasis on … the knowledge part of it … rarest of the rare conditions and if you knew that you were a good medical student … Here … people were much more tuned on what is the most commonest thing they are going to see rather than what's the rarest thing they are going to see … . In that respect … we were slightly behind … When we came here … the conditions were so different: there, it was mostly infectious diseases we used to see. Whereas when we came here we saw some … conditions we had never seen in our lives. So … we had to relearn.[17]

Hasmukh Joshi's balancing of the benefits of the practical application of skills in India against a tendency to overemphasise the arcane and the need to acquire skills in a British context gives his account a quality that goes beyond that of a narrative simply claiming professional superiority over counterparts. Taking this sort of approach can form the basis for a critical discussion of how the NHS was shaped by different medical cultures. Whilst gaining an understanding of the precise nature of cultural transfer in the NHS is beyond the scope of this study, it is certainly intriguing to note that South Asian doctors perceived themselves to be a different kind of physician.

Although medical education on the Indian subcontinent was in many respects modelled on that received in Britain, the professional identity of a number of South Asian GPs is for instance based on notions of being a 'hands on', interventionist doctor, able to respond to the pressures generated by the social context in which medicine is practised:

> The practical aspect, the clinical aspect was very good because we had much more turnover than ... what we see in this country ... and even the European countries ... because the population is high, the turnover is high, so you get more chance of hand-on experience. And you see more variety of things, the clinical problems ... which was quite stimulating.[18]
>
> It was not only medicine we learned ... we learned lots of things which ... a future doctor ... ought to know: bedside manners and other things ... And ... try and rely on ... clinical judgment rather than sending bloods to the paths [pathology] lab and wait for the results. That was another ... difference between ... the way we were taught and the way things were taught in England ... My two children studied here, they were born here and I think our teaching was much better.[19]

The claim that a subcontinental medical education was better than one obtained in Britain serves as a reminder that medicine remains an art as well as a science and that debates about which model produces superior doctors can only ultimately be sterile. What seems important to take from these accounts is a sense that South Asian medical graduates cultivated a distinctive professional identity. This notion of being a 'hands on' doctor was reflected in the way that doctors talked about their approach to general practice:

> To have to wait for a week or two weeks for ... results to come back from somewhere and the consultant won't probably be able to see a patient

for weeks on end is something that was difficult to get used to. Because, looking back at where I came from, Dhaka ... you could go and see ... a doctor, you could get immediate ... treatment and ... investigations done—if you had money. If you didn't have money then of course you only got treatment in the hospital outpatients. So I had then realised that this is something GPs need to do themselves to improve their lot.[20]

When I came to this country and GP work ... I used to say to myself 'What is this?' You don't do anything yourself! You send everything to the hospital ... urine, blood. 'What is this?' While in India you do whatever you can yourself, because it's expensive to send blood to the path [ology] lab.[21]

The repetition of the question 'What is this?' emphasises the intensity of Shirin Kutar's feelings of surprise, practically shock, when she encountered a different way of working in Britain, in a way that is reminiscent of doctors' surprise at the poor quality of practice premises. It also serves to link her interview to an emotional reaction at a time when she was starting out as a doctor. Her account conveys a sense of an encounter located in the past with an aspect of British medical practice that struck her as deeply alien rather than appearing as having been subsequently constructed to fit with British understandings of general practice.

There was a synergy between such notions concerning the roles of doctors and moves to reform British general practice. The one research participant whose initial ambition was to become a GP (albeit in India rather than in Britain) described a conception of the general practitioner with additional qualifications and special interests which fitted closely with the emerging notion of the GP in British primary care developing specific areas of expertise:

I thought ... I'm going to do general practice in India, my father had a ... general ... practice, I have done DA [Diploma in Anaesthetics] which will help me, and I have done Diploma in Tropical Medicine and Hygiene ... but before I go to India I want to do general practice.[22]

The desire to gain additional skills and/or have careers as specialists was of course the reason that the majority of participants gave as an explanation for their initial decisions to come to Britain. In many cases they had spent a great deal of time working in the hospital system before opting to become general practitioners. In addition to being

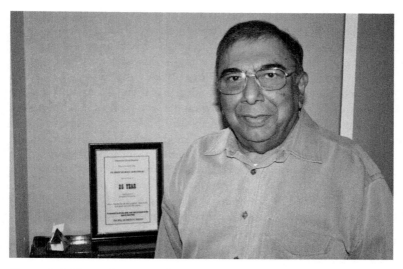

**Figure 9** Self-staged portrait of Gloucester GP Arup Chaudhuri, in front of a mock certificate stating that he had survived 'a 25-year sentence as a hospital practitioner'.

the products of their South Asian backgrounds, doctors still retained strong specialist/hospital doctor identities even after decades spent working as GPs. One doctor, in the context of this study of the development of general practice, chose to frame the portrait that was made of him in a way that identified him primarily as a hospital practitioner (Figure 9). This is not to deny the possibility that chance played a part in the production of this portrait. It does however resonate with other interviews and played its part in constructing a wider picture and helping to develop a deeper appreciation of the dynamics shaping South Asian doctors' professional identities. The latter continued to be tied into their aspirations to have careers in hospitals decades after their moves into general practice:

> I still call that am a trained surgeon and it is a professional suicide I committed. But then ... in the same ... breath, I will say that I ... selected the general practice which I am proud of it. I have contributed to ... the betterment of ... my fellow citizens of the country.[23]

The availability of this South Asian medical workforce supported
Britain's ability to develop primary care services which took on some
of the responsibilities which had previously been the preserve of secondary care. The movement towards the provision of a wider range
of treatments in primary care settings was one that many participants
recall actively embracing. The very fact that they talk about it in such
detail strongly suggests that they were not as a group simply bypassed
by change. It is perfectly conceivable to think that the vast majority
of South Asian doctors interviewed might have described providing
a reactive service, prescribing and referring, locating themselves in
the process on the margins of change in British general practice. After
all, they admit to being on the periphery of the activities of the Royal
College of General Practitioners as we will see later. The development
of the British model of primary care was supported by a cohort of South
Asian doctors who identified with the notion of a more interventionist
GP, were prepared to engage in prevention, run clinics and establish
relationships with hospitals.

Whilst it is impossible to come to any definitive conclusions without
comparing the experiences of South Asian doctors to those of white
British-trained doctors, it is conceivable that the presence in British
general practice of a cohort of doctors who felt their hospital careers
were thwarted as a result of institutional discrimination served to support this process. It was certainly intriguing that a number of doctors
described some of their work as GPs as a quasi-continuation of hospital
careers in the context of general practice:

> That was ... one of my ambitions ... to ... do some surgery, so I did
> the minor ops session in surgery when I was in ... general practice, but
> only minor ops ... which didn't need any general anaesthetic ... *Why
> were you keen to do minor surgery in general practice?* ... Because I always
> wanted to do surgery, knife and a scalpel was my ambition. I couldn't
> achieve that ambition while in hospital so I thought I will do something
> in general practice. So I did ... minor ops, like ... removal of cysts ... I
> asked the ... Medical Defence Union and they said you are not covered
> for any major surgery in general practice, so I dared not do it.[24]

In the above scenario, it is notable that only concerns about insurance
prevented this doctor from carrying out major operations. Once more,
the aim here is not to say South Asian doctors were unproblematically

enabling progress. It is to portray them as actors of a process of change that had a range of effects. Ruban Prasad, a thwarted hospital doctor like many South Asian GPs, gave a sense of striving to recreate a hospital environment in his surgery:

> I established minor surgical procedures which wasn't a thing to be thought in general practice in those days. I established a theatre ... in my practice ... hospitals were built and they used to discard the old equipments ... as nobody's business and I could get hold of an operating table, I could get hold of some things, some instruments were bought ... from the surgical manufacturers ... and then we were doing all sorts of minor surgery.[25]

A significant number of doctors interviewed continued to work in hospitals after they became GPs and spoke of having good relationships with consultants with whom they felt able to communicate 'at the same level'[26] and whom they socialised with.[27]

The evolution of the roles of general practitioners was not however solely linked to the provision of surgical procedures and the transposition of hospital methods into GP surgeries. The development of a primary care system reliant on prevention as well as treatments outside of hospital is also reflected in the accounts South Asian GPs give of the type of initiatives they were taking in the 1970s:

> We provided every service, every service one could think of. My wife was very keen, with our practice manager, family planning service ... intrauterine coil she used to fit ... cervical smear ... immunisation we used to do ... I used to do medical examinations as well ... *So what years would we be talking about here, roughly?* Well, since we moved into our new premises, '79 onwards. Every service was provided, medical services ... I used to do minor op ... [28]
>
> We started providing services that were never provided ... in the primary care before that. Our practice was the first one, certainly in Bolton, and ... there can't be very many like that ... when we actually started providing diabetic clinics ... in the medical centre. *In what year was that?* Oh, I'm going back to 1983 ... . There were no, certainly to my knowledge, within my area or anywhere else, there were not any diabetic clinics or heart clinics placed within the primary care centres. So we started diabetic clinic and shortly after that, my interest in diabetes took me into this diabetes in primary care and I was for a while chair of the Diabetes in Primary Care Group UK – DIPC ... [In 1977] I started also working

as clinical assistant in cardiology ... Inevitably then I started looking at starting a clinic for the people suffering from the heart diseases.[29]

At least some South Asian doctors therefore embraced the emergence of a new general practice. Satish Ahuja's recollection of having, along-side his wife Raj, provided 'every service we could think of' certainly goes beyond any sense of carrying out a tick box exercise to meet basic obligations. Krishna Korpilara's description of how he became involved in the treatment of diabetes in primary care and specialised in cardi-ology is suggestive of a deep-seated desire to be part of these develop-ments, rather than a sense of having to go with the flow of professional change.

The contemporaneous development of increased teamwork in gen-eral practice is equally reflected in participants' descriptions of how work in their practices changed up to the early 1980s.[30] It is hard to imagine a more proactive process of change in a practice than that which was described by a participant who worked in a deprived inner-city area in northern England. The level of detail and strength of feeling conveyed in interviews can only serve to underline doctors' familiarity with these issues and contribution to the development of British gen-eral practice:

In 1970s we started to bring in changes within our own practice ... Anybody who came to surgery aged forty or above, we automatically checked his blood pressure and flagged the notes with a marker ... we were looking for high blood pressure in the ... community ... Recognising undiagnosed diabetes—the incidence of diabetes in this place in the books was mentioned at what two per cent of which one per cent was known and one per cent was unknown. It was trying to bring these unknown cases to light and start treatment ... as early as possible ... So we already had a diabetes register ... and ... good screen-ing ... programme. We took vaccination very, very seriously ... The ini-tial uptake in the population was something like twenty per cent ... we increased that to ... over sixty per cent within a few years ... I remem-ber ... identifying the people who had not been vaccinated and asked them to take ... the notes out and go the weekend when I had time and visit families and do the vaccination at their home ... even when I was not on call ... Preventive medicine produces ... results which serves the community's health more than hospitals can do, so that's the right way around ... I felt fairly strongly ... about this. We also developed ...

doing minor surgeries in our own surgery ... premises ... that took the
load off the ... hospitals.[31]

The emergence of the practices which characterise the renaissance
of British general practice in terms of the nature of the care provided
by GPs was therefore supported and shaped by South Asian doctors.
Whilst oral history accounts can be expected to be framed in terms that
put forward an attachment to a professional ethos rather than financial
gain, one can of course speculate on the extent to which changes to GP
remuneration following the adoption of the Family Doctors' Charter
in the 1960s might also serve to partly explain doctors' interest in this
agenda. The proportion of payments based on capitation (i.e. related to
the number of patients) diminished following its implementation and
greater emphasis was placed on the delivery of preventive medicine.[32]
Irrespective of what their deep-seated motivations may have been,
a number of South Asian doctors were however playing their part in
making these shifts in policy a reality when it came to the day-to-day
delivery of primary care.

In addition, even if this is not always explicitly articulated, the development of certain clinical interests can be linked in some instances to
personal background. If the interest in minor surgery in primary care
can be connected to doctors' experiences in South Asian healthcare
systems and their time spent in British hospitals, it is worth noting that
heart conditions and diabetes, which a number of doctors mentioned
taking a special interest in, are particularly common in South Asian
populations. That roots in the Indian subcontinent could encourage
doctors to pursue certain interests and as a result influence the development of care in Great Britain was made explicit by one participant. His
explanation of the process whereby he became specialised in diabetes
merges frustrated professional ambitions and sublimation of hospital
ambitions into research in the context of the evolution of general practice on one hand, with a sense of responsibility linked to ethnic belonging on the other hand:

> It [general practice] was a new ... specialised branch of medicine ... and
> people ... were encouraged to take and build up their own experience of
> specialty as well in those days. And I think that inspired me more ... that
> I could take my interest in ... diabetes ... Because I couldn't become a
> consultant, so I said OK, if I can move into general practice and if I get

a chance to ... keep my special interest in the subject going ... slowly, I just developed my interest in the subject ... *What led you to ... develop that particular interest in diabetes?* I think there are two reasons. a) It was my initial opening you could say when I was doing medicine, and the second thing was it was just awareness was being raised at that stage ... it was I think in early '80s, the early study which came from Southall ... by Hugh Mather and other colleagues, that the prevalence was much more high in the Asian community and there was very little awareness amongst the community ... plus, visiting back home I was introduced to some of the families which were diabetics as well and they were craving for some kind of help or something so all those, putting two and two together ... my interest which initially started earlier, I just wanted to explore it and go further ahead into it.[33]

## Engaging with the professionalisation of general practice

Participants also talk of their engagement with the ongoing professionalisation of the culture of general practice. Greater emphasis was placed during this period on vocational training and on research, with the discipline being recognised as a specific area of expertise and academic departments of general practice being set up.[34] An 'ideology of general practice' was developed which drew in particular on a 'biopsychosocial' model of the discipline which sought to distinguish general practice from reductive biomedical approaches.[35] Interviewees described embracing this model and their interviews suggest they built cultural variations of it. The professionalisation of general practice also provided an opportunity for doctors marginalised by the NHS system to obtain the type of status within medicine that they aspired to. A number of South Asian doctors talk with enthusiasm of the recognition of general practice as a specialty in its own right and the associated increase in the prestige of the profession.

Whilst the conclusions presented here rely mainly on oral history interviews, there is also archival evidence that migrant doctors were actively involved in these developments. The ODA expressed concern in 1978 that migrant GPs were being denied the opportunity to become trainers in their chosen field.[36] As noted in the previous chapter, the ODA was also working to improve training opportunities for its members and published a guide to passing the MRCGP examination.

These are not the actions of a group whose membership had little or no connection to the ongoing professionalisation of general practice. The embracing of the emergence of new conceptions of the role of the GP provided an opportunity to gain respect and achieve professional status in a racist and heterophobic system. Doctors absorbed the new culture of general practice, contributed to its dissemination and at times can arguably be seen to subject it to the influence of their background and experiences.

For some doctors who found themselves working as GPs after aspiring to careers in the hospital system, the fact that general practice was acquiring greater status within British medicine was described as an opportunity to define a professional niche within the NHS. The quest for status which general practitioners as a whole were engaged in at the time thus intersected with a quest for status of South Asian doctors within the racist and heterophobic context of the NHS:

> It's ... a quest for professional satisfaction. I really wanted to get away, this was my obsession if you like, that we must move out of that public image that these GPs are the third-rate doctors who just give the sick notes or give what the patients want. Two, we had to move from that position to the doctors being able to clinically examine, to judge and to think what is right and guide the patients on what is required rather than referring anything other than sick notes to the hospitals. So I think that was my quest for professional pride in what I'm doing.[37]
>
> In my early part of my career I felt I wasn't very well supported by our local consultants, because we were always looked down ... We weren't one of them. Very rarely if ever they called you by your first name ... If you go to a medical meeting you are like lemon on a stick ... sitting ... in a corner, talking to other Asians because nobody will come and talk to you. And if you try and talk to them they will just absolutely ignore you. So that's ... what it was, those days and I wanted to beat that ... I decided the only way to do it is to ... start developing yourself and go from there ... *Why did you decide to join the Royal College of General Practitioners?* ... I just wanted to prove a) that I was a good doctor and I wanted to be assessed by my peers ... I think ... I also felt that there will be a day when if you wanted to do general practice you had to be the member of the College ... That didn't happen for best part of thirty-odd years ... But I saw the writing on the wall ... The most important thing was ... to prove to myself that ... the care that I was giving to my

patients was equivalent to any other doctor who became the member of the ... College of GPs.[38]

The engagement of a number of doctors with the emerging culture of general practice can therefore be linked to a desire for professional identity and status which was common to South Asian doctors and to GPs irrespective of ethnicity. Although it was admittedly produced in the room at the RCGP where he was interviewed, Hasmukh Joshi's decision to frame his portrait with paintings of eminent doctors in the background is perhaps not coincidental in this context (Figure 10). As with P. L. Pathak's portrait in front of the plaque marking the opening of her surgery, it can be seen as laying claim to a place amongst those who shaped British general practice. Syed Ahmad Ali Gilani's description of applying for a training position at the University of Manchester is, thirty years on, suggestive of a desire to understand the nature of developments in an emerging field, of pride in being familiar with the names of prominent figures and their work and of satisfaction at the resulting pleasure of finding a place in British medicine. It is probably

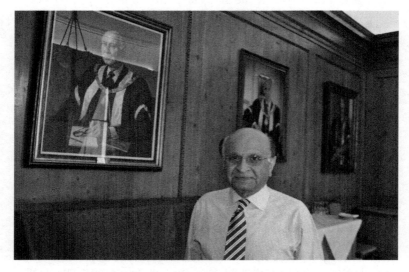

**Figure 10**  Self-staged portrait of Hasmukh Joshi in a meeting room at the Royal College of General Practitioners.

not insignificant that a liberating burst of laughter punctuates occasions in the interview when obstacles are overcome, intimate knowledge of the field having been demonstrated, as well as the end of the anecdote when the self-described 'outsider' has proven to himself that his understanding of the dynamics of the interview process was superior to that of a local candidate:

> In Manchester ... Professor Byrne ... he started this idea of training in general practice for doctors. And in fact the first chair of professors in general practice was created in Manchester. And he had written ... two books: *Learning to Care* and *The Future General Practitioners* [*The Future General Practitioner*]. And I ... became interested in that ... Then they advertised positions, the deanery decided we need to have trainers ... properly qualified trainers. So they advertised positions of trainers. I applied, I remember ... we went for interview, there were six of us ... I was the only one who was outsider ... and five were English doctors ... When my turn came ... there was a board of about ten or twelve interviewers ... chaired by Professor Byrne ... One of them asked me: 'If you were selected as a trainer, how will you set about ... putting a programme of training together?' I said 'Well, if you read the book *Learning to Care* written by Professor Byrne he has given a beautiful ... flow chart in that, I think I'll follow that' (laughter) ... There was another consultant sitting there he said 'Well ... most of your experience and qualifications are in surgery, how are you going to treat people in general practice?' I said 'Well sir, if you look at the statistics, in fact sixty per cent of the cases who come to general practitioners, they have got some surgical problems' (laughs). Then the other chap asked me 'Have you done any teachers' training course?' It just so happened I had done teachers' training course at the University of Manchester ... and that was the first course ever started in that discipline ... I didn't realise the importance of this question until I met one English short-listed candidate doctor, who was very senior, we were in a dinner and he asked me 'Oh, did you get the job?' I said 'Yes' ... 'You know they turned me down'. I said 'Why?'. He said 'I don't know, they asked me "Have you done a teachers' training course?", I said "No, I don't need to do teachers' training, I've been teaching students for a long time."' (laughs) So he didn't get it.[39]

The active embracing of the emerging specialty of general practice by South Asian practitioners is illustrated by the fact that some doctors talk of enthusiastically opting into professional courses instead of immediately starting to work—this before vocational training became mandatory:

> I could have joined as a partner, I could have just started in ... a des-
> ignated area but I wanted to ... do a training and give a good ... start
> because it was a totally a change direction ... I'm really delighted that
> I did that one year training, because that gave me a good insight not
> only of the business of general practice but also the whole system of
> the NHS.[40]

The culture of general practice can therefore be seen as a natural sub-
stitute for the prestige of a senior hospital job that many doctors had
originally aimed for. Understanding the attachment of South Asian
doctors to the improved status of general practitioners in this way helps
to explain how the introduction of compulsory specialised training for
GPs could be seen by one doctor as not just a welcome development,
but as a source of personal joy and fulfilment:

> I was a ... trainer for twenty years and I have been involved ... with
> the ... VTS [Vocational Training Scheme] training at Leeds right
> from the beginning ... One of my happiest day was that when VTS
> was actually made a permanent feature—you know that you couldn't
> go into general practice without training ... And that was absolutely
> wonderful.[41]

As has already been pointed out, change in general practice was not a
homogenous process and many South Asian doctors remained outside
of the RCGP and disconnected from its activities. However, a number
of interviewees not only spoke enthusiastically about the need for general practice to evolve but also became involved in the provision of GP
training when such programmes were still in their infancy. Syed Ahmad
Ali Gilani's familiarity with the names of those who were leaders in the
field at the time gives his account a credibility that it would not have if
it were simply a general declaration of being enthusiastic about change
uttered years after the events. The reference that he kept, attesting to
his role as a GP trainer in the 1970s, also places him at the forefront of
processes of change (Figure 11).

The imprint of the 'new ideology of general practice' described
by Charles Webster is also detectable in doctors' memories of their
work. Their actions and conceptions of their roles are at times clearly

Gateway House,
Piccadilly South,
Manchester, M60 7LP

Tel: 061—236 9456, Ext............317

Dean of Post-graduate Medical Studies
R.M. Stirland. M.A., M.D. (Cantab.), F.R.C.Path.
Regional Adviser in General Practice
James Roberts, M.B.Ch.B., D.R.C.O.G., F.R.C.G.P.

Admin. Asst. to Dean of Post-graduate Medical Studies
Leslie Scott

JR/MF

22nd. September 1980

Dr. S.A.A. Gilani
Corby Willowbrook Health Centre
Cottingham Road
Corby
Northants. NN17. 2UR

Dear Dr. Gilani,

I am writing to confirm that for a period of five years, from 1974 until 1979, you worked for this department as a trainer in general practice. This was remunerated employment involving the active use of person to person teaching methods in addition to taking part in group discussion and giving an occasional lecture.

During the tenure of your appointment you attended two courses, each lasting one week, to give you practice and instruction in the skills required.

During the time that you worked for this department we were very satisfied with your capabilities and achievements.

I wish you well.

Yours sincerely,

J. ROBERTS
Regional Adviser for General Practice

**Figure 11**  Reference obtained by S. A. A. Gilani for having acted as a trainer in general practice in the 1970s.

embedded in 'renaissance' notions of general practice, which they contributed to disseminating. As well as being defined as distinct from hospital medicine, this new culture presented a challenge to the hierarchical culture of hospitals, with doctors engaging in research, learning alongside others rather than dispensing knowledge, and using new pedagogical methods:

> We used to meet in the … medical institute … on Thursdays and exchange notes and occasionally I used to present a case in the medical institute of some interest to my colleagues. I did that because as a teacher which I said … I became [from the 1970s] … a teacher and trainer … we used to meet as trainers in the medical institute and … it's so wonderful to … have a little chit-chat with your colleagues … *Were these informal meetings or were these organised by the RCGP at the time?* Oh, these were organised by RCGP, yes, yes, they were. We used to meet … once a week … As I said I did the trainership … and I made sure I used to have trainees who, like me, had done the FRCS or MRCP … but then they had change of mind to become a GP … I used to say well look, you are a surgeon or a physician, but general practice is very different. Because I … knew both sides, having done both kind of qualifications … Every one of my trainee eventually … became a member of the college, MRCGP. For which I am very pleased. We … used to involve them in … medical research. In fact, some of the articles were published in one chapter in the book [about a specific aspect of practice] … And we used to have … television coverage in the trainees' room and my room … Once or twice a week we used to sit down and look at the tapes, as to what you have done, what I have done and … that … was a very, very useful thing … in general practice … I wouldn't say it's teaching, it's learning from each other.[42]
>
> We started to take medical students and also … postgraduates [in the 1970s] … *Why did you do that, what made you interested in that?* Well these are all challenges of life … I was always interested in teaching … The interest in teaching has always been there and this was ideal opportunity which presented and I took the challenge … If you are using undergraduate and postgraduate students, they monitor you, so you have to produce … quality in practice.[43]

The notion of doctors learning from one another, for instance, clearly subverts the traditionally strict and top-down hierarchies of hospital medicine. General practice appears here, to quote Mathers and Rowland again, as a 'post-modern medical specialty',[44] with different versions of truth competing with each other, hence the need for people to learn together and to improve by being monitored by those less senior than they were. At the time, this was a radical notion within medicine.

The absorption of the defining characteristics of British general practice as it developed from the 1950s onwards is equally evident in the way doctors talk about their work. The holistic approach to general practice derived from Michael Balint's research was important to defining a separate identity for general practitioners in the early years of the College of General Practitioners. It emphasised the need for a biopsychosocial approach to care which promotes engagement with biological factors of disease but also social context and psychological considerations and can be found reflected in participants' conceptions of their roles as GPs:

> *Can you describe to me what your status in the community was as a doctor?*
> Oh, very popular, very highly respected ... I got confidence and respect and ... they used to come, you know ... he's a 'friend, philosopher and guide' (laughs), that's the slogan ... They used to come for various reasons, for advice on this and that unconnected with your practice ... [45]
>
> One of my patients said he is my God, he is my Bhagwan,[46] he is my father, he is my brother, he is my sister, any problem I go to him. So, that makes me happy if my patient ... give me that esteem. But the question is this: general practice is not only medicine ... it's a whole approach of whole life ... When patient come to you in most cases, they have ... more than an illness. They're depressed, they have broken relationship, they're financially broken, their children have had something wrong ... So this is ... an art ... it's a human side to it ... I always tell my partner ... there's no denying that you are a good clinician, but be a ... good person as well ... Understand their problem ... a few words doesn't take anything from you. You are going to treat his illness anyway, why not ... go to his soul as well (laughs) ... that has been my approach.[47]

Hearing a doctor conceive of their role in such terms is suggestive of connections between the traditional roles that doctors might have expected to assume as senior community figures and the agenda of British general practice at the time. At times, cultural transfer was more immediately apparent. Whilst it is not inconceivable that some white British-trained doctors might have studied their ethnic minority patients' culture and taken similar initiatives, the following account shows how doctors' cultural hinterland could have a direct impact on their clinical practice:

> Postnatal depression was very common in ... Asian women ... because ... they were losing their extended family, there was nobody here for them ... I used to use a very interesting method ... For Asians ... if

some elder man blesses when the child arrives they think it's a very happy thing. I used to carry one pound coins in my pocket and I used to go and visit the ... women who delivered and I used to take the baby in my lap and put a coin ... in the baby's little palm—and mothers used to feel happy ... So I created that sort of atmosphere in my practice ... that's ... how it should be done, it's a holistic approach.[48]

South Asian doctors thus (consciously or not) absorbed the biopsychosocial discourse of general practice and could integrate it into their own belief systems.

The fact that doctors had migrated from the Indian subcontinent was not an obstacle to them conceiving of their roles in ways which are considered typical of the development of British general practice at the time. The 'renaissance' of British general practice was supported by a reliance on South Asian practitioners, who had their own agendas and distinct professional, social and cultural backgrounds. In addition, if there was indeed a form of 'renaissance' in general practice in the 1960s and 1970s, it is one that was supported by the racist and heterophobic structures of the NHS, which had led migrant doctors to work in general practice, and by the way in which they responded to finding themselves in that position. It was also defined by the marginalisation of many South Asian doctors.

### 'Deprived patients and deprived doctor': 'renaissance', marginalisation and retreat

If South Asian doctors shaped the 'renaissance' of general practice by supporting it, the form taken by this rebirth was also to a degree the product of the fact that they could find themselves on the margins of processes of change. If to a certain extent, the marginalisation of South Asian doctors is a reflection of an uneven engagement with the Royal College and change amongst all British general practitioners at the time, irrespective of origin, it also appears as the product of discrimination and of doctors' avoidance of environments where they might be subjected to it. Racism and heterophobia in the NHS led doctors to retreat from engagement with contexts in which changes were discussed and implemented.

The marginalisation of South Asian doctors from the process of 'renaissance' of general practice is most in evidence in the way in which they talk about their relationship with the Royal College of General

Practitioners. Questioning doctors on this subject frequently led to curt replies, a degree of derision and a desire to move the conversation on to other subjects:

> *Were you involved at all in the work of the … RCGP?* No, no, I was not. *Why do you think that was? …* Royal College of General Practitioners— I was not a member there … I was not invited anyway so there wasn't any contact with them.[49]
>
> *What sort of relationship—if any—did you have with the Royal College of General Practitioners? …* None … I had no, no role at all to play, I wasn't a member. *Why was that?* I never did the exam. (silence) I didn't do the exam, no.[50]
>
> I would read the literature … I would read the … *British Medical Journal* and you know one is able to keep abreast with the latest issues. What the Royal College did, I don't even know really … *Why do you think that was, that you … saw it in that way? …* No reason, really, I never wanted to go in there, it probably would mean giving them an extra 100–200 pounds a year what for I don't know (laughter).[51]

It is striking that doctors who worked as GPs in the NHS for decades could say they had no contact with the RCGP or that they did not know what it did. The detachment of a number of practitioners from the NHS system in which they operated as well as from the main professional organisation representing general practitioners is also apparent in the accounts they give of their professional lives. This cannot solely be attributed to a desire to simply be 'left alone' in the words of Julian Tudor Hart. M. A. Salam, who mentioned having had no contact with the RCGP and not being invited to become involved in its activities also expressed frustration at not being able to access support when running his practice:

> *How would you describe your relationship with the NHS generally?* (pause) … Of course, we were … self-employed … in general practice, we were slightly aloof from the hustle bustle of … management but they were not greatly helpful … They could be more helpful to help their practices to develop more but they weren't … we had to manage ourselves. *What sort of support did you feel that you could have got that you didn't get? …* Possibly for the management of the practice, possibly for financial management or … development of surgeries, development of staff, those are the … areas the GPs were at that time not very good at. Because it was more of a managerial aspect than a clinical aspect … In those

days they called Family Practitioners' Committee [Family Practitioner Committee] they said 'Oh, you are self-employed, you do whatever you like, you just carry on, we are not … involved'. So I thought possibly if they had some liaison officer, they could come and advise us that … this is the best way to do it, develop a surgery, develop a building … employ a practice manager, employ a few more nurses … that would have been much, much better in those days … but that was not forthcoming.[52]

Such views about the NHS and the RCGP should not necessarily be seen as being specific to South Asian practitioners. The work of the Royal College was also received with scepticism by a number of British-trained doctors. The terseness of the responses given to questions about the RCGP does however suggest that it may have played a specific part in marginalising South Asian doctors. It is telling that, as recounted in Chapter 4, Hasmukh Joshi, its vice-chair at the time of being interviewed, described encountering blatant racism in postgraduate courses that it ran. Professionalisation is founded on exclusion and further research exploring the extent to which the professionalisation of general practice involved the marginalisation of South Asian doctors would undoubtedly raise interesting questions.

It is also possible that the lack of support described by M. A. Salam was typical of the experience of doctors working in the Welsh Valleys, and of the lack of resources in an area of high need, rather than a direct result of his origins. Origins are, however, as has been shown, closely linked to the professional trajectories that determined the geographical location of practices where doctors found work. Location and background could in effect become mutually reinforcing factors in the marginalisation of doctors. Another GP from the Valleys, Rupendra Kumar Majumdar thus described his lack of involvement with the RCGP as resulting both from his location in South Wales and the fact that he was not as he put it a 'local' doctor:

*Were you involved in the work of the Royal College of General Practitioners?* No. If I … would have practised in big cities, Manchester, Liverpool I could have but they won't listen anything of this … area … they think it's … one or two people are here goes to … Royal College of General Practitioners but mostly they are local, local who had influence in BMA. *When you say local you mean white doctors?* Yes, white, not any … I practised in … not a very good, big area or champion area or whatever it may be ... unattractive area it's very hard ... and you have got so many problems to tackle and to go to politics, if I have a partner or anyone to look after my practice, I should slip to London or Manchester and spend the week-end ... it's not possible here.[53]

If working in particular types of practice in specific areas could contribute to marginalising South Asian doctors, the fact that a significant number of participants talk about feeling isolated from the mainstream of medical developments of the time should not be disassociated from their ethnicity. South Asian doctors were working, as has been shown, within a racist and heterophobic system. Some of them clearly felt at a disadvantage as a direct result when it came to engaging with the professional environment they found themselves in.

As befits perhaps a 'post-modern' specialty, no definitive over-arching narrative is discernible when it comes to doctors' relationship with the renaissance of general practice. Some felt in a position to shape it, others believed that the obstacles that they were presented with were overwhelming:

The whole attitude is wrong ... no good ... premises, no good computers, not enough staff. They ... still treat us as second rate citizens ... I wish they wouldn't ... I've tried to tell them ... it's in their interests, the worse ... health they have, they are a danger to the society ... *Do you feel that that's because you are an Asian doctor, because you are a female doctor, because your patients are Asian, because your patients are working class, a mixture of all of that, other reasons?* Everything—you name it, it matters ... Victimisation is their best quality (laughs) ... I don't think they can see in the right light. If you point out, they think that you are being ... rude ... On one hand we say that we should tell them so that they can improve on the other hand they think that 'Oh, now they are telling us what to do' ... *Would you feel you were treated differently to white doctors?* ... In white doctors they wouldn't even question and they would pay them, with us, they would keep on questioning till they find excuses not to pay ... *Can you give me an idea of what sort of relationship you had with your FPC?* I think that has been a very negative relationship ... I am a proper Indian female who can fight anything, so I just keep on doing it. Till today that has been the case ... I'm the last person to be trained and last person to be maintained for the computers ... So it's been ... deprived patients and deprived doctor (laughs), that sort of thing.[54]

Although the above experience was not particularly representative of the group of doctors I interviewed, I have quoted from it at length here as it may be typical of the perspective of a wider group of migrant doctors who did not take part in the study. Doctors whose view on their career was that they were victimised and targeted and who saw their relationship with local medical structures as 'very negative' may well have been more reluctant than most to reflect on professional lives they saw as fundamentally unsatisfying. This doctor's account also suggests once more that a specific focus on the experience of female migrant doctors might well reveal additional layers of discrimination and greater marginalisation as a result. As the gendered dimensions of the experiences of South Asian doctors were not the primary focus of my work I can only highlight this as an area ripe for further research rather than offer definitive conclusions.

If a sense of discrimination being a reality that could be negotiated and to a degree overcome was more commonly encountered in interviews, they did also convey a sense of being kept at arm's length from institutions run by white British doctors. Krishna Korlipara, in spite of being a prominent medical politician, one of the leaders of the ODA and a long-standing member of the GMC was for instance ambivalent about the role of the RCGP during the period that provides the focus for this book:

> I think the relationship [with the RCGP] has improved ... I hope it'll continue—that momentum of improvement—so that the overseas doctors and the British doctors, together or separately, can feel at home and can feel welcomed by the Royal College. I don't really have any great complaint now, as things are ... *But do you think that there was an issue in terms of Asian doctors feeling welcomed by the ... Royal College?* Oh, without any doubt, going back to the '70s and the early '80s ... there were these comments, snide comments, that overseas doctors were not particularly ... good at speaking English, that they can't really communicate with the patients and the ... implication was that they are not as good doctors without the communication skills. Until people like me challenged and then there was some backtracking.[55]

Several other participants spoke of attempts by the local medical establishment and those responsible for NHS structures to dissuade them or even prevent them from establishing or developing a practice.[56] If some doctors could see the hostility that they encountered as a challenge to be surmounted,[57] others simply chose to avoid or withdraw from environments in the mainstream of British medicine where they expected to be subject to discrimination:

> I was in [Manchester] LMC [in 1980–82 approximately] also ... you tell anything, you are banging with the head. Whatever they wanted, they will do it ... so I stopped that thing also ... Whatever we have a problem we used to discuss in LMC ... When there is a local doctor it is always cover. When there is Asian doctor, it was highlighted a lot. So it's always there. And you always one or two people in LMC or three people ... you can't do much. You raise your point, and ... tell them, please note.[58]
>
> Discrimination ... there has always been. And that is much more visible in higher you go, the clearer it is ... I did my membership exam in 1977. The majority of the FRCGPs ... are called to Fellowship. But then they ... made ... assessment. The assessment is to keep unwanted people out ... Previously it is ... MRCGP, MRCS, MRCP, they are all called to fellowship by selection. If you have worked in that branch for so many years, if you have good reputation ... you are normally made fellowship which is honorary ... it's just recognition. But they stopped that as well so I have not been made, I have not been made (laughs) the, the fellow of Royal College of General Practitioner. And I thought I won't ... do the test because they again do the same thing: they will say 'Oh, your accent is that' ... and that sort of things ... this is what the situation is.[59]

Laughter appears once more as a means of defusing tension associated with a subject that might have been difficult for the participant to broach—in this instance as it concerns a form of professional humiliation. The fact that the manifestation of laughter coincides with the mention of the processes associated with the obtention of the Fellowship of the Royal College of GPs points not just to a disconnect between the College and migrant doctors but to the fact that this was not necessarily the result of a lack of awareness of ongoing developments or a symptom of a lack of interest. It should also be seen as the product of the disengagement of many migrant practitioners from the professional environment they found themselves in at the time. After all, M. S. Kausar was clearly engaged enough with the professionalisation of general practice to sit his membership examination well before it became compulsory for GPs to do so. His cynicism towards the Fellowship examination cannot simply be attributed to a lack of willingness to subject himself to the scrutiny of his peers. If many South Asian doctors became involved in promoting change, the history of general practice in this period is also defined by the barriers that practitioners faced in their relationships with the NHS and professional bodies. The 'renaissance' of general practice was shaped by the agency and the cultural, social and professional background of South Asian doctors. The form it took was also the product of racism and heterophobia which led a number of South Asian doctors to retreat from some of the contexts in which change was being discussed and implemented.

## Notes

1  Horder, 'Conclusion', p. 278.
2  Wendland, *A Heart for the Work*, pp. 21–4.
3  Collings, 'General practice in England', p. 580.
4  S. K. Ahuja interview with author.
5  H. Joshi interview with author.
6  'Ambitious plan for £250,000 medical centre', *Evening News* (18 July 1981), p. 8
7  Private papers of Dr Hira Lal Kapur, Letter dated 5 May 1972.
8  R. N. Rao interview with author.
9  Anonymous interview with author.
10 Smith, *Overseas Doctors*, pp. 20–1.
11 M. N. I. Talukdar interview with author.
12 D. Ray interview with author, 5 December 2008.
13 L. R. M. Kamal interview with author.
14 Berridge, *Health and Society*, pp. 42–3; Fry & McLachlan, 'The future', p. 246.
15 Fry & McLachlan, 'The future', p. 246.
16 This argument applies of course only to the thirty-seven participants who were trained on the Indian sub-continent rather than the three who migrated as children. It is possible that those doctors were influenced by the thinking of parents trained on the Indian subcontinent but this question was not explored in detail by this study.
17 H. Joshi interview with author.
18 Anonymous interview with author.

19 Anonymous interview with author.
20 L. R. M. Kamal interview with author.
21 BLSA, C648/28/01–06, 'Oral History of General Practice 1936–1952', S. Kutar interviewed by M. Bevan, 1993.
22 S. K. Ahuja interview with author.
23 S. Pande interview with author, 23 November 2009.
24 Anonymous interview with author.
25 R. Prasad interview with author.
26 Anonymous interview with author.
27 F. B. Kotwall interview with author.
28 S. K. Ahuja interview with author.
29 K. Korlipara interview with author.
30 Two anonymous interviews with author; H. Joshi interview with author.
31 Anonymous interview with author.
32 M. Drury, 'The GP and professional organisations', in Loudon et al. (eds), *General Practice under the National Health Service*, p. 210.
33 Anonymous interview with author.
34 Howie, 'Research in General Practice: Perspectives and theories', in Loudon et al. (eds), *General Practice under the National Health Service*, pp. 147 & 164; Pereira Gray, 'Postgraduate training', pp. 182–93; Fry & McLachlan, 'The future', p. 246.
35 Bosanquet & Salisbury, 'The practice', p. 61; Berridge, *Health and Society*, p. 43; M. J. Gavin, 'A crisis of legitimacy? The clinical role, intellectual status and career motivations of general medical practitioners' (PhD dissertation, The University of Manchester, 2004), pp. 62–4.
36 National Archives, BS 6/2893, Royal Commission on the NHS. Oral Evidence from the Overseas Doctors' Association, 22 May 1978.
37 K. Korlipara interview with author.
38 H. Joshi interview with author.
39 S. A. A. Gilani interview with author, 30 June 2010.
40 S. Pande interview with author, 23 November 2009.
41 L. R. M. Kamal interview with author.
42 Anonymous interview with author.
43 Anonymous interview with author.
44 Mathers & Rowland, 'General practice'.
45 R. K. Majumdar interview with author.
46 Hindi word meaning god, which can also be employed as a term of respect when applied to an individual.

47  M. S. Kausar interview with author.
48  S. Venugopal interview with author.
49  M. A. Salam interview with author.
50  Anonymous interview with author.
51  H. L. Kapur interview with author.
52  M. A. Salam interview with author.
53  R. K. Majumdar interview with author.
54  Anonymous interview with author.
55  K. Korlipara interview with author.
56  Anonymous interview with author; M. S. Kausar interview with author;
    P. L. Pathak interview with author.
57  H. Joshi interview with author.
58  N. Shah interview with author.
59  M. S. Kausar interview with author.

# Conclusion: historicising a 'revolution'

One of my aims in this book was to contribute to a different way of thinking about the history of immigration. This involves seeing it as a component of wider social change rather than focusing exclusively on identity, culture and difference or 'problematic' migrants subject to public hostility and/or government and professional controls. In 1991, Orin Starn wrote a seminal article critiquing his fellow anthropologists' approach to the study of Andean populations; in his view their perspective was distorted by what he called 'Andeanism'—the notion that contemporary highland peasants in South America were outside the flow of modern history.[1] He argued that this helped explain how, in spite of the presence of dozens of researchers carrying out fieldwork in Peru's Southern Highlands at the time, the start of the violent Maoist Shining Path insurrection in 1980 'came as a complete surprise'.[2] Hence the title of his article: 'Missing the revolution'. I agree with Starn that it is not the function of scholars to predict revolutions and that their inability to do so should not be held against them. I also share his view that such episodes enlighten us as to the nature of scholars' gaze and should encourage a critical reflection around their priorities. It is helpful to bear his critique in mind when thinking about how historians engage with the contemporary history of migration.

When it comes to the role of migration in post-war Britain, much research so far has missed the fundamental impact of population movement on everyday life. This is not to prescribe one way of doing history over another or to deny legitimacy to studies dedicated to the exploration of identity or Westminster political intrigues. It is to argue for more space for histories that engage with the interface between migrants and the mainstream, that chart the lives of middle-class migrants, and map the less conflictual interactions between incomers and the environment that they find. The history of migrants and work, leisure and politics all offer rich terrain to explore in this respect.

This study provides an illustration of the extent to which such an approach can prove fruitful. When I started researching the history of migrant South Asian doctors in the NHS a decade ago, I was struck by the contrast between their numerical importance and the lack of historical interest in their roles. When they were mentioned in historical accounts, it was mainly in the form of statistics concerning their numbers. In the context of the NHS, avoiding a reflection around the impact of medical migration is tantamount to missing a revolution in post-war Britain. By focusing on one group of migrants, I have shown how the history of the NHS cannot be disentangled from Britain's imperial past, which helps to account for the post-war flow of doctors to Britain. I have highlighted the structural dependency of British general practice on the labour of migrant doctors prepared to take on specific roles within the NHS. I have drawn attention to the agency of migrants who were able to shape their social and professional environment. This book has brought to the fore the influence of racism and discrimination on the grounds of difference on the development of British medicine. It has highlighted that medical migrants need to be recognised as agents of the development of healthcare as they are in a position to shape its nature—in ways that are, so far, little understood.

Looking at migration history from a different angle and exploring questions such as these is important not just because it adds to our historical understanding but also because it can help us to think differently about the place of migrants in modern British society and elsewhere. This at a time when political debates around this question abound, without critical histories of population movement having any discernible role to play in them. The role of the historian at this level is not in my view to be prescriptive. History can however serve to undermine assumptions, reveal contradictions and point to different ways of approaching policy questions. I will explore in this conclusion what the account I have given of the working lives of South Asian GPs in the NHS between the 1940s and the 1980s might contribute to ongoing debates with regards both to healthcare and wider issues concerned with migration in Britain.

## Migrant doctors, medical margins and medical cultures

At the beginning of this book, I noted that the NHS is often perceived as epitomising Britishness. It should by now be apparent that such a view is only tenable if one embraces a conception of Britishness that encompasses the impact of migration and empire. If the NHS is indeed a typically British institution, it is partly in the sense that was sarcastically suggested by Zaki, one of the characters in Hanif Kureishi's screenplay for the film *My Beautiful Laundrette*: it is 'typically English' to get someone else to do the work.[3]

The imperial legacy, the availability of a workforce of migrant doctors willing to take on particular roles and their impact on British medicine and society as well as the field of general practice are, as has been shown, a central and formative part of the history of the NHS. I should reiterate here, for the sake of avoiding any confusion, that my aim was not to write a celebratory history. It was to engage critically with the social reality of immigration and its importance to Britain in the post-war period. I gave this book the title *Migrant Architects of the NHS* because that is an accurate description of the role of South Asian doctors in the organisation and because it offers a challenge to scholarly and public understandings of the NHS that marginalise the role of migrants and minorities in its development. Zaki's ironic remark is amusing but like much humour reveals an underlying truth. We should take seriously the notion that it is 'typically English [or British]' to delegate tasks to others and rely on their labour. In terms of our historical understanding that means interrogating the legacies of empire, which by definition depended on establishing forms of domination over other societies, and reflecting on the nature of the roles performed in British society by migrants who are frequently relied upon to take on specific types of work.

The history of South Asian GPs in the NHS can only appear to be a cause for celebration if we restrict our horizons to the British context and view the NHS as an unmitigated good. Although it has achieved a particular symbolic status in Britain, it is ultimately simply the national system for the delivery of healthcare. Whether it is superior to other such systems is a moot point. It is probably reasonable to assume that patients in rural South Asia where doctors are in short supply would find little to celebrate in this story of South-Asian trained doctors, socialised in a medical system shaped by empire, who helped to build the British medical system. This history also raises fundamental questions about the culture of medicine and the gap between the needs of the NHS, British governments' willingness to invest in it and the aspirations of the British medical profession. Martin Powell, in his analysis of the geographical distribution of doctors in England and Wales in the 1930s, concluded that 'before the NHS, doctors were magnetically attracted to areas of wealth. They were drawn to coasts and repelled by coalfields.'[4] As has been shown, this pre-war flight from coalfields and industrial areas was still relevant to understanding the context in which healthcare was delivered post-war and why British policy objectives of widening access to care were as a result highly dependent on migrants. Focusing on the influence of overseas doctors on the social mainstream raises questions both about the roles of migrants and the reasons why their labour is necessary, as well as highlighting the integral part that they played in the development of modern societies. In this case, it points to an ongoing gap between professional agendas and the needs of the welfare state, highlighting that a creation that might be viewed as typical of a specific post-war British agenda was in fact fundamentally the product of transnational forces. Focusing on the interaction between migrants and the mainstream thus highlights not just migrant agency and the importance of engaging with the concept of cultural transfer in the context of medicine but also particular characteristics of the mainstream.

The NHS has never been self-sufficient in medical labour and there are clearly structural reasons for this which cannot be addressed by simply training more doctors. Migrant doctors have frequently been located in parts of Britain experiencing doctor shortages and worked with populations such as the elderly, the mentally ill, and the urban poor. The fact that migrant doctors have historically taken on these functions in effect adds an additional dimension to the 'inverse care law' formulated by Julian Tudor Hart.[5] This posits that resources dedicated to healthcare provision tend to be more scarce where the need for care is the greatest. One can add to this that the concentration of migrant professionals will most likely be higher.[6]

Moreover, as has been shown, this dependency on migrants has been historically associated with their construction as a problem rather than a resource. History has a role to play in questioning the logic of such discourses. Medical self-sufficiency may be a legitimate political goal, but depending on migration while at the same time stigmatising migrants (the dominant narrative of British policy in this respect) is, as Christopher Kyriakides and Satnam Virdee have argued, somewhat paradoxical.[7] More generally, this history shows that medical training in the UK has never been adequately aligned to the needs of the NHS. UK medical schools have not succeeded in bringing about a training system that over the long term has ensured that new cohorts of doctors contain sufficient numbers of graduates willing to fill all available posts. As an Oxfam report published in 1970 noted, the UK will remain a 'doctor deficit' country unless there is radical change.[8] This could for instance involve giving greater responsibilities to nurses, exploring the merits, as suggested in the same report, of a system of 'medical auxiliaries', or investing more in prevention and public health.[9] Alternatively, governments could intervene more directly in medical training, for instance by offering reductions in tuition fees in exchange for commitments to work in certain specialties or parts of the country. In the absence of reforms of this type, it would seem logical to acknowledge that the UK is in effect dependent on medical migration and plan accordingly. This could involve taking further steps to ensure that doctors are adequately supported when starting to work in the NHS.

Similarly, if we recognise that the diversity of the medical profession is a factor when it comes to the development of healthcare systems, we have much to gain from seeking to understand what the implications of this might be. What, for instance, is the significance of the fact that some South Asian doctors state that they identify with South Asian patients and their concerns? Do such attitudes then shape the research interests of doctors as suggested directly by one participant and serve to improve care for particular populations? In which case what could be the consequences for sections of the population under-represented in the medical profession? If migrants are able to drive change as has been seen, are their skills employed to best effect? In the same way that examples of good medical practice might be sought overseas, is appropriate use made of the specific knowledge that migrant doctors bring with them? To what extent might racism and heterophobia and particular social attitudes be imported by doctors when they migrate and what impact does this have on care? There is some evidence that migrant doctors in the UK might have less positive attitudes towards patients with HIV-AIDS than their British-trained counterparts.[10] Another study found both that doctors of South Asian ethnicity were more likely to describe themselves as having a strong attachment to a religious faith and that doctors who described themselves as non-religious tended to provide different treatments to dying patients.[11]

Recognising that doctors are vectors of social and cultural norms, not just of skills acquired in westernised medical settings, opens the way for a more detailed consideration of the effect this might have on British healthcare and a greater awareness of the need to manage the potential benefits and downsides brought about by the cultural diversity of practitioners working in Great Britain. By extension, similar insights could be gained in other medical systems where migrants play a significant role and in contexts other than healthcare. Particular types of medical work have been constructed as undesirable, although we have limited understanding of how these attitudes have developed in different places at different periods.

## Histories of migration and immigration policy

Histories that explore the interaction between migrants and the societies that they settle in can give us a better sense of how immigration has, over time, shaped the modern world. These insights are of value at a time when immigration has increasingly come to be presented as a problem to be contained rather than a reality to be engaged with and a resource to be managed. History as a field simply cannot remain neutral when it comes to immigration debates. Minimising the importance of the transformative impact of immigration effectively lends support to discourses that portray migrants as outsiders. By engaging critically with the legacies of migration, historians can contribute to ongoing discussions around immigration policy. As the Parekh report noted over a decade and a half ago:

> A state is not only a territorial and political entity, but also, it has been said, an imagined community ... A sense of national identity is based on generalizations and involves a selective and simplified account of a complex history.[12]

Whilst it might be tempting to academic researchers to think that such criticisms should be principally directed to public and popular representations of history, it is important for all historians to reflect on the extent to which their own personal subjectivity, shaped by their upbringing and experiences, influences the writing of history. Donna Gabaccia has highlighted the connection between national discourses on immigration and the importance afforded to migrants in historical work.[13] She notes that in Germany, for instance, where foreign workers have been 'excluded from the nation' there has also been a tendency to ignore them in national histories.[14] This contrasts with the American notion of a 'nation of immigrants' which, while not being above all criticism, does at least open up a space where it is possible to discuss the roles of migrants in the development of nations.[15] Historians working in nations where population movement has traditionally not been considered a central part of the national story could therefore gain from reflecting on the extent to which this state of affairs has shaped national historiographies of immigration and what might be done to generate a more balanced perspective.

History is subject to political uses and psychologists have demonstrated that a group's sense of its history serves to shape its values.[16] The past is appropriated in the construction of what Benedict Anderson calls the 'imagined communities' that form nations.[17] Historical research therefore has an important contribution to make to ongoing contemporary debates on immigration, by serving to ground them in a critical understanding of the past. Political discourses and national narratives that emphasise continuity and ethnic homogeneity are supported by the sidelining of migrants in general histories of Britain and in histories of organisations such as the NHS, which are perceived as being constitutive of British national identity. A history that reintegrates discontinuities, transnational dimensions, and international influences back into national narratives can inform ongoing political debates on immigration. If historians do not seek to inform such debates, who will?

By adding to our understanding of how migrants have made the UK what it is today, they can contribute to the emergence of, in Lucassen's words, the 'Ellis Islands', the symbols of the presence of migration in the national landscape that have the potential to encourage the UK to be more aware of its past and more reflective and perceptive of the possibilities of immigration, as well as its costs, when it comes to making choices in the present.[18] This is not simply about writing popular or public histories. It is about taking seriously history's role as a social science—as a means of understanding the development of societies. If, for instance, the NHS is seen as central to national identity, and migration is then recognised as being central to the history of the NHS, this can serve to disrupt national narratives that construct migrants as non-British. Writing history in this way therefore has the potential to contribute to a national discussion on what a different 'imagined community' might look like; an 'imagined community' that would be grounded in a greater awareness of the impact of immigration on the development of an institution viewed as a central part of British national identity.

I did not seek in this study to answer all of the questions that one might pose in relation to the role of migrant South Asian doctors in the NHS. Future work would benefit from exploring the obvious diversity within this group of doctors. A more specific focus on the trajectories of doctors from Pakistan, India, Bangladesh, Sri Lanka or East Africa as well as the experiences of other migrant doctors would most likely produce different insights. The gender of doctors as well as their social background are hinted at in interviews as factors which shape the personal and professional trajectories of participants. The relevance of religion is another factor to be considered: are Muslim doctors treated differently; could coming from a particular Hindu caste have a bearing on medical careers in Britain? It is also the case that this study has primarily engaged with doctors who settled in Britain and had careers in general practice. An analysis of the trajectories and experiences of doctors who returned to the Indian subcontinent or moved on to other countries would cast further light on the history of international medical graduates.

Whilst the research I have presented here was concerned with doctors who migrated from the Indian subcontinent, this story is connected to a wider history of British-born South Asian doctors, which remains, so far, largely unexplored despite its central role in modern British medicine. According to GMC figures for 2016 there are roughly similar numbers of doctors with the surname Patel (1,656) and the common British surname Smith (1,705) registered to work as doctors in the UK.[19] Whilst many doctors with South Asian names are undoubtedly migrants, many others are the children of migrants, including migrant doctors. The long-term legacy of empire and post-war population movement continues to shape British medicine today.

Finally, the history of migrants in the NHS is not limited to doctors or indeed to nurses who have also been the subject of some research interest. Other groups of migrants have underpinned the functioning of the NHS since its inception. If the paucity of historical research devoted to migrant doctors in the history of the NHS is deserving of criticism, what of migrant cleaners, porters or cooks? One of the challenges of the task of writing migrants back into the history of the NHS is to avoid offering recognition solely to those having attained a particular professional and class status. It would also be instructive to reflect on how time overseas might have influenced the practice of British healthcare workers—be they doctors, nurses or administrators—who returned to work in the NHS.

Undertaking such a task in the context of the NHS could contribute to highlighting the importance of asking such questions about the impact of migration on the mainstream in other contexts. How for instance have Irish priests and Polish worshippers shaped the development of the Catholic Church in Britain? What part have migrant fruit pickers played in the development of British agriculture? How has low paid migrant labour contributed to making London the city that it is today? There are undoubtedly other architects of the NHS, and other architects of a range of aspects of modern Britain whose stories have yet to be told. By engaging with this dimension of the past, historians would deepen our appreciation of the transformative effect population movement has had on the development of modern Britain. They would also offer a different lens through which to examine the terms of reference of contemporary immigration debates.

## Notes

1 O. Starn, 'Missing the revolution: Anthropologists and the war in Peru', *Cultural Anthropology*, 16:1 (1991), p. 64.
2 Starn, 'Missing the revolution', p. 63.
3 H. Kureishi, *My Beautiful Laundrette* (London: Faber & Faber, 2000), p. 35.
4 Powell, 'Coasts and coalfields', p. 263.
5 J. T. Hart, 'The inverse care law', *The Lancet,* 297:7696 (1971).
6 J. M. Simpson & A. Esmail, 'The UK's dysfunctional relationship with medical migrants: The Daniel Ubani case and reform of out-of-hours services', *British Journal of General Practice*, 61 (2011); Simpson et al., 'Providing "special" types of labour'.

7  Kyriakides & Virdee, 'Migrant labour'.

8  Oxfam Public Affairs Unit, *The Doctor-Go-Round. Health Care in Britain and the Developing World: Medical Manpower, Migration and Aid* (London: Oxfam, 1976), p. 17.

9  Oxfam Public Affairs Unit, *The Doctor-Go-Round*, p. 18.

10 Shapiro, 'General practitioners' attitudes'.

11 C. Seale, 'The role of doctors' religious faith and ethnicity in taking ethically controversial decisions during end-of-life care', *Journal of Medical Ethics*, 36 (2010).

12 *The Future of Multi-Ethnic Britain*, Report of the Commission on the Future of Multi-Ethnic Britain [The Parekh Report] (London: Profile Books, 2000), pp. 15–16.

13 D. R. Gabaccia, 'Nations of immigrants: Do words matter?', *The Pluralist*, 5:3 (2010); D. R. Gabaccia, 'Nomads, nations and the immigrant paradigm', in Spickard (ed.), *Race and Immigration in the United States*, pp. 36–7.

14 Gabaccia, 'Nations of immigrants', pp. 26–7.

15 Gabaccia, 'Nations of immigrants', p. 27.

16 J. H. Liu & D. J. Hilton, 'How the past weighs on the present: Social representations of history and their role in identity politics', *British Journal of Social Psychology*, 44 (2005), p. 1.

17 B. Anderson, *Imagined Communities: Reflections on the Origin and Spread of Nationalism*, revised edition (London, New York: Verso, 2006); J. H. Liu, C. G. Sibley, L. L. Huang, 'History matters: Effects of culture-specific symbols on political attitudes and intergroup relations', *Political Psychology*, 35:1 (2014).

18 Lucassen, *Immigrant Threat*, p. 13.

19 GMC, 'List of Registered Medical Practitioners'. Accessed 7 November 2016 at: www.gmc-uk.org/doctors/register/LRMP.asp.

# Bibliography

## Primary sources

*Oral history interviews conducted by author, in order of first interview*

Dipak Ray 5 December 2008 and 19 March 2010
Rooin Boomla 5 December 2008 and 16 September 2009
Darius Boomla 15 September 2009
Krishna Korlipara 24 September 2009
Sri Venugopal 5 November 2009
Shiv Pande 23 November 2009 and 9 December 2009
Muhammad Noorul Islam Talukdar 1 December 2009
S. K. Ahuja 8 December 2009
L. R. M. Kamal 8 March 2010
M. A. Salam 18 March 2010
Rupendra Kumar Majumdar 18 March 2010
Arup Chaudhuri 30 March 2010
Mohammed Abu Khaled 2 April 2010
Ruban Prasad 20 April 2010
Hasmukh Joshi 27 April 2010
P. L. Pathak 14 May 2010
Urmila Rao 28 May 2010
Raman N. Rao 28 May 2010
Nanalal Shah 7 June 2010
Anup Kumar Sen 10 June 2010
Muhammad Fazlul Haque 16 June 2010
Sir Netar Mallick 23 June 2010
Syed Ahmad Ali Gilani 30 June 2010 and 10 November 2010.
F. B. Kotwall 11 October 2010
M. S. Kausar 26 October 2010

Hira Lal Kapur 5 January 2010
Raj Chandran 7 March 2011
Sir Donald Irvine 7 April 2011
K. S. Bhanumathi 16 April 2011
Sir Liam Donaldson 9 May 2011
S. M. Qureshi 20 May 2011
Ajeet Gulati 24 May 2011
Jangu Banatvala 9 July 2015

(Details of an additional 12 interviews are withheld in order to preserve
the anonymity of research participants who did not wish to be identified.)

## Archives

British Library Newspaper Archive
British Library Sound Archive
British Medical Association Archives
General Medical Council Archives
Manchester Archives and Local Studies
Museum of London
Royal College of General Practitioners Archives
Runnymede Collection at Middlesex University
UK National Archives

## Personal collections

Personal papers of H. L. Kapur
Personal papers of K. Korlipara
Personal papers of D. Ray
Personal papers of Dr Satya Chatterjee and Mrs Enyd Chatterjee

## Journals, newspapers, newsletters and magazines

*Andhra Medical Graduates' Reunion* (UK) Silver Jubilee Edition: a retrospective
*BMJ*
The *Daily Mail*
The *Daily Telegraph*
*Doctor*
*Eastside Community Heritage Newsletter*
*Economic Review*
The *Guardian*

*Hindustan Times*
*Hospital Doctor*
*The Lancet*
*Medical World*
*Medicos*
*ODA News*
*Pulse*
*The Times*
*TUC In Touch* e-bulletin
*West Indian World*

## Memoirs and accounts of doctors' lives

Bhowmick, B., *You Can't Climb a Ladder with Your Hands in Your Pockets* (Warboys, Cambridgeshire: Biograph, 2006).
Chatterjee, S., *All my Yesterdays* (Stanhope: The Memoir Club, 2006).
Chowdhary, S., *I Made my Home in England* (Basildon: published by Savitri Chowdhary and printed by Grant-Best Ltd, 1962?).
Lawrence, R. A. A. R., *A Fire in his Hand* (London: Athena Press, 2006).
Prem, D. R., *The Parliamentary Leper: A History of Colour Prejudice in Britain* (Aligarh, India: Metric Publications, 1965).
Sayeed, A., *In the Shadow of my Taqdir* (Stanhope: The Memoir Club, 2006).

## Official publications

Great Britain, Department of Health and Social Security, On the state of public health: The annual report of the Chief Medical Officer of the Department of Health and Social Security for the year 1975 (London: HMSO, 1976).
Great Britain, Department of Health and Social Security, On the state of public health: The annual report of the Chief Medical Officer of the Department of Health and Social Security for the year 1976 (London: HMSO, 1977).
Great Britain, Department of Health and Social Security, On the state of public health: The annual report of the Chief Medical Officer of the Department of Health and Social Security for the year 1979 (London: HMSO, 1980).
Hansard
Report of the Committee of Inquiry into the regulation of the medical profession [Merrison report] (London: HMSO, 1975).
Department of Employment, The role of immigrants in the labour market: Project report by the unit for manpower studies (London: Department of Employment, 1976).

## Films and documentaries

Asquith A., *The Millionairess*, Twentieth Century Fox, 1960.
Eastside Community Heritage, *Living in Barking: Hidden from History*, 2010 (?).
Foot, J., *Time shift: From the Raj to the Rhondda*, BBC, 2003.
Suri, S., *I for India*, Fandango and Zero West, 2005.
Thomas, R., *Doctor in the House*, Group Film Productions Limited, 1954.

## Websites

BBC: www.bbc.co.uk (accessed 26 May 2017).
Birmingham City Council: www.birmingham.gov.uk (accessed 26 May 2017).
Centre for the History of Science, Technology and Medicine, The University of Manchester: www.chstm.manchester.ac.uk (accessed 8 April 2013).
The *Daily Telegraph*: www.telegraph.co.uk (accessed 8 December 2012).
General Medical Council: www.gmc-uk.org (accessed 7 November 2016).
Kannada Balaga UK: www.kannadabalaga.org.uk/ (accessed 23 November 2015).
Margaret Thatcher Foundation: www.margaretthatcher.org (accessed 12 April 2017).
Oral History Society: www.ohs.org.uk (accessed 26 May 2017).
The Shipman enquiry: www.the-shipman-inquiry.org (accessed 1 May 2012).

## Secondary sources

Abel-Smith, B., 'Foreword', in F. Honigsbaum, *The Division in British Medicine: A History of the Separation of General Practice from Hospital Care 1911–1968* (London: Konan Page, 1979).
Abel-Smith, B. & K. Gales (with the assistance of Gillian MacFarlane), *British Doctors at Home and Abroad*, Occasional papers on social administration No.8 (Welwyn, England: Published for the Social Administration Research Trust by the Codicote Press, 1964).
Afonso, A., 'Permanently provisional: History, facts and figures of Portuguese immigration in Switzerland', *International Migration*, 53:4 (2015).
Ahmad, W. I. U., E. E. M. Kernohan, M. R. Baker, 'Patients' choice of general practitioner: Influence of patient's fluency in English and the ethnicity and sex of the doctor', *Journal of the Royal College of General Practitioners*, 39 (1989).

Ahmad, W. I. U., M. R. Baker, E. E. M. Kernohan, 'General practitioners' perceptions of Asian and non-Asian patients', *Family Practice*, 8:1 (1991).

Ali, L., 'West Indian nurses and the National Health Service in Britain 1950–1968' (Master of Arts by Dissertation, University of York, 2001).

Alkhudairy, S. I., 'International labour migration to Saudi Arabia: A case study of the experiences of medical doctors in Riyadh' (PhD dissertation, University of Essex, 2001).

Anderson, B., *Imagined Communities: Reflections on the Origin and Spread of Nationalism*, revised edition (London, New York: Verso, 2006).

Anwar, M. & A. Ali, *Overseas Doctors: Experience and Expectations* (London: Commission for Racial Equality, 1987).

Armstrong, J., 'A system of exclusion: New Zealand women medical specialists in international medical networks, 1945–1975', in L. Monnais & D. Wright (eds), *Doctors Beyond Borders: The Transnational Migration of Physicians in the Twentieth Century* (Toronto: University of Toronto Press, 2016).

Aspin, J., 'Tuberculosis among Indian immigrants to a Midland industrial area', *BMJ*, 1962, 1: 5289 (1962).

Baggott, R., *Health and Healthcare in Britain*, third edition (Baskingstoke & New York: Palgrave Macmillan, 2004).

Bammer, A. and R.-E. Boetcher Joeres (eds), *The Future of Scholarly Writing: Critical Interventions* (Basingstoke: Palgrave, 2015).

Barnett, J. R., 'Foreign medical graduates in New Zealand 1973–79: A test of the "exacerbation hypothesis"', *Social Science and Medicine*, 26:10 (1988).

Benencia, R., 'Apéndice: La inmigración limítrofe' in F. Devoto *Historia de la inmigración en la Argentina* (Buenos Aires: Sudamericana, 2009) (Spanish).

Ben-Shlomo, Y., I. White, P. M. McKeigue, 'Prediction of general practice workload from census based deprivation scores', *Journal of Epidemiology and Community Health*, 46 (1992).

Berridge, V., *Health and Society in Britain since 1939* (Cambridge: Cambridge University Press, 1999).

Berridge, V., 'Public or policy understanding of history?', *Social History of Medicine*, 16: 3 (2003).

Berridge, V., 'Thinking in time: Does health policy need history as evidence?' *The Lancet*, 375: 9717 (2010).

Berridge, V. & J. Stewart, 'History: A social science neglected by other social sciences (and why it should not be)', *Contemporary Social Science: Journal of the Academy of Social Sciences*, 7:1 (2012).

Bivins, R., 'Coming "home" to (post) colonial medicine: Treating tropical bodies in post-war Britain', *Social History of Medicine* 26: 1 (2013).

Bivins, R., *Contagious Communities: Medicine, Migration, & the NHS in Post-War Britain* (Oxford: Oxford University Press, 2015).

Bornat, J. & H. Diamond, 'Women's history and oral history: Developments and debates', *Women's History Review*, 16: 1 (2007).

Bornat, J., L. Henry, P. Raghuram, '"Don't mix race with the specialty": Interviewing South Asian overseas-trained geriatricians', *Oral History*, 37: 1 (2009).

Bornat, J., L. Henry, P. Raghuram, 'The making of careers, the making of a discipline: Luck and chance in migrant careers in geriatric medicine', *Journal of Vocational Behavior*, 78 (2011).

Bosanquet, N. & C. Salisbury, 'The practice', in I. Loudon, J. Horder, C. Webster (eds), *General Practice under the National Health Service 1948–1997* (London: Clarendon Press, 1998).

Brown, C., 'Reflections on oral history and migrant communities in Britain', *Oral History*, 34: 1 (2006).

Burton, A., *After the Imperial Turn: Thinking With and Through the Nation* (Durham, North Carolina and London: Duke University Press, 2003).

Butler, J. R. & R. Knight, 'The choice of practice location', *Journal of the Royal College of General Practitioners*, 25 (1975).

Butler, J. R. (in collaboration with J. M. Bevan and R. C. Taylor), *Family Doctors and Public Policy* (London: Routledge and Kegan Paul, 1973).

Buxton M. J. & R. E. Klein, 'Population characteristics and the distribution of general medical practitioners', *BMJ*, 1 (1979).

Cargill, D., 'Recruitment to general practice in Essex and Birmingham', *The Lancet*, 1: 7596 (1969).

Cartwright, A., *Patients and Their Doctors: A Study of General Practice* (London: Routledge and Kegan Paul, 1967).

Cartwright, A. & R. Anderson, *General Practice Revisited: A Second Study of Patients and Their Doctors* (London: Tavistock Publications, 1981).

Castles, S. & M. J. Miller, *The Age of Migration: International Population Movements in the Modern World*, fourth edition (Basingstoke: Palgrave Macmillan, 2009).

Chakrabarti, P., *Medicine and Empire 1600–1960* (Basingstoke & New York: Palgrave Macmillan, 2013).

Chanchal, J., N. Narayan, K. Narayan, L. A. Pike, M. E. Clarkson, I. G. Cox, J. Chatterjee, 'Attitudes of Asian patients in Birmingham to general practitioner services', *Journal of the Royal College of General Practitioners*, 35 (1985).

Clover, D. U., 'Out of the dark room: Participatory photography as a critical, imaginative and public aesthetic practice of transformative education', *Journal of Transformative education*, 4 (2006).

Coker, N. (ed.), *Racism in Medicine: An Agenda for Change* (London: King's Fund Publishing, 2001).

Coleborne, C., *Insanity, Identity and Empire: Immigrants and Institutional Confinement in Australia and New Zealand, 1873–1910* (Manchester: Manchester University Press, 2015).

Collings, J. S., 'General practice in England today: A reconnaissance', *The Lancet*, 255: 6604(1950).

Consterdine, E., 'Community versus Commonwealth: Reappraising the 1971 Immigration Act', *Immigrants and Minorities*, 35:1 (2017).

Cox, P., 'The future use of history', *History Workshop Journal*, 75:1(2013).

Creighton, S., 'Harbans Lal (1) Gulati'. Unpublished talk (no date).

Dadabhoy, S., 'The next generation, the problematic children: A personal story', in N. Coker (ed.), *Racism in Medicine: An Agenda for Change* (London: King's Fund Publishing, 2001).

Davenport-Hines, R., 'Ruxton, Buck (1899–1936)', *Oxford Dictionary of National Biography* (online) (Oxford: Oxford University Press, 2004).

Delap, L., S. Szreter, P. Warde, 'History and policy: A decade of bridge-building in the United Kingdom', *Scandia*, 80:1 (2014).

Dickinson, T., *'Curing Queers': Mental Nurses and Their Patients 1935–74* (Manchester: Manchester University Press, 2014).

Digby, A., 'The British National Health Insurance Act, 1911', in M. Gorsky & S. Sheard (eds), *Financing Medicine: The British Experience since 1750* (Abingdon and New York: Routledge, 2000).

Donaldson, L. J., 'Health and social status of elderly Asians: A community survey', *BMJ*, 293 (1986).

Doyal, L., G. Hunt, J. Mellor, 'Your life in their hands: Migrant workers in the National Health Service', *Critical Social Policy*, 1 (1981).

Doyal, L., F. Gee, G. Hunt, J. Mellor, I. Pennell (with the support of N. Parry), *Migrant Workers in the National Health Service: Report of a Preliminary Survey* (Polytechnic of North London, Department of Sociology, 1980).

Drakeman, D., *Why we Need the Humanities: Life Science, Law and the Common Good* (Basingstoke and New York: Palgrave Macmillan, 2016).

Drury, M., 'The GP and professional organisations', in I. Loudon, J. Horder, C. Webster (eds), *General Practice under the National Health Service 1948–1997* (London: Clarendon Press, 1998).

Esmail, A., 'Asian doctors in the NHS: Service and betrayal', *British Journal of General Practice*, 57 (2007).

Esmail, A., 'Racial discrimination in medical schools', in N. Coker (ed.), *Racism in Medicine: An Agenda for Change* (London: King's Fund Publishing, 2001).

Esmail, A. & S. Everington, 'Racial discrimination against doctors from ethnic minorities', *BMJ*, 306 (1993).

Evans, R. J., *In Defense of History* (London: Granta Books, 2000).

Evans, R. J., *Telling Lies about Hitler: The Holocaust, History and the David Irving Trial* (London and New York: Verso, 2002).

Fanon, F., *Peau noire, masques blancs* (Paris: Editions du Seuil, 1952). (French)

Farooq, G. Y., 'A study of overseas-trained South Asian doctors in England and Wales' (PhD dissertation, University of Manchester, 2014).

Ferris, P., *The Doctors* (London: Victor Gollancz, 1965).

Fisher, M. H., S. Lahiri, S. Thandi (eds), *A South Asian History of Britain: Four Centuries of Peoples from the Indian Sub-Continent* (Oxford and Westport, Connecticut: Greenwood World Publishing, 2007).

Freeman, G. K., H. Rai, J. J. Walker, J. G. R. Howie, D. J. Heaney, M. Maxwell, 'Non-English speakers consulting with the GP in their own language: A cross-sectional survey', *British Journal of General Practice*, 52 (2002).

Frenz, M., *Community, Memory and Migration in a Globalizing World: The Goan Experience, c. 1890s–1980* (New Delhi: Oxford University Press, 2014).

Fry, J. & G. McLachlan, 'The future', in J. Fry, Lord Hunt of Fawley, R. J. F. H. Pinsent (eds), *A History of the Royal College of General Practitioners – The First 25 Years* (Lancaster, Boston and The Hague: MTP Press Limited, 1983).

The Future of Multi-Ethnic Britain: Report of the Commission on the Future of Multi-Ethnic Britain [The Parekh Report] (London: Profile Books, 2000).

Gabaccia, D. R., 'Nations of immigrants: Do words matter?', *The Pluralist*, 5:3 (2010).

Gabaccia, D. R., 'Nomads, nations and the immigrant paradigm', in P. Spickard (ed.), *Race and Immigration in the United States* (New York and London: Routledge, 2012).

Garner, J. S., 'The great experiment: The admission of women students to St Mary's Hospital Medical School, 1916–1925', *Medical History*, 42 (1998).

Gavin, M. J., 'A crisis of legitimacy? The clinical role, intellectual status and career motivations of general medical practitioners' (PhD dissertation, The University of Manchester, 2004).

Gibson, R., *The Family Doctor: His Life and History* (London: George Allen & Unwin, 1981).

Gill, P. S., 'General practitioners, ethnic diversity and racism', in N. Coker (ed.), *Racism in Medicine: An Agenda for Change* (London: King's Fund Publishing, 2001).

Gilles, M. T., J. Wakerman, A. Durey, ' "If it wasn't for OTDs, there would be no AMS": Overseas-trained doctors working in rural and remote Aboriginal health settings', *Australian Health Review*, 32:4 (2008).

Gish, O., *Britain and the Immigrant Doctor* (Institute of Race Relations, 1969).

Gish, O., 'Emigration and the supply and demand for medical manpower: The Irish case', *Minerva*, 7:4 (1969).

Gish, O., 'British doctor migration 1962–67', *British Journal of Medical Education*, 4 (1970).

Gish, O., 'Overseas-born doctor migration 1962–66', *British Journal of Medical Education*, 5 (1971).

Goddard, M., H. Gravelle, A. Hole, G. Marini, 'Where did all the GPs go? Increasing supply and geographical equity in England and Scotland', *Journal of Health Services Research Policy*, 15:1(2010).

Goldacre, M. J., J. M. Davidson, T. W. Lambert, 'Country of training and ethnic origin of UK doctors: Database and survey studies', *BMJ*, 2004, doi: 10.1136/bmj.38202.364271.BE.

Goldacre, M. J.,T. W. Lambert, J. M. Davidson, 'Loss of British-trained doctors from the medical workforce in Great Britain', *Medical Education*, 35 (2001).

Gorman, M., 'Introduction of western science into colonial India: Role of the Calcutta Medical College', *Proceedings of the American Philosophical Society*, 132:3 (1988).

Gorsky, M., 'The British National Health Service 1948–2008: A review of the historiography', *Social History of Medicine*, 21:3 (2008).

Green, A., 'Continuity, contingency and context: Bringing the historian's cognitive toolkit into university futures and public policy development', *Futures*, 44 (2012).

Green, A., 'History as expertise and the influence of political culture on advice for policy since Fulton', *Contemporary British History*, 29:1 (2015).

Green, A., *History, Policy and Public Purpose: Historians and Historical Thinking in Government* (London: Palgrave, 2016).

Greenwood, A. & H. Topiwala, *Indian Doctors in Kenya, 1895–1940: The Forgotten History* (Basingstoke: Palgrave, 2015).

Grosvenor, I., 'Prem, Dhani Ram (1904–1979)', *Oxford Dictionary of National Biography* (online) (Oxford: Oxford University Press, 2013).

Hann, M. & H. Gravelle, 'The maldistribution of general practitioners in England and Wales: 1974–2003', *British Journal of General Practice*, 54 (2004).

Hannay, D., 'Undergraduate medical education and general practice', in I. Loudon, J. Horder, C. Webster (eds), *General Practice under the National Health Service 1948–1997* (London: Clarendon Press, 1998).

Harrington, V. E., 'Voices beyond the asylum: A post-war history of mental health services in Manchester and Salford' (PhD dissertation, The University of Manchester, 2008).

Harrison, M., 'Science and the British Empire', *Isis*, 96:1 (2005).

Harrison, S. & R. McDonald, *The Politics of Healthcare in Britain* (London, Thousand Oaks, New Delhi and Singapore: SAGE Publications, 2008).

Hart, J. T., 'The inverse care law', *The Lancet*, 297:7696 (1971).

Hart, J. T., *A New Kind of Doctor: The General Practitioner's Part in the Health of the Community* (London: Merlin Press, 1988).

Hing, B. O., *Defining America Through Immigration Policy* (Philadelphia: Temple University Press, 2004).

Hobsbawm, E., 'From social history to the history of society', *Daedalus*, 100:1(1971).

Hobsbawm, E., *How to Change the World: Tales of Marx and Marxism* (London: Little, Brown, 2011).

Holmes, C., *John Bull's Island: Immigration and British Society 1871–1971* (Basingstoke, London: Macmillan Education, 1988).

Horder, J., 'Conclusion', in I. Loudon, J. Horder, C. Webster (eds), *General Practice under the National Health Service 1948–1997* (London: Clarendon Press, 1998).

Howie, J., 'Research in general practice: Perspectives and themes', in I. Loudon, J. Horder, C. Webster (eds), *General Practice under the National Health Service 1948–1997* (London: Clarendon Press, 1998).

Hutt, P., I. Heath, R. Neighbour, *Confronting an Ill Society: David Widgery, General Practice, Idealism and the Chase for Change* (Oxford and San Francisco: Radcliffe Publishing, 2005).

Iredale, R., 'Luring overseas trained doctors to Australia: Issues of training, regulating and trading', *International Migration*, 47:4 (2009).

Jeffery, R., 'Recognizing India's doctors: The institutionalisation of medical dependency, 1918–39', *Modern Asian Studies*, 13:2 (1979).

Jeffery, R., *The Politics of Health in India* (Berkeley, Los Angeles and London: University of California Press, 1988).

Jefferys, M. & H. Sachs, *Rethinking General Practice: Dilemmas in Primary Medical Care* (London and New York: Tavistock Publications: 1983).

Johnson, M. R. D., M. Cross, S. A. Cardew, 'Inner city residents, ethnic minorities and primary health care', *Postgraduate Medical Journal*, October, 59 (1983).

Johnson, T. J. & M. Caygill, 'The British Medical Association and its overseas branches: A short history', *The Journal of Imperial and Commonwealth History*, 1:3 (1973).

Jones, E. L. & S. J. Snow, *Against the Odds: Black and Minority Ethnic Clinicians and Manchester, 1948 to 2009* (Lancaster: Carnegie, 2010).

Jones, G., '"A mysterious discrimination": Irish medical emigration to the United States in the 1950s', in L. Monnais & D. Wright (eds), *Doctors Beyond Borders: The Transnational Migration of Physicians in the Twentieth Century* (Toronto: University of Toronto Press, 2016).

Jones, R. & S. Menzies, *General Practice Essential Facts* (Abingdon: Radcliffe Medical Press, 1999).

Jordanova, L., *History in Practice* (London: Hodder Arnold, 2006).

Keely, C. B., 'Effects of the immigration act of 1965 on selected population characteristics of immigrants to the United States', *Demography*, 8:2 (1971).

Keulen, S. & R. Kroeze, 'Back to business: A next step in the field of oral history – The usefulness of oral history for leadership and organisational research', *The Oral History Review*, 39:1(2012).

Kirby, R. K., 'Phenomenology and the problems of oral history', *The Oral History Review*, 35:1 (2008).

Klein, R., *The New Politics of the National Health Service*, sixth edition (Oxford and New York: Radcliffe Publishing, 2010).

Knox, P. L., 'The intraurban ecology of primary medical care: Patterns of accessibility and their policy implications', *Environment and Planning A*, 10 (1978).

Kondapi, C., *Indians Overseas 1838–1949* (New Delhi, Bombay, Calcutta, Madras and London: Indian Council of World Affairs, Oxford University Press, 1951).

Kramer, A., *Many Rivers to Cross: The History of the Caribbean Contribution to the NHS* (London: TSO, 2006).

Kumar, A., *Medicine and the Raj: British Medical Policy in India, 1835–1911* (New Delhi, Thousand Oaks and London: SAGE Publications, 1998).

Kureishi, H., *My Beautiful Laundrette* (London: Faber & Faber, 2000).

Kushner, T., *Remembering Refugees: Then and Now* (Manchester, New York: Manchester University Press, 2006).

Kushner, T., 'Great Britons: Immigration, history and memory', in K. Burrell & P. Panayi (eds), *Histories and Memories: Migrants and Their History in Britain* (London and New York: Tauris Academic Studies, 2006).

Kyriakides, C. & S. Virdee, 'Migrant labour, racism and the British National Health Service', *Ethnicity and Health*, 8:4 (2003).

Lahiri, S., *Indians in Britain: Anglo-Indian Encounters, Race and Identity, 1880–1930* (London: Frank Cass, 2000).

Lewis, J., 'The medical profession and the state: GPs and the GP contract in the 1960s and the 1990s', *Social Policy and Administration*, 32:2 (1998).

Liu, J. H. & D. J. Hilton, 'How the past weighs on the present: Social representations of history and their role in identity politics', *British Journal of Social Psychology*, 44 (2005).

Liu, J. H., C. G. Sibley, L. L. Huang, 'History matters: Effects of culture-specific symbols on political attitudes and intergroup relations', *Political Psychology*, 35:1 (2014).

Logan, R. F. L., J. A. Roberts, P. Stockton, 'General practice – The immigrant doctor in N.E.T.R.H.A.', *Medicos*, 4: 1(1979).

Loudon, I. & M. Drury, 'Some aspects of clinical care in general practice', in I. Loudon, J. Horder, C. Webster (eds), *General Practice under the National Health Service 1948–1997* (London: Clarendon Press, 1998).

Loudon, I., J. Horder, C. Webster (eds), *General Practice under the National Health Service 1948–1997* (London: Clarendon Press, 1998).

Lucassen, L., *The Immigrant Threat: The Integration of Old and New Migrants in Western Europe since 1850* (Urbana and Chicago: University of Illinois Press, 2005).

Luker, K. A., 'Reading nursing: The burden of being different', *International Journal of Nursing Studies*, 21:1 (1984).

Lynd, S., 'Historical past and existential present', in T. Roszak (ed.), *The Dissenting Academy: Essays Criticizing the Teaching of the Humanities in American Universities* (London: Pelican, 1969).

Mathers, N. & S. Rowland, 'General practice – a post-modern specialty?', *British Journal of General Practice*, 47 (1997).

Matthews, H. & J. Bain, *Doctors Talking* (Edinburgh: Scottish Cultural Press, 1998).

McCarthy, A., 'Migration and madness at sea: The nineteenth- and early twentieth-century voyage to New Zealand', *Social History of Medicine*, 28:4 (2015).

McDermott, R. F., L. A. Gordon, A. T. Embree, F. W. Pritchett, D. Dalton (eds), *Sources of Indian Traditions: Modern India, Pakistan and Bangladesh*, third edition (New York: Columbia University Press, 2014).

McDowell, L., *Working Lives: Gender, Migration and Employment in Britain, 1945–2007* (Chichester: Wiley-Blackwell, 2013).

McManus, I. C. & R. Wakeford, 'PLAB and UK graduates' performance on MRCP (UK) and MRCGP examination: Data linkage study', *BMJ*, 348 (2014).

Mejia, A., 'Migration of physicians and nurses: A world wide picture', *International Journal of Epidemiology*, 7:3 (1978).

Memmi, A., *Le racisme: Description, définitions, traitement*, nouvelle edition revue. (Paris: Gallimard, 1994). (French)

Mohan, P. R. L., 'Asian doctors in England: Their professional experiences and social life (A case study in Sandwell)' (Master of Social Sciences thesis, University of Birmingham, 1979).

Mold, A., *Making the Patient-Consumer: Patient Organisations and Health Consumerism in Britain* (Manchester: Manchester University Press, 2015).

Monnais, L. & D. Wright (eds), *Doctors Beyond Borders: The Transnational Migration of Physicians in the Twentieth Century* (Toronto: University of Toronto Press, 2016).

Moorhead, R., 'Hart of Glyncorrwg', *Journal of the Royal Society of Medicine*, 97 (2004).

Morrell, D., 'Introduction and overview', in I. Loudon, J. Horder, C. Webster (eds), *General Practice under the National Health Service 1948–1997* (London: Clarendon Press,1998).

Mullally, S. & D. Wright, 'La grande séduction? The immigration of foreign-trained physicians to Canada c. 1954–76', *Journal of Canadian Studies*, 41:3 (2007).

Nava, M., 'Sometimes antagonistic, sometimes ardently sympathetic: contradictory responses to migrants in postwar Britain', *Ethnicities*, 14:3 (2014).

Noiriel, G., *Le creuset Français* (Paris: Editions du Seuil, 1988). (French)

Noiriel, G., *Introduction à la socio-histoire* (Paris: Editions La Découverte, 2006). (French)

OECD, *International Migration Outlook 2015* (Paris: OECD Publishing, 2015).

Olusoga, D., *Black and British: A Forgotten History* (London: Macmillan, 2016).

Oxfam Public Affairs Unit, *The Doctor-Go-Round. Health Care in Britain and the Developing World: Medical Manpower, Migration and Aid.* (London: Oxfam, 1976).

Panayi, P., *An Immigration History of Britain: Multicultural Racism since 1800* (Harlow: Pearson, 2010).

Pereira Gray, D., 'Postgraduate training and continuing education', in I. Loudon, J. Horder, C. Webster (eds), *General Practice under the National Health Service 1948–1997* (London: Clarendon Press, 1998).

Perks, R., 'The roots of oral history: Exploring contrasting attitudes to elite, corporate, and business oral history in Britain and the U.S.', *The Oral History Review*, 37: 2 (2010).

Portelli, A., 'What makes oral history different?', in R. Perks & P. Thomson, *The Oral History Reader*, second edition (London and New York: Routledge, 2008).

Porter, A., 'Empires in the mind', in P. J. Marshall (ed.), *The Cambridge Illustrated History of the British Empire* (Cambridge: Cambridge University Press, 1996).

Powell, M., 'Coasts and coalfields: The geographical distribution of doctors in England and Wales in the 1930s', *Social History of Medicine*, 18:2 (2005).

Raghuram, P., 'Asian women medical migrants in the UK', in A. Agrawal (ed.), *Migrant Women and Work*. (New Delhi: SAGE, 2006).

Raghuram, P., J. Bornat, L. Henry, 'Ethnic clustering among South Asian geriatricians in the UK: An oral history study', *Diversity in Health and Care*, 6 (2009).

Raghuram, P., J. Bornat, L. Henry (2011) 'The co-marking of aged bodies and migrant bodies: Migrant workers' contribution to geriatric medicine in the UK', *Sociology of Health and Illness*, 33: 2 (2011).

Ramamurthy, A., *Black Star: Britain's Asian Youth Movements* (London: Pluto Press, 2013).

Ramanna, M., *Western Medicine and Public Health in Colonial Bombay 1845–1894* (London: Sangam Books, 2002).

Ranasinha, R., 'Introduction', in R. Ranasinha (ed.), *South Asians and the Shaping of Britain 1870–1950* (Manchester and New York: Manchester University Press, 2012).

Rivett, G., *National Health Service history* [online]. Available at: www.nhshistory.net/ (accessed 30 April 2012).

Roberts, P. D., H. James, A. Petrie, J. O. Morgan, A. V. Hoffbrand, 'Vitamin B12 status in pregnancy among immigrants to Britain', *British Medical Journal*, 3 (1973).

Robinson, V. & M. Carey, 'Peopling skilled international migration: Indian doctors in the UK', *International Migration*, 38:1 (2000).

Rosenberg, C. E., 'Anticipated consequences: Historians, history and health policy', in R. A. Stevens, C. E. Rosenberg, L. R. Burns (eds), *History and Health Policy in the United States: Putting the Past Back In* (New Brunswick, New Jersey and London: Rutgers University Press, 2006).

Rowbotham, S., *Hidden from History: 300 Years of Women's Oppression and the Fight Against It* (London: Pluto Press, 1977).

Ryan, L., 'Who do you think you are? Irish nurses encountering ethnicity and constructing identity in Britain', *Ethnic and Racial Studies*, 30 (2007).

Said, E. W., *Culture and Imperialism* (London: Vintage Books, 1994).

Schwartz, B., '"The only white man in there": The re-racialisation of England, 1956–1968', *Race and Class*, 38:1(1996).

Seale, C., 'The role of doctors' religious faith and ethnicity in taking ethically controversial decisions during end-of-life care', *Journal of Medical Ethics*, 36 (2010).

Seaton, A., 'Against the "sacred cow": NHS opposition and the Fellowship for Freedom in Medicine, 1948–72', *Twentieth Century British History*, 26:3 (2015).

Shapiro, J. A., 'General practitioners' attitudes towards AIDS and their perceived information needs', *BMJ*, 298 (1989).

Shaunak, S., S. R. Lakhani, R. Abraham, J. D. Maxwell, 'Differences among Asian patients', *BMJ*, 293:6555 (1986).

Sherif, J., A. Altikriti, I. Patel, 'Muslim electoral participation in British general elections: An historical perspective and case study', in T. Peace (ed.), *Muslims and Political Participation in Britain* (Abingdon: Routledge, 2015).

Sidel, V. W., M. Jefferys, P. J. Mansfield, 'General practice in the London borough of Camden: Report of an enquiry in 1968', *Journal of the Royal College of General Practitioners*, 22 (Suppl. 3) (1972).

Simpson, J. M., 'Gulati, Harbans Lall (1896?–1967)', *Oxford Dictionary of National Biography* (online) (Oxford: Oxford University Press, 2012).

Simpson, J. M., 'Diagnosing a flight from care: Medical migration and "dirty work" in the NHS', Policy Papers, *History and Policy* (2014) [online]. Available at: www.historyandpolicy.org/policy-papers/papers/diagnosing-a-flight-from-care-medical-migration-and-dirty-work-in-the-nhs (accessed 26 May 2017).

Simpson, J. M., 'Reframing NHS history: Visual sources in a study of UK-based migrant doctors', *Oral History*, 42:2 (2014).

Simpson, J. M. & A. Esmail, 'The UK's dysfunctional relationship with medical migrants: The Daniel Ubani case and reform of out-of-hours services', *British Journal of General Practice*, 61 (2011).

Simpson, J. M. & J. Ramsay, 'Manifestations and negotiations of racism and "heterophobia" in overseas-born South Asian GPs' accounts of careers in the UK', *Diversity and Equality in Heath and Care*, 3–4 (2014).

Simpson, J. M. & S. J. Snow, 'Why we should try to get the joke: Humor, laughter and healthcare history', *Oral History Review*, 44:1 (2017).

Simpson, J. M., A. Esmail, V. S. Kalra, S. J. Snow, 'Writing migrants back into NHS history: Addressing a "collective amnesia" and its policy implications', *Journal of the Royal Society of Medicine*, 103:10 (2010).

Simpson, J. M., S. J. Snow, A. Esmail, 'Providing "special" types of labour and exerting agency: How migrant doctors have shaped the UK's National Health Service', in L. Monnais & D. Wright (eds), *Doctors Beyond Borders: The Transnational Migration of Physicians in the Twentieth Century* (Toronto: University of Toronto Press, 2016).

Sinclair, G. & C. A. Williams, ' "Home and away": The cross-fertilisation between "colonial" and "British" policing, 1921–85', *The Journal of Imperial and Commonwealth History*, 35:2 (2007).

Small, S. & J. Solomos, 'Race, immigration and politics in Britain: Changing policy agendas and conceptual paradigms 1940s–2000s'. *International Journal of Comparative Sociology*, 47 (2006).

Smith, D. J., *Overseas Doctors in the National Health Service* (London and Thetford: Policy Studies Institute, 1980).

Smith, G. & M. Nicolson, 'Re-expressing the division of British medicine under the NHS: The importance of locality in general practitioners' oral histories', *Social Science and Medicine*, 64 (2007).

Smith, G., F. Ferguson, E. Mitchell, M. Nicolson, G. C. M. Watt, *Speaking for a Change: An Oral History of General Practice*. School of Health and Related Research (ScHARR), University of Sheffield, ScHARR Report Series No.17, 2007. Available at: http://personal.rhul.ac.uk/usjd/135/indexgp.htm (accessed 1 May 2012).

Snow, S. & E. Jones, 'Immigration and the National Health Service: Putting history to the forefront', *History and Policy* (2012) [online]. Available at: www.historyandpolicy.org/papers/policy-paper-118.html (accessed 26 January 2014).

Solomos, J., *Race and Racism in Britain* (Basingstoke and New York: Palgrave Macmillan, 2003).

Spickard, P., 'Introduction: Immigration and race in United States history', in P. Spickard (ed.), *Race and Immigration in the United States* (New York: Routledge, 2012).

Starn, O., 'Missing the revolution: Anthropologists and the war in Peru', *Cultural Anthropology*, 16:1 (1991).

Stevens, R. A., 'Fifty years of the British National Health Service: Mixed messages, diverse interpretations', *Bulletin of the History of Medicine*, 74:4 (2000).

Stevens, R. A., C. E. Rosenberg, L. R. Burns (eds), *History and Health Policy in the United States: Putting the Past Back In* (New Brunswick, New Jersey and London: Rutgers University Press, 2006).

Stewart, J., 'Angels or aliens? Refugee nurses in Britain 1938 to 1942', *Medical History*, 47 (2003).

Stewart, J., 'The political economy of the British National Health Service, 1945–75: Opportunities and constraints?', *Medical History*, 52:4 (2008).

Stoller, P., 'Looking for the right path', in A. Bammer and R.-E. Boetcher Joeres (eds), *The Future of Scholarly Writing: Critical Interventions* (Basingstoke: Palgrave, 2015).

Szreter, S., *Health and Wealth: Studies in History and Policy* (Rochester: University of Rochester Press, 2007).

Tabili, L., *Global Migrants, Local Culture: Natives and Newcomers in Provincial England, 1841–1939* (London: Palgrave Macmillan, 2011).

Taylor, D. H. Jr & A. Esmail, 'Retrospective analysis of census data on general practitioners who qualified in South Asia: Who will replace them as they retire?', *BMJ*, 318 (1999).

Thane, P. M., 'Oral history, memory and written tradition: An introduction', *Transactions of the Royal Historical Society*, 6:9 (1999).

Thane, P., 'History and policy', *History Workshop Journal*, 67:1 (2009).

Thompson, A., *The Empire Strikes Back? The Impact of Imperialism on Britain from the Mid-Nineteenth Century* (Harlow: Pearson Education Limited, 2005).

Thompson, E. P., *The Making of the English Working Class* (London: Penguin Books, 1991).

Thompson, P., 'Oral history and the history of medicine: A review', *Social History of Medicine*, 4:2 (1991).

Thompson, P., *The Voice of the Past: Oral History*, third edition (Oxford: Oxford University Press, 2000).

Thomson, A., 'Making the most of memories: The empirical and subjective value of oral history', *Transactions of the Royal Historical Society*, 6:9 (1999).

Thomson, A., 'Four paradigm transformations in oral history', *The Oral History Review*, 34:1 (2007).

Tosh, J., *Why History Matters* (Basingstoke: Palgrave Macmillan, 2008).

Verghese, A., *My Own Country: A Doctor's Story of a Town and its People in the Age of AIDS* (London: Phoenix, 1995).

Visram, R., *Asians in Britain: 400 Years of History* (London: Pluto Press, 2002).

Watkins, S., *Medicine and Labour: The Politics of a Profession* (London: Lawrence and Wishart, 1987).

Webster, C., *The Health Services since the War*: Volume I (London: HMSO, 1988).

Webster, C., *The Health Services since the War*: Volume II (London: HMSO, 1996).

Webster, C., *The National Health Service: A Political History* (Oxford and New York: Oxford University Press, 1998).

Weekes-Bernard, D. (with interviews by Klara Schmitz, Saher Ali & Valentina Migliarini), *Nurturing the Nation: The Asian Contribution to the NHS since 1948* (London: The Runnymede Trust, 2013).

Weindling, P., 'The contribution of Central European Jews to medical science and practice in Britain, the 1930s–1950s', in W. E. Mosse (coordinating ed.), J. Carlebach, G. Hirschfeld, A. Newman, A. Paucker, P. Pulzer (eds), *Second Chance: Two Centuries of German-Speaking Jews in the United Kingdom* (Tübingen: J. C. B. Mohr (Paul Siebeck), 1991).

Weindling, P., 'Medical refugees and the modernisation of British medicine, 1930–1960', *Social History of Medicine*, 22:3 (2009).

Weindling, P., 'Medical refugees in Britain and the wider world 1930–1960: Introduction', *Social History of Medicine*, 22:3 (2009).

Wendland, C. L., *A Heart for the Work: Journeys through an African Medical School* (Chicago and London: The University of Chicago Press, 2010).

Whiting, R., 'The Empire and British politics', in A. Thompson (ed.), *Britain's Experience of Empire in the Twentieth Century* (Oxford: Oxford University Press, 2016).

Winkelmann-Gleed, A. & J. Eversley, 'Salt and stairs: A history of refugee doctors in the UK', in N. Jackson & Y. Carter (eds), *Refugee Doctors: Support, Development and Integration in the NHS* (Oxford & San Francisco: Radcliffe Publishing, 2004).

Woolcock, M., S. Szreter, V. Rao, 'How and why does history matter for development policy', *Journal of Development Studies*, 47:1 (2011).

Wright, D. & S. Mullally, '"Not everyone can be a Gandhi": South Asian-trained doctors immigrating to Canada, c. 1961–1971', *Ethnicity and Health*, 21:4 (2016).

Wright, D., N. Flis, M. Gupta, The "brain drain" of physicians: Historical antecedents to an ethical debate', *Philosophy, Ethics and Humanities in Medicine*, 3:24 (2008).

Wright, D., S. Mullally, M. C. Cordukes, '"Worse than being married": The exodus of British doctors from the National Health Service to Canada, c. 1955–75', *Journal of the History of Medicine and Allied Sciences*, 65:2 (2010).

# Index